KAUSHIK SUNDER RAJAN

Pharmocracy

Value, Politics & Knowledge in Global Biomedicine

Duke University Press   Durham and London   2017

Library of Congress Cataloging-in-Publication Data
Names: Sunder Rajan, Kaushik, [date] author.
Title: Pharmocracy : value, politics, and knowledge in global
biomedicine / Kaushik Sunder Rajan.
Other titles: Experimental futures.
Description: Durham : Duke University Press, 2017. | Series:
Experimental futures | Includes bibliographical references and index.
Identifiers: LCCN 2016035907 (print)
LCCN 2016037764 (ebook)
ISBN 9780822363132 (hardcover : alk. paper)
ISBN 9780822363279 (pbk. : alk. paper)
ISBN 9780822373285 (e-book)
Subjects: LCSH: Pharmaceutical industry—Management. |
Pharmaceutical industry—Economic aspects. |
Pharmaceutical industry—India. | Papillomaviruses—
Vaccination—India—Case studies.
Classification: LCC HD9672.I42S68 2017 (print) |
LCC HD9672.I42 (ebook) | DDC 338.8/8716151—dc23
LC record available at https://lccn.loc.gov/2016035907

COVER ART: Design and illustration by Matthew Tauch.

Pharmocracy

Experimental Futures

Technological lives, scientific arts, anthropological voices

A SERIES EDITED BY MICHAEL M. J. FISCHER AND JOSEPH DUMIT

For Q.
HOW NOW?

CONTENTS

ACKNOWLEDGMENTS

Acknowledgments are both a pleasure and impossible to write. This book has been a decade in the making, and in the process I have accumulated a large number of debts. The people who have made this book possible are too numerous to list, and in many cases these debts cannot be adequately repaid with mere thanks. But there are a few people who deserve special mention.

No ethnographic work is possible without the interlocutors in the domains one is researching who make it so. This project has benefited from conversations with scientists, clinicians, members of the pharmaceutical and clinical research industry in India and the United States, public health practitioners, patient advocates, bureaucrats, politicians, journalists, lawyers, judges, and activists fighting for access to essential medicines or against unethical clinical trials. A few interlocutors deserve special thanks. Brajesh Regal and Karen Haneke allowed me my first introduction to the work of clinical research organizations. Raghu Cidambi and Yusuf Hamied have been especially important in shaping my understanding of the histories and strategies of the Indian pharmaceutical industry. Nilotpal Basu, Amitava Guha, and Brinda Karat have taught me about the histories of involvement of the Communist Parties of India in pharmaceutical politics. I thank Ahn Gi Jong, Mi-Ran Kwon, Chul Won Jung, Hee Seob Nam, and Seoc-Kyun Woo for their conversations and insights on the politics of Gleevec in South Korea; and Sang-Hyun Kim, Youngyung Paik, and Seo-Young Park for facilitating introductions to key actors in Korea, and for acting as translators as I conducted my interviews there. Katy Athersuch, Krista Cox, and Judit Rius have given me important insights on global civil society advocacy for access to essential medicines, while Justice Prabha Sridevan has taught me much about Indian judicial cultures. Conversations with Allyson Pollock have been invaluable in alerting me to debates within the public health community around the HPV vaccine studies. Rachna Dhingra, Rashidabi, and Satinath Sarangi have discussed clinical trials conducted on Bhopal gas victims in light of longer struggles for health and justice in Bhopal. I have learned much about the comparable (and incomparable) political issues around pharmaceuticals in West Africa from Morenike Folayan. While that is not a part of the world that I empirically focus on in my research, getting a sense of how political economies have been shaped there has been invaluable to my understanding of the political economies that I trace out of India.

And then there are those interlocutors who have truly become comrades, whose struggles and advocacy I feel accountable to. I am grateful for the tireless work of Lawyers Collective, the Access to Medicines and Treatment Campaign of Médicins sans Frontières, and to Sama Resource Group for Women and Health, not just for their constant presence as intellectual resources through this project, but for their inspiration and solidarity. I am especially grateful to Kajal Bharadwaj, K. M. Gopakumar, Leena Menghaney, Anand Grover, S. Pratibha, and N. Sarojini for comradeship and camaraderie; Vineeta Bal and Satyajit Rath, additionally, have been models of thinking and doing biological and biomedical research out of commitments to and involvements with feminist and people's health and science movements. I can only hope that this book does some justice to the work and praxis of these individuals and groups, and their allies.

I have benefited greatly from the intellectual communities that I have been privileged to be a part of while researching and writing this book: the Anthropology Department at the University of California, Irvine, and the Anthropology Department at the University of Chicago. Long-term fieldwork was enabled by a grant from the American Institute for Indian Studies. I thank audiences at the various institutions where I have presented some of this work as talks. I am especially grateful to students in my Health, Value and Politics seminar at Chicago, who read and commented upon this manuscript as it was being revised for publication. They will see the marks of their engagement in the final product.

Some of my academic colleagues, friends, and teachers deserve special thanks. I have been in conversation throughout the past decade and more with Joe Dumit and Kristin Peterson, whose own important books on pharmaceutical political economies have been published in recent years. My thinking and writing has been indelibly shaped by them. Melinda Cooper, Mohan Rao, and Catherine Waldby have been vital resources for helping me think about economies of clinical trials in relation to those of reproductive labor. Sheila Jasanoff has always been a vital resource for helping me understand relationships between science and the law, while Brenna

Bhandar and Mario Biagioli have taught me much about critical thinking in relation to intellectual property. Michael Fischer, Kim Fortun, and George Marcus have taught me what I know about conducting ethnographic research on global political economic systems, and have generatively and continuously reinforced their lessons as I have worked on this book. Etienne Balibar and Joe Dumit have taught me to read and think with Marx, a lesson that never exhausts itself. Tim Choy has helped me think about value, and about so much else. My colleagues in the Knowledge/Value collective have provided me much food for thought over the past few years; I especially thank Gail Davies, who has engaged my work with the eyes of a geographer, and Sabina Leonelli, who has done so with the eyes of a philosopher of science. These are perspectives that have meaningfully thickened my ways of understanding the world, even if they do not find full (or even adequate) expression in these pages.

I thank those who have read through the entirety of this manuscript and provided feedback to me on the whole. This includes two anonymous referees for Duke University Press, and also Joe Dumit, Michael Fischer, Sunil Maulik, and Rajeswari Sunder Rajan. In addition, I have benefited greatly from feedback on different portions of the manuscript from a number of people. Heartfelt thanks are due to Naira Ahmad, Jean-Paul Gaudilliere, Sabina Leonelli, Kelly Mulvaney, Priya Nelson, Dina Omar, Kristin Peterson, Natalie Porter, Amber Reed, Emilia Sanabria, Lisa Wedeen, and Winnie Wong. Ken Wissoker and Elizabeth Ault at Duke University Press have supported and stewarded this process through its various stages of writing and production. Ch'ava Cafe (which alas, no longer exists) provided the space and fluid for sustenance and inspiration through much of my writing.

There are three people who deserve special thanks. Perhaps more than anyone else, Naira Ahmad has taught me to understand the perspectives and rationalities of the multinational pharmaceutical industry, sometimes argumentatively but always with kindness and generosity. She has been a font of knowledge and a pillar of strength in so many ways. I have for many years learned from the work and practice of my mother, Rajeswari Sunder Rajan. While writing this book, I have realized just how close the intellectual and political connections are between the politics of health that I trace here and the histories of feminist theory and praxis in and from India. It is not just the content of my mother's work that I have learned from; she models the kind of academic I wish to be. And finally, thanks to my father, N. Sunder Rajan, bureaucrat and romantic. He taught me that bureaucracy is not just about red tape, but about a quiet and understated ethical investment in democracy itself. His relentless curiosity and gregarious humility have set an example that I can never live up to, but that I will always aspire to and be grateful for. This book is dedicated to him.

A SHORTER version of chapter 1 was published in *South Atlantic Quarterly* 111 (2). A shorter version of chapter 3 was published in *Social Research* 78 (3). The first part of chapter 3 and the initial parts of chapter 4 are part of a chapter in *Science and Democracy: Making Knowledge and Making Power in the Biosciences and Beyond*, edited by Stephen Hilgartner, Clark Miller, and Rob Hagendijk (Routledge).

Value, Politics, and Knowledge in the Pharmocracy

SAN DIEGO, 2008—I was at a life science investment conference devoted to investment opportunities in India and China organized by Burrill and Co., one of the world's leading life science investment funds. Important figures in the Indian biotechnology and pharmaceutical industries were in attendance. The focus of the conference concerned innovation in Indian biomedicine: the need for it, and the lack of it. One speaker was explicit that the biggest challenge to India becoming "innovative" was that it is a democracy. According to her, this led to a "democratic lag." The contrast was drawn to China, which happily could just foist innovation upon its population.

As I listened, I considered the market contradictions that emerged in this conversation. There was talk about the importance of India making novel therapeutics rather than focusing on the prevalent model of reverse engineering generic versions of drugs already on the market, but there was no discussion of how these novelties would be priced to be affordable to the Indian population. There was talk about building global partnerships with multinational drug companies to foster innovative capabilities among Indian companies, but no explanation of the nature of a partnership with powerful entities who are your direct competitors, in a global playing field that is anything but level. And no reflection on how it was possible to talk about innovation without talking about universities. Pricing strategies, competitive landscapes, and enabling technologies are all fundamental market issues that were being elided, in the name of an innovation that was out there, all powerful, all ready to bestow its enormous benefits upon an ignorant, suspicious, or resistant population.

It was repeatedly emphasized by the investors at the meeting that this innovation was necessary to help the rural poor.

BHOPAL, 2011—Santosh was living in the slums near Qazi Camp in Bhopal. He was fourteen when I met him. His entire life had been lived in the aftermath of December 3, 1984: the night when Bhopal became the focus of global attention because of the deadly leak of methyl isocyanate from a factory owned by the chemical company Union Carbide. I met Santosh at a meeting of gas survivors planning a *rail roko*, an agitation that would involve their lying on railway tracks to stop trains going through Bhopal, to mark the twenty-eighth anniversary of the disaster. Many of the people at the meeting were women in their eighties, who were explaining to others the bodily techniques of lying on railway tracks: how to hold hands together, how to become flaccid when the police came so that they would find it difficult to lift the protesters, how to come back to the tracks once removed, how to congregate. After the meeting, Santosh and I walked as we talked. There was a lake nearby. It was bright green, toxic sludge. Santosh said that no water that the slum dwellers drink is untainted by chemicals and poison; all the water that their animals drink is poison.

In 2010 and 2011, the Central Drugs Standard Control Organisation of India (CDSCO) conducted site inspections of the Bhopal Memorial Hospital and Research Centre to audit three clinical trials that had been conducted there from 2004 to 2008. The hospital was set up in 2004 as part of the 1989 Indian Supreme Court settlement of the 1984 Union Carbide gas tragedy in Bhopal as a tertiary care hospital that would provide free care to gas victims. Since its establishment, it has morphed into a two-tiered hospital. While it still provides free care to victims, it is also a for-profit hospital that makes money by charging private patients who are not designated as victims. The CDSCO reports created a furor, because they suggested that victims of the Bhopal gas tragedy, who had since 1984 been denied any kind of justice or rudimentary provisions for health care, had now been made experimental subjects in clinical trials in the very hospital that had been set up as part of a court settlement to care for them. Furthermore, these were global clinical trials, sponsored by American biotechnology or pharmaceutical companies.

Hence there was a sense not just of violation, but of continued violation by multinational corporate interests.

One resident of the slums told me that he does not go to the hospital anymore, because "they do trials there, and we come out dead."[1] Satinath Sarangi, who runs a free clinic in the slums for the gas victims, subsequently described this to me as a continuation of the "circle of poison" that started with chemical companies and continues to be propagated by pharmaceutical companies.[2] He reminded me that a pharmaceutical company is just another kind of chemical company. Santosh told me, as our conversation continued, that he wants to become a biologist when he grows up, because he wants to do research that can improve the health of people like his who live in the slums.

BOMBAY, 2008—I was talking to Yusuf Hamied, the chairman of Cipla, India's oldest surviving pharmaceutical company. I asked him about the impact of World Trade Organization (wto)-imposed patent regimes on access to medicines in India. His response: "What a silly question, Professor Sunder Rajan. What we are witnessing is selective genocide."[3]

Representations of Health

It is an obvious truism that there are investments in health across social positions. These investments are variously monetary, bodily, and affective. But what health might mean, how health might be achieved, and what imaginations of social relations and relations of production underlie various conceptions of health differs depending on institutional location, social hierarchy, and power relations. Clinical trials are thought of as benefiting humanity even as they are considered scandalous; hospitals are seen as spaces of cure but also in certain situations as spaces of death; intellectual property rights are argued for as necessary for innovation even as they are decried as being genocidal.

This book seeks to understand the political economy of health in contemporary India as it operates in relation to global biomedicine. It concerns emergent biomedical regimes of experimentation on the one hand, and therapeutic production, circulation, and access on the other. These regimes are operating in political economic environments that are highly capitalized, albeit through different mechanisms, business models, and industrial forms. In turn, these capitalized political economies foreground forms of biomedicine that focus on pharmaceutical production, access, and consumption, rendering forms of care that are not so commodity- and artifact-driven less visible as a matter of policy or political concern. This capitalization operates at national and global scales, and is not without contestation. Arguments and considerations pertaining to value—both market value and ethical value—come to be front and center in these politics.

Further, the politics at stake is a representative politics, one whose forms and spaces are emergent and contingent, but that nonetheless operate within and in relation to structures of power and modes of production that are enduring. With their invocations about helping India's rural poor, the investors at the Burrill conference in San Diego were not shy about taking on the role of representatives promoting public health—just as Satinath Sarangi has been doing by providing free care for gas victims through his clinic in Qazi Camp in Bhopal, even as he has been at the forefront of the more than three-decade struggle for justice for the victims; as Yusuf Hamied has been doing, as a vanguard nationalist industrial leader who was one of the pioneers of the Indian pharmaceutical industry as a nationally viable industry that could reverse engineer generic versions of drugs to sell in domestic markets at competitive cost, and who in the early 2000s became a major player in global politics of access to essential medicines by selling generic antiretrovirals in African markets at a fraction of the price that Euro-American companies were selling their patented medications. Indeed, even as Santosh was aspiring to do, in his hopes of becoming a biologist who could contribute to the health of the people of his community.

And so, the democracy that investors at the Burrill conference lamented is neither an abstract philosophical concept nor simply a formal macropolitical exercise in choosing leaders; nor even just an expression of popular or community sentiment. Rather, it speaks to particular kinds of representative relationships: individuals and institutions acting on behalf of the marginalized, the vulnerable, or the disenfranchised in the cause of a more public health. But they suggest radically different conceptions of how health, value, and politics might be conceptualized, in and of themselves and in relation to one another.

While I was in Bhopal conducting research on clinical trials conducted on gas victims, I interviewed an oncologist who was at the time running trials on forty cancer patients, many of whom were gas victims. We were sitting in his outpatient office. He pointed to an old man sitting hunched next to me and said, "Look at him. He is a gas victim. He has stage IV pancreatic cancer. Either I enroll him in a clinical trial to give him experimental medication, or he dies."[4] The image of that scene has stayed with me, of a man whose only chance of living was to be on experimental medication. But what I remember most is not the man himself, but rather the pointing finger of the doctor—directed at a dying man sitting in front of him, as he talked about that man to a stranger in English, a language he could not understand. He was pointing not just to a dying man, but to the situation of treating gas victims as their tissues turned malignant, in a context that has been marked by a failure of both health care and the law for over three decades. The doctor was engaging simultaneously in experimentation, therapeutic intervention, and representation, even as he was involved in a deeply politicized situation that had already been rendered scandalous.

How do we think about value that emerges here, in such spaces and through such relationships? How do we think about the politics that emerges here? How do we think about the health that emerges here? How do we think about the democracy that emerges here? I ask such questions by following ways in which health, value, and politics are constituted globally, in and through speculative metrics of value established on Wall Street, or pharmaceutical corporate lobbies in Washington, DC, or through local, national, and global civil society advocacy around health issues as they play out in high courts in India, in the calculations of brokers in clinical research located in Seattle and Hyderabad, North Carolina, and Northern Andhra Pradesh, in the investments of Indian capitalists with nationalist inheritances attempting to be global health players, in trade negotiations happening behind closed doors within bilateral and multilateral forums, in the pages of public health journals, or in legislative debates in the Indian Parliament. These are questions of pharmocracy.

Pharmocracy

In early 2005, the Indian government passed two consequential pieces of legislation for the pharmaceutical sector. Both involved bringing national laws in line with global regulatory frameworks, a process referred to as harmonization. One involved an amendment to Schedule Y of India's Drugs and Cosmetics Rules of 1945, in order to harmonize guidelines for the conduct of clinical trials with those mandated by the International Conference on Harmonisation of Technical Requirements for Registration of Pharmaceuticals for Human Use (ICH), the purpose being safe, efficient, and ethical processes for the testing, approval, and registration of drugs for market. The second change was to India's patent laws to make them compliant with the mandates of the Trade-Related Aspects of Intellectual Property Rights (TRIPS) agreement, enshrined under the aegis of the World Trade Organization (WTO), which would involve a radical amendment of India's 1970 Patent Act. These "global" frameworks were both Euro-American ones, and the term *harmonization* suggests their normative value and benevolent nature.

This book argues as its point of departure that in fact such policy moves are not about harmony as much as they are about hegemony. *Pharmocracy* is a term I coin to refer to the global regime of hegemony of the multinational pharmaceutical industry. It describes the ways in which the Euro-American research and development (R&D)-driven pharmaceutical industry operates to institute forms of governance across the world that are beneficial to its own interests. I argue that the global harmonization of clinical trials and intellectual property regimes must be understood in terms of this expansion of multinational corporate hegemony. Third World national regulations are now being instituted to facilitate First World corporate interests. This has consequences for state policy, industrial competitiveness, and public health that materialize in specific ways in different national contexts.

The policies that India implemented in 2005 could be interpreted in radically different ways. An interpretation that emphasizes the harmonic aspects of these policies would highlight their social benefit. After all, a strong regulatory environment for the conduct of clinical trials is one that would provide adequate protections to individuals subject to potentially risky biomedical experimentation. Equally, an environment that strongly protects intellectual property is seen as a spur to innovation, providing monopolistic protections that are essential to incentivize the high-risk, capital-intensive venture that novel drug development is.[5] Meanwhile, an interpretation that focuses on the hegemonic aspects of these changes would recognize the perversity of synchronous legislation that constructs India as a global hub of clinical experimentation at the same time as it renders access to medicines potentially more difficult.

What are the logics, forces, and relations of production that allow us to make sense of this hegemony that is naturalized as harmony? This could simply be seen as the naked exercise of power by corporations with global reach and influence, cynically manufacturing ethical justifications for their profit-driven actions. But that still begs the question: Where does their power come from? Through what kinds of institutional and political mechanisms does it act? And how is it naturalized, such that it can be portrayed as the story of an industry pushing for more innovation and acting with ethical consciousness? Answering these questions involves understanding the nuanced notion of power represented by the idea of hegemony.

As Antonio Gramsci emphasized, hegemony does not imply a simple relationship of coercive dominance.[6] Rather, it involves a contestation for the "common-sense" of a society at a given moment in time. Gramsci uses "common-sense" to allude to naturalized sensibilities about politics, economy, and culture that prevail within social formations under given historical situations. These sensibilities develop within the context of prevalent modes and relations of production, of structures of political economy. Following Gramsci, it is worth asking: What are the structures, situations, and sensibilities that give shape to this moment of policy harmonization in India? Whose norms are being established, at whose expense? Within what kinds of power hierarchies do these policies operate? Through what regimes of governance are they instantiated? And what might that tell us about global pharmaceutical production, circulation, and consumption today?

Acknowledging the power of the multinational pharmaceutical industry is important, but understanding its hegemony involves moving beyond simple explanations grounded in a purely cynical reasoning of their actions. To be sure, pharmaceutical corporations—and not just large Euro-American ones but also smaller, nationally located, Global Southern ones—are strategic actors involved in profit maximization, influencing state regulation, and manipulating public perception to their advantage. Mapping their machinations is an essential empirical and political task. But pharmocracy is constituted in more complex ways than merely rational, strategic, or cynical action on the part of corporate actors. I argue that we must additionally understand the mechanisms by which health gets appropriated by capital, in order to instantiate forms of political economic value that are dictated by logics of capital; how these logics of capital materialize through regimes of governance; and how they are contested and rendered political. In the process, the notion of health itself as it gets constituted in relation to emergent forms of experimentation and therapy comes to be at stake. Health is no longer just an embodied, subjective, experiential state of well-being or disease; it can be abstracted and grown, made valuable to capitalist interests.

One part of the task of understanding pharmocracy then is to elucidate the political economy of the appropriation of health by capital. At stake here is a conceptualization of value. The complementary part of this task is to recognize that logics of capital are not seamless. They materialize differently in different places and times through different forms of capitalism and often consequent to deep contestation. At stake here is a conceptualization of politics. Undergirding and articulating forms of and relations between value and politics are ways of knowing, and questions of what kinds of authorities are vested in particular ways of knowing. At stake here is a conceptualization of knowledge in its interactions with value and politics. These conceptualizations cannot occur in the abstract. They have to emerge out of concrete empirical substance: historical trajectories, critical events, institutional structures, political economic formations. The moment of synchronous policy harmonization in relation to experimentation and therapeutic access in 2005 in India provides a useful starting point in this regard because it reflects major shifts in the political economy of global biomedicine happening along two tracks.

One concerns the harmonization of the regulation of clinical trials, which are required to certify a new drug molecule as safe and efficacious for the market.[7] This set of practices serves in its rationale as a regulatory watchdog to prevent the market from being flooded with unsafe or spurious medication.[8] In the United States, the clinical trials procedure is an elaborate one, conducted in a number of stages and contributing to the immense time, risk, and expense of the drug development process. First, there is preclinical toxicological testing of a potential new drug molecule. This is usually performed on animals, in order to determine whether the molecule being tested is safe enough to put into a living system. The second stage is dosage studies, designed to come up with a metric for the dose of the drug to be administered. Predictably, the efficacy of a drug increases with its dose, but so too does its toxicity; the aim is therefore to find an optimum range within which efficacy is maximized without too greatly compromising safety.

If the drug is too toxic when tried on animals, the trial will not proceed any further, but if acceptable dose ranges can be determined, the third stage is a three-phase trial in humans. Phase 1 trials are conducted on a small number of healthy volunteers to test the drug's basic safety, since drugs that seem safe in animals may still show adverse effects in humans. Phase 2, which serves as a bridge, involves larger, scaled-up efficacy and safety trials on as many as a few hundred subjects, who may be either patients or healthy individuals. Phase 3 involves large-scale randomized trials on several thousand people, usually patients suffering from the ailment for which the therapy has been developed. These trials are frequently coordinated across multiple centers, increasingly on a global scale.

The sponsors for trials are generally biotechnology or pharmaceutical companies, since drug development in the United States and most other parts of the world is undertaken largely by the private sector. Universities and publicly funded laboratories play a major role in the early stages of discovery—the identification of potential lead molecules and the conduct of preclinical tests—but the institutional structure of drug development is such that they increasingly license promising molecules to corporations that take them through clinical trials. These later stages of drug development have come to be significantly privatized over the past forty years. According to the Healthcare Financial Management Association's newsletter, "[In the late 1970s], 80 per cent of clinical research trials were conducted through academic medical centers. In 1998, estimates indicated the number of [these] centres as investigator sites had dropped to less than half" (Jones and Zuckerman 2007). This means that the biomedical and experimental rationales for clinical trials are entwined with the market value these companies see in the drugs that eventually get developed, and with the market risk that attends the drug development process. The increasing complexity of clinical trials over this period has however meant that it has been difficult for pharmaceutical companies themselves to manage them, leading to the emergence of an entirely new sector devoted to the management and administration of clinical trials. These companies, known as clinical research organizations (CROS), are now an integral part of the overall biomedical economy.[9]

This is the context in which to situate the ICH as a multilateral institutional framework to govern the global conduct of clinical trials. It was initially established in 1990 as a conference between pharmaceutical regulatory authorities in the United States, Europe, and Japan to devise uniform guidelines for the conduct of clinical trials and their evaluation for drug approval to market.[10] While this was an attempt to ensure ethical clinical trials conducted in accordance with what is known as good clinical practice, it must also be seen in the light of this broader emergent trajectory of the privatization and globalization of trials and the concomitant actual and potential expansion of pharmaceutical markets for the Euro-American industry.

The second track along which major shifts toward harmonization/hegemony in global biomedicine has occurred concerns the regulation of intellectual property rights, specifically drug patents. Current regimes that govern patenting pharmaceuticals emerged out of structures involved in the regulation of global trade, specifically the General Agreements on Tariffs and Trade (GATT), a post–World War II multilateral agreement. Seven rounds of negotiations under GATT occurred between 1949 and 1979. The eighth round (referred to as the Uruguay Round) commenced in 1986 in Punta del Este, Uruguay. It included 123 countries and deliberations continued for the next eight years, leading eventually to the establishment of a new multilateral regulatory organization for global trade, the WTO, in 1995. The Uruguay Round departed from all previous rounds by bringing intellectual property into the purview of free trade negotiations for the first time. This was enshrined in the TRIPS agreement. Hence, while it is a trade regulatory authority, the WTO's significance lies in its power to enforce uniformity in intellectual property regimes across its member nations.

At its simplest, TRIPS enforces regimes that approximate those already prevalent in the United States and Europe. In the case of pharmaceuticals, this entails the establishment of product patent regimes by all member nations of the WTO. Before becoming a signatory to TRIPS, India operated under a Patent Act passed in 1970 that allowed only process and not product patents on pharmaceuticals. This meant that one could not patent a drug molecule itself, only its method of manufacture. This was a spur to India's local drug industry, which developed expertise in reverse engineering generic versions of medications patented in the West. It also led to a market terrain that allowed for free market competition in drugs, as opposed to the monopolistic terrain of patented medication prevalent in the West. Consequently, drug prices in India since the 1970s have been among the lowest in the world (Chaudhuri 2005, 53–58). Under TRIPS, India had to relinquish its process patent regime and replace it with one that allowed patents on drug molecules. It also had to extend the duration of patent validity, from seven years as stipulated in its 1970 Act to twenty years, the same period as exists in the United States. The new patent laws therefore instituted patent monopolies of the sort prevalent in the United States and Europe. As a less developed country, India was allowed a ten-year transition period to modify its laws. This meant that Indian laws had to be TRIPS compliant by 2005, by which time any drug developed after 1995 would qualify for a twenty-year product patent in India. Any drug developed before 1995 would however still only be eligible for a process patent as under the 1970 Act.

This new patent regime, enshrined in law in 2005, would have implications for India's largely generic drug industry. But there was also concern about its implications for drug prices in India, which over the previous three decades were largely controlled through free market competition. Like the United States (but unlike most European countries, or indeed most other countries in the world), India does not have a system of nationalized therapeutic access except for central government and defense employees, and its state regulatory mechanisms for controlling drug prices have proven inconsistent. Hence, the control of drug prices in India since the 1970s, while extremely successful, has almost entirely been a function of free market competition in generic drugs. Meanwhile, TRIPS compliance on India's part would have potentially beneficial implications for that section of the global pharmaceutical industry that depends upon patent medications for revenue generation. This includes companies that are mostly Euro-American and multinational and that have based their business models on R&D into novel therapeutics (and are therefore referred to as R&D-based companies). Indeed, this industry lobbied powerfully to ensure that intellectual property would come under the purview of Uruguay Round negotiations in the first place.[11]

The trajectories of harmonization/hegemony that resulted in the legislative changes in India in early 2005 therefore concern two simultaneous movements of global agreement and compliance, those of ethical regimes on the one hand and of intellectual property regimes on the other. The harmonization of clinical trials regulation facilitates the outsourcing of trials away from the United States and western Europe to parts of the world where they are cheaper to perform. Meanwhile, the 1970 Indian Patent Act, in allowing for a strong national pharmaceutical industry, squeezed the multinational industry out of the country; but now the multinational, R&D-driven industry can enjoy monopoly protection on its patented medication in India, which emerges as a potentially lucrative market to return to (albeit with limits, as I elaborate in chapter 1). Thus the legislations of 2005 allow experiments to travel (to use Adriana Petryna's [2009] phrase), even as they allow patented medications to travel.

The harmonization of clinical trials and intellectual property regimes are both a function of logics of global capital touching down in India. However, the contestations around the kinds of hegemony they represent would come to develop through different forms of politics, within distinct institutional spaces and adopting different discursive modalities running in parallel. Issues concerning clinical trials have been rendered political largely by means of publicity around the ethical imperatives underlying the proper conduct of trials and the often scandalous failure to conform to such ethics. Those concerning access to medicines meanwhile have been significantly judicialized, such that the constitution of the political has tended to happen largely in and through the courts.[12] I am interested in each of these biomedical domains and political trajectories in their own right, but also in their confluence, which sees the opening of borders for clinical experimentation at the very moment that access to essential medicines has become potentially more difficult through the institution of monopolistic patent regimes. It is in thinking about these two domains together that one can conceptualize broader structures of global pharmaceutical political economy. What interests me is precisely the fact that in the same place (India), at the same time (the 2000s), in the same industrial sector (concerning pharmaceuticals and health), one can have such different trajectories of political contestation, which intersect and interact with globally hegemonic movements in political economy.

This is the empirical conundrum that allows me to enter into a further discussion of how I conceptualize the emergent phenomenon of pharmocracy. This is a complex phenomenon, operating across scales, locales, histories, and events. I do not wish to present a simplified picture of this phenomenon for the sake of analytical clarity; but I also do not want to allude to the massive complexity of this phenomenon without a concerted attempt to unpack it.[13] This will necessarily be partial, following certain threads that I feel are significant, and focusing largely on Indian events and circumstances. But through a multiplicity of such partial perspectives, juxtaposed and set in historical, geographical, epistemic, and sectoral relationship to one another, I hope to generate elements of a broader and more comprehensive structural elucidation of contemporary biomedicine, contemporary capital, contemporary globalization, and contemporary Indian politics.

I enter into an empirically grounded analysis of pharmocracy through the case: significant events in India that have structured terrains of global biomedicine even as they highlight elements of that terrain. The two cases that are central to this book concern clinical studies of vaccines against human papilloma virus (HPV) infection conducted in the Indian states of Andhra Pradesh and Gujarat (the focus of chapter 2), and patent disputes in India around an anticancer drug, Gleevec, developed by the Swiss pharmaceutical company Novartis for the treatment of chronic myelogenous leukemia (the focus of chapter 3). Alongside that, I unpack the critical concepts of value, politics, and knowledge, to show how complex and multifaceted each one is. I next elaborate these two parallel routes through which I elucidate elements of pharmocracy as they have materialized in contemporary India.

Elements of Pharmocracy (1): A Tale of Two Trials

The year 2005 saw the coincidence of critical pieces of legislation being passed in India in the domains of clinical trials and intellectual property rights respectively. These changes must be located within larger trajectories and contexts of global harmonization/hegemony that facilitate capital flows. How does one think of the relationship between these *longue durée* institutional reconfigurations and the particularity of a legislative event? Or more simply: how might we see structures of pharmocracy through the lens of these esoteric and coincidental regulatory moments?

One way I do so is by focusing on two significant events that played out over a longer time horizon (months and years) rather than a single moment of policy formulation. The first event concerns a scandal that erupted consequent to the death in 2010 of seven teenage girls who had been enrolled in a clinical study of vaccines against HPV, developed by the American multinational company Merck (whose vaccine was called Gardasil) and the British multinational GlaxoSmithKline (which developed a comparable counterpart, Cervarix). The second concerns the Indian Patent Office's denial in 2005 of a patent on the anticancer drug Gleevec, developed by the Swiss multinational pharmaceutical company Novartis, and the long judicial appeals and judgments that followed in Indian courts.[14] The former case exemplifies the politicization of clinical trials in India through public scandal, while the latter exemplifies the judicialized politicization of intellectual property rights and issues concerning access to essential medicines.

The scandal of the deaths of seven girls in the HPV studies unfolded as follows. The new vaccines were considered revolutionary advances in the prevention of cervical cancer, for which HPV is a primary causal agent.[15] Phase 3 clinical trials for these vaccines had already been conducted (though never in India), so these were not studies to demonstrate the safety and efficacy of the vaccines. Rather, they were demonstration studies being conducted by the Seattle-based Program for Appropriate Technology in Health (PATH), a global health nonprofit whose major donor is the Bill and Melinda Gates Foundation, in collaboration with the Indian Council of Medical Research (ICMR), which is the apex public body for the formulation, coordination, and regulation of biomedical research in India. The purpose of the studies was to consider inclusion of these vaccines in India's national immunization program. It could not eventually be established that the girls had died because of the vaccines, but the controversy that arose subsequent to the deaths provided an impetus for civil society mobilization against unethical clinical trials in India.

The second case I discuss relates to Gleevec, a revolutionary treatment for chronic myeloid leukemia. It directly targets the protein *bcr-abl*, known to cause the cancer. Therefore it provides a more targeted, less dangerous therapy than the possibilities that had existed earlier (either treatment with interferon or bone marrow transplantation). In this regard, Gleevec provides one of the earliest examples of rational anticancer therapy that directly addresses the cause of the disease and not just the symptoms of out-of-control cell division.[16] The basis of the Gleevec patent denial in India was a public health flexibility incorporated into the amended, WTO-compliant 2005 Patent Act, which prevented what is known as pharmaceutical evergreening. Evergreening is a common practice in the United States and Europe, whereby a patent holder on a drug modifies it slightly as it approaches the end of its patent term and claims a new twenty-year product patent for the new drug that is thus produced. The Indian legislation by contrast included a provision under Section 3(d) that prevented a patent on a modification of an already known substance unless it conferred significantly enhanced efficacy on the prior molecule. The core molecule that would subsequently be developed by Novartis, imatinib, was patented in the United States and Canada in 1993. A crystalline salt isoform of this molecule, β-imatinib mesylate, was the subsequent marketed iteration of this molecule for which patent protection was being sought in India. It was determined that this was not a new molecule, simply a modification of an existing patented molecule, which came under the purview of the 1970 Act since it had already been patented prior to 1995 and hence was not eligible for a product patent. Novartis disputed this denial by embarking upon a seven-year legal battle, first in the Madras High Court (2006–2007) and then in the Indian Supreme Court (2009–2013). It lost both cases and the denial of the Gleevec patent stands in India.

What was at stake in the legal adjudication of the Gleevec patent was not just the patentability of a single drug, but the very question of how the new Indian patent legislation would be interpreted, especially as intellectual property rights had to be balanced against considerations of public health. The 2005 Act came to be rendered an interpretive matter, even as the politics of intellectual property and access to essential medicines came to be judicialized. Indeed, subsequent to Gleevec becoming a subject of legal contestation, a slew of drugs have had their patent status questioned in India through judicial and quasi-judicial appellate procedures. The law has provided a terrain by which intellectual property rights have become politically contestable. Meanwhile, following the HPV vaccine controversy, the capacity building for global clinical trials that had been envisaged in the 2005 Schedule Y amendments has come to be mired in controversy and scandal, as further cases of possibly unethical clinical studies have come to light and the general absence of adequate regulation of experimentation on human subjects has been questioned. This controversy has become a nodal point around which the conduct of clinical trials in India more generally has come to be politicized, largely through the register of public scandal. At the same time, the gendered dimensions of biomedical intervention came to be especially evident through this case, as connections were explicated between emergent regimes of clinical research and longer histories of reproductive politics.[17]

Just as the ways in which the two cases have become politically contested have been different, so too has the configuration of actors involved in each.[18] The Gleevec case saw Novartis pitted against a host of Indian pharmaceutical companies that had started manufacturing generic versions of the drug; the patient group Cancer Patients Aid Association (CPAA), which was involved in procuring generic medication and subsidizing its availability to poor cancer patients; an Indian legal advocacy group, Lawyers Collective, which represented CPAA throughout the legal trajectory of Gleevec; and the Access to Medicines and Treatment Campaign of Médicins sans Frontières (MSF), which had been established with Nobel Peace Prize money in 1999 and emerged as a major global advocate for affordable medication. These legal actors were joined by other civil society actors, especially HIV-AIDS groups in India and global civil society groups involved in battles around access to knowledge and access to medicines, in the terrain of popular and policy advocacy around Gleevec.

Meanwhile, mobilization against the HPV vaccine studies was initially orchestrated by feminist groups, including the All India Democratic Women's Association, which is affiliated with the Communist Party of India (Marxist), and Sama, an advocacy group for women and health based in Delhi. They joined together with medical ethicists, people's health movements, and advocates concerned with the proper regulation of scientific and medical activities in India. It was less clear in this case who the adversaries were: even though the vaccines in question belonged to Merck and GlaxoSmithKline, their responsibility for the studies seemed to have been outsourced along with the vaccine itself. Questions were asked of PATH, which was notably absent in answering any of them. Much of the immediate ire therefore ended up being directed at the Indian state, specifically the ICMR. If the Gleevec case targeted the multinational corporation as the hegemonic global capitalist adversary, the HPV case showed how difficult identifying such an adversary could be in situations where global capital flowed through dispersed and multiply outsourced brokerage economies operating under the sign of public-private partnerships.

I elaborate upon the controversy surrounding the HPV studies in chapter 2 and upon the Gleevec case in chapter 3. These speak to two distinct meanings of *trial*, one biomedical and the other legal. The first is concerned with movements of pharmaceutical clinical trials and concomitant politics consequent to their progressive privatization and globalization, while the second refers to the judicialization of pharmaceutical politics, which describes the playing out of politics of access to essential medicines in the courts (see Biehl and Petryna 2011).[19] I situate these in relation to a third, everyday use of *trial* to describe any kind of problem, difficulty, or trouble, in the sense of the structure of constitutive crisis under which both the Euro-American R&D-driven pharmaceutical industry and the Indian generic industry operate. Taken together, the HPV and Gleevec cases become emblematic of and signify a broader political terrain in their own right, and are therefore events that function beyond themselves.[20] They demand conceptualization that goes beyond just pointing to the contingency of their own happening, and allow for a thicker insight into the structural trajectories informing the legislative moment of 2005 while also signifying this moment as a site for the theorization of value, politics, and knowledge. But what do these terms mean, and what are these structural trajectories? I next discuss how I analyze value, politics, and knowledge in this book. This involves disaggregating them into multiple registers through which they operate, and thinking about the articulations and contradictions between these registers.

Elements of Pharmocracy (2): Theorizing Value, Politics, and Knowledge

This book traces the hegemonic structures and operations of pharmocracy. One of the nuances of Gramsci's notion of hegemony is that while it refers to a state of (naturalized or legitimated) domination, it is fluid. Hegemonies can be established, contested, overturned, or reconfigured. Battles over hegemony constitute politics, while politics comes to be the means of establishing hegemony. I argue that the establishment of regimes of value becomes a means through which hegemonies can be naturalized or reconfigured, such that value itself becomes the ground upon which further politics plays out. Value and politics become mutually constituting and reinforcing. Further, questions of knowledge often come to be at stake or mediate various articulations of value and politics. Yet none of value, politics, or knowledge is a singular thing, and each requires disaggregation and conceptualization in its own right.

Certain elements of value, politics, and knowledge have emerged as constitutive to contemporary global biomedical economies as they have materialized in India. I consider value in four registers: as an abstraction that has material consequences; as surplus value for capital; in terms of norms and ethics; and as an antinomy, something that is in contradictory relationship to itself. This in turn leads me to think of five sites through which value in all of its registers comes to be explicitly articulated through and as politics: (1) the speculative value of financial capital (chapter 1); (2) the bioethical value that underlies the establishment of good clinical practice for biomedical experimentation (chapter 2); (3) the constitutional values that underlie modes of judicial interpretations of intellectual property law in India (chapter 3); (4) philanthropic values that rationalize corporate monopoly (chapters 4); and (5) postcolonial values that contest Euro-American corporate and state hegemony through both market and state intervention (chapter 5).

Additionally, I consider politics in terms of six emergent forms of and spaces for representation:

1   the conjuncture of policy harmonization as creating openings for flows of global capital and for political mobilizations of global civil society around access to essential medicines and against unethical clinical trials (as summarized in this chapter and elaborated through the HPV and Gleevec cases in chapters 2 and 3);

2   logics of financialized capital and the spaces of crisis that they create, leading to structural contradictions requiring political reconfiguration of multiple sorts, including more intense forms and strategies of financialization (chapter 1);

3   civil society advocacy as activated and mobilized through scandal (chapter 2);

4   judicialization and the fight to make patents incentivize the public good (chapter 3);

5   competing forms of social responsibility, as articulated through corporate philanthropy and as demanded of the state (chapter 4); and

6   corporate alliance making with civil society groups for access to medicines in the context of imperialist geopolitics (chapter 5).

Some of these political forms establish hegemonic modes and relations of production, while others contest this hegemony.

Finally, I think through the ways in which articulations between value and politics are mediated by knowledge, which itself is neither pure nor static. Rather, knowledge gets appropriated into different domains and to various ends, rendered instrumental, serviceable, or commodified as it moves across domains and geographies. In other words, knowledge can be mobilized in a variety of ways to configure value, politics, and their relationships; in the process, forms of knowledge can themselves be coproduced with those of value and politics. Some of the manifestations and mobilizations of knowledge that concern me the most in this book are

1 the actual kinds of scientific and medical knowledge required in drug discovery and development, ranging from the organic synthetic chemistry required in much small-molecule drug manufacture to the pharmacological knowledge that goes into establishing drug dosage, the clinical knowledge involved in establishing safety and efficacy profiles in clinical trials, and the knowledge of cellular and molecular mechanism required in ventures of rational drug development of which Gleevec is exemplary;
2 the epidemiological knowledge that underlies public health interventions, or broader population-based targeting of therapeutic markets;
3 various kinds of anticipatory knowledge that operate in different domains, ranging from financial markets to clinical research to patent law; and
4 knowledge as process and strategy of making meaning, modalities of reasoning and interpretation that operate in particular situations or domains with more or less authority.

But further, knowledge matters not just when it explicitly becomes valuable or political (or renders particular articulations of value and politics), but also when value and politics manifest through erasing, silencing, or obscuring knowledge, or in situations in which knowledge operates through uncertainty or indeterminacy.

What results, then, is a more complex, elaborated, and differentiated structure of pharmocracy, something that looks like figure 1.1.

Value

The most important abstraction that this book is concerned with is value. In order to elaborate how I think about value, I find it particularly useful to turn to the way in which Karl Marx analytically conceptualized it in relation to labor and capital. Marx insisted that any proper understanding of capital has to come from beginning the analysis with the question of value.[21] And for capital, value has no meaning unless it is surplus value. For money to be capital, it must have the potential for generating surplus within it as it circulates in processes of commodity exchange. In relation to the situation of European (especially English) industrial capitalism that Marx was writing

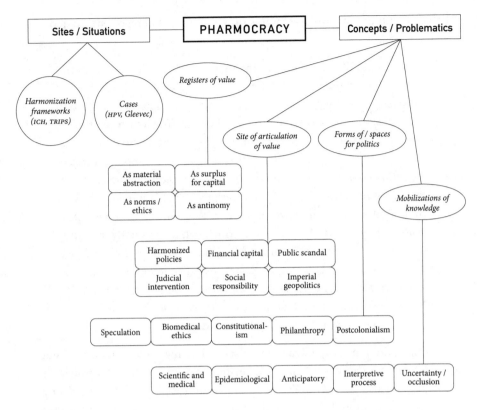

FIGURE I.1

about, this potential comes from what he called labor power—the potential for the worker to generate more labor than that rendered adequate by wage. The question of whether and to what extent the labor theory of value is applicable to all places and times is of less interest to me than the methodological insight it provides into an analysis of how capital generates value through an exploitation of bodily potential, even as the generation of value becomes an end in itself.[22] Further, value is that which allows the commodity, which is always the product of specific and concrete human labor, to figure as abstract labor. At the core of Marx's critique of political economy is his insistence that value is an abstraction device.

Therefore, on the one hand, value is simply an attribute (something that a commodity has: its utility, its beauty, its ability to be worn or eaten; something that money has: its ability to circulate itself, to mediate and measure other kinds of circulations, to quantitatively express circulation itself). But on the other hand, value itself performs the various materializations and abstractions of those things that it is simply supposed to represent. To quote Marx:

> In the circulation M-C-M both the money and the commodity function only as different modes of existence of value itself, the money as its general mode of existence, the commodity as its particular or, so to speak, disguised mode. It is constantly changing from one form into the other, without becoming lost in this movement; it thus becomes transformed into an *automatic subject*. If we pin down the specific forms of appearance assumed in turn by *self-valorizing value* in the course of *its life*, we reach the following elucidation: capital is money, capital is commodities. In truth, however, *value is the subject [i.e., the independently acting agent]* of a process in which, while constantly assuming the form of money and commodities, it ... *valorizes itself independently*. For the movement in the course of which it adds surplus-value is its own movement, its valorization is therefore self-valorization. . . . *By virtue of being value, it has acquired the occult ability to add value to itself.* (Marx [1976] 1867, 255, emphases added)[23]

This definition of capital in terms of self-valorizing value is significant, but is not the point at which Marx's explanation runs out. Rather it signifies, in Spivak's terms, "the possibility of an indeterminacy" (1985, 78). The ability to "add value to itself" is precisely that which renders capitalist value appropriative—of labor (turning it into surplus), but also, in other situations, of health (turning it into surplus), or of ethics (turning it into surplus). It is also that which renders the generation of capitalist value political, a politics that plays out through both the consolidation and the contestation of modes and relations of power and production. Hence an ethnographic elucidation of these relations and of their consolidation and contestation allows us to work backward toward a conceptualization of the capitalist value form itself.

How does this relate to health? The most literal answer to this question has been provided by Joseph Dumit (2012a, 2012b), who developed the notion of surplus health as an analogy to Marxian surplus labor.[24] This refers to the market value that pharmaceutical capital gains from the potential for future illness of those who might one day consume drugs, which includes anyone with the buying power to constitute a market for therapeutics and crucially excludes those without. Empirically, Dumit (2012a) studied the growth of pharmaceutical marketing in the United States in the second half of the twentieth century and its imbrication with the growth of clinical trials, a trajectory that has resulted in the progressive growth of prescription rates in the country with no signs of stopping. Analytically, he substituted Marxian labor-related keywords with health-related keywords in volume 1 of *Capital* (Dumit 2012b).[25] In the process, Dumit generated a "health theory of value" that is literally analogous to Marxian labor theory, showing how value creates health that is appropriate to and appropriable by capital, alienated from embodied healthiness. Value thus is that which allows the symptom, which is always the product of specific and concrete human health, to figure as abstract health.[26] Even as health itself comes to be at stake, so too does labor, as biomedical economies engender both multiplications and divisions of labor, seen especially in the various proliferations and dislocations of experimental subjectivity in clinical trials.[27]

There is a further tangle here, because value is never just about surplus; it also refers to the ethical and the normative. Often, pharmaceutical corporate capital is contested by taking recourse to seemingly opposed value systems grounded in ethics and morality: for instance, by an insistence on the ethical conduct of clinical trials and human-subject experimentation based on principles of good clinical practice; or by demands for equitable and broad access to essential medicines for people who do not have the purchasing capacity to buy them on the market; or by attempts to hold states accountable to their responsibility to ensure the health and care of their populations. In other words, one could envisage a value that is not just defining of capital but (in its ethical registers) also an alternative normative framework to capital. And yet corporations are perfectly capable of enfolding these concerns into their own value-generating enterprises.[28] Hence, these latter forms of value are never entirely outside the fold of capital but are always appropriable by it. Ethics can be potentially opposed to surplus value but also deeply tangled within its logics.

There are enmeshed conceptual relationships between the ethical and the norm as well, given that the norm also inflects in two ways, implying either the normative or the normal (Hacking 1990). To the extent that the normal is normative in a given situation, ethics is the norm; to the extent that the normal falls short of the normative in a given situation, ethics is precisely not the norm but an improvement upon it. And so, the ethical can come to be the grounds for political contestation around the norm itself. One saw this transpire in the Gleevec case, as Novartis's lawyers argued for the product patent, among other things, on grounds that this drug was patented in forty other countries. Hence, they claimed that granting a patent on the drug was the normal thing to do, and that the Indian Patent Office's denial was unethical, preventing as it did a legitimate monopoly that had already been established in other jurisdictional contexts. The opposition, on the other hand, argued for an ethics based in normativity, claiming that what was normal had no bearing on what was appropriate, which was adhering to the standard of invention as established under Indian law with its public health flexibilities that prevented pharmaceutical evergreening. If the former position established the authority of the norm by taking recourse to a patent claim that had already been held valid in multiple other contexts, then the latter did so by taking recourse to legislative history that rendered the normative constitutional ordering of how invention was to be understood in India as a higher standard to be met than normal standards of patentability prevalent in other countries.

What is at stake, through and through, are the antinomies of value in its multiple registers. An antinomy is a contradiction between two beliefs or conclusions that are in themselves reasonable. Resolution or consensus is often impossible; what is at stake is living within the mutual incompatibility. Value, in the contested, conjoined, multiply jointed senses of market/surplus value and ethical/normative value, precisely because of its inherent indeterminacy, constitutes the terrain of politics. My investments therefore do not lie in defining what value really is, and certainly do not correspond in any straightforward way to what people say or believe value really is. I am not interested in finding an ontology of value that manages a transhistorical reconciliation of its contradictory manifestations, nor am I attempting an elucidation of cosmologies of value that describe the ways in which actors resolve these contradictions for themselves.[29] Rather, I stay attentive to the articulations and antinomies of value as it is rendered political.

Politics

Without a doubt, global pharmaceutical politics has come to be deeply contested, often with polarized positions around a range of issues. I have already introduced the polarization around global harmonization, which is projected as being about ethics and innovation by its cheerleaders and about the hegemony of multinational corporate capital by its detractors. But beyond this, there are all sorts of situated alliances across adversarial positions, just as there are major disagreements among actors who are otherwise in positions of structural solidarity.

Even among those who oppose the appropriation of health by capital, there is a range of different positions. There are those who respond to the problem of unethical clinical trials by adopting an antiscience position toward clinical research, while others insist upon the importance of clinical research for public health even as they oppose the ways in which it has been institutionalized; there are those who decry the conduct of clinical research on the poor and vulnerable, just as others believe that any genuinely progressive public health practice must include research on more marginal populations within its ambit; there are those who believe that civil society has the right and the responsibility to shape public health agendas, while others who believe in the paramount importance of scientific autonomy free from such dictation; there are those who believe that access to medicines cannot be achieved without a pragmatic engagement with the multinational pharmaceutical industry, including the provision of incentives, while others insist that genuine transformation in political economies of health cannot happen as long as one is wedded to privileging the institutional capacities of the most powerful corporate players; there are huge disagreements around specific mechanisms of enabling access, or around the relationship between pharmaceutical access and primary health infrastructure development.

Of course, there are deep divisions among capitalist interests as well, especially between Euro-American innovator industries involved in R&D and Indian companies who have primarily been involved in reverse engineering generic drugs; but even those divisions are fluid as Indian companies strategically align themselves in certain instances with multinational pharmaceutical corporations, just as the latter seek out national generic competitors as potential targets of acquisition. Different kinds of clinical trials brokers act in concert when it comes to driving regulatory harmonization even as they compete with each other to construct market terrains according to their perception of strategic interest.

The state too is an inherently conflicted actor. If capital is defined by its incessant drive toward surplus, then the state in its liberal democratic form is caught within its own fundamental antinomy, accountable both to the interests of local, national, and global capital on the one hand and on the other to its citizens. What this division means and how its different representative functions get activated becomes an important empirical question.[30] Political orientation toward the state on the part of both corporate and civil society interests is immediate and constant, in a context in which what the state is, which arms of it are activated, and how it emerges as a differentiated entity that is often acting at odds with itself all come to be at stake and contested. This is so even—perhaps especially—as the place of the state as a primary institution of governance comes to be in question with the growth of parastatal, nongovernmental, multilateral, or corporate governance regimes.

Part of the task of conceptualizing politics then is empirical, tracking and mapping the content of heterogenous positions, strategic alliances, and situated articulations in relation to different biomedical domains. But further, this book focuses on different forms of and spaces for politics in the context of health. Similarly to my engagement with value, my attempt here is not to generate some authoritative definition of the political as much as it is to show the situated intersection and interaction of particular modalities of politics that emerge within certain economic and governance structures and out of specific historical conjunctures.

This book considers the constitution of the forms of and spaces for politics as health comes to be appropriated by capital. I think of constitution in two mutually reinforcing but opposing senses. The first is in terms of the ways in which these forms and spaces are constituted. This speaks to an active sense of constituting, of putting in place. Constituted entities are not static or given; they are almost by definition historically enacted, culturally endowed, in formation, even as they are emplaced and located. This is a concern with emergent forms of and spaces for politics (Fischer 1980, 2003). At the same time, there is a sense of the constitutional as related to the constitutive—that which is inherent to or defining of a political order. This refers to institution-alized codes, legal and normative, that get held up as defining prescribed codes of action and governance; taking the form perhaps of a Constitution (with a capital *C*), a foundational (often national-state) document that goes beyond prescription to signifying the ethos of "a people" (Ackerman 1991). But it could also imply constitution with a small *c*; the multiple sites of regu-lation and governance within which rules and norms come to be enshrined (Jasanoff 2003, 2011).

Hence, this book locates its analysis within a fundamental tension that exists between the variant trajectories of the materialization of value and the normative consolidation of the appropriation of health by capital; but also within the tension that exists between the content of a politics around health and the forms and spaces of its emergent and constitutive articula-tions, which are at once unsettled and deeply normed, constantly contested but also variously constrained and naturalized. What is at stake here is not simply the generation of a catalog of different emergent political forms, but rather the question of relationships between different constitutive and emer-gent forms of and spaces for politics. Which ones get activated, and which are suppressed, contested, and denaturalized? Which imaginaries fall out and lose salience? Which ones sediment to become the grounds upon which naturalized assumptions get made?[31] Imbricated in these forms of and spaces for politics is a third register of the constitutional, referring to health, to the body and its overall well-being.[32]

If a conceptualization of value has implications for an understanding of the reconfigurations of health as it gets appropriated by global capital, then I argue that tracing these forms of and spaces for politics in the context of value-laden health is equally consequential for a conceptualization of democracy. It is useful to think here of two important modalities of theorizing the democratic. One considers it in terms of rational communicative action with the eventual goal of consensus, going beyond goal-directed strategic action for one's own benefit (for instance, Habermas 1984, 1985). Another conceptualizes it in more organic terms, as the expression of popular sentiments and actions that can never be completely constrained or represented by the macropolitical form of the state (for instance, Chatterjee 2004, 2011). My own stakes in the democratic go beyond both formulations. The Habermasian ideal of rational communicative action as the means and consensus as the ends of an ideal democratic situation is, certainly in an Indian context, an empirical absurdity, and Chatterjee provides a more productively realist formulation.[33] But there are empirical limits to this formulation as well, because it locates the site of the political outside formal structures of the law, outside corporatized modes and relations of production. Hence, the sites of the political come to be rendered outside structures of representative power or hegemonic modes of production. Chatterjee's theorization of democracy occurs largely within what he calls political society; capital itself, or law itself, or civil society itself, get evacuated of empirical and explanatory thickness.[34]

This book traces political struggles for ethical clinical trials or access to medicines that occur resolutely within civil society (and indeed, are involved in constructing domains of civil society across scales, as seen with global civil society movements for access to medicines); follows the law as it comes to be the site for the instantiation of judicial sensibilities that have cultural and historical specificity and resonance; and conceptualizes capital in its most corporatized, monopolized, financialized forms, containing its own sectoral, national, and situational sensibilities. Hence, it theorizes democracy not in terms of what Chatterjee calls the politics of the governed, but rather in terms of the politics of governance. Chatterjee locates democratic politics within the realm of popular reason; this book correspondingly does so within representative domains that see the constitution and contestation of public reason

(Jasanoff 2013). Representative politics are not just ideological constructs of liberal political philosophy; they speak to political forms and spaces that are central to the configuration of contemporary democracy in ways that demand empirical attention in their own right.[35]

Knowledge

Questions of value and politics, of global hegemonies and their contestations, often come to be at stake around questions of knowledge. When, how, and on whose terms does knowledge come to matter in the articulations of value and politics in global biomedicine? Biomedicine is, among other things, a knowledge-producing activity, even as it produces artifacts, institutional structures, and subjective states around something called health. The centrality of knowledge production to biomedical research and production has perhaps become more explicit throughout the second half of the twentieth century, through the growth of evidence-based medicine (Timmermans and Berg 2003). But knowledge practices are consequential not just internally to the practice of biomedicine. As part of its very rationale and practice, biomedicine interacts with regimes of value shaped by representative forms of politics. Clinical research for instance might be a constitutive part of the apparatus of evidence-based medicine, but it is equally and immediately also about the experimental subjection of humans (and animals) and therefore about the apparatus of ethical norms and regulatory frameworks under which such subjection can occur. Intellectual property is integral to many practices of drug discovery and development, increasingly globally, but it also concerns philosophical and legal questions of what constitutes invention and which jurisdictional frameworks apply in deciding the answers to such questions.

And so my interest in knowledge is not as something that can be purified and thought of in its own terms, but rather as something that is coproduced with and mobilized in relation to value and politics.[36] Sheila Jasanoff (2004) describes coproduction in terms of the mutually determining ways in which scientific knowledge and social order come to be produced. Following Jasanoff, my attempt is to understand the coproduction of knowledge with value and politics in a context in which health comes to be appropriated by capital in ways that put democracy at stake. One cannot think of knowledge in global biomedicine devoid of value and politics; one cannot contemplate the stakes of changing modes and relations of knowledge production in biomedicine without considering its stakes for democracy. Value and politics do not emerge, as it were, after the fact, but are conjoined with it.

I attend to such coproduction by looking at how knowledge comes to be mobilized across domains and geographies in global biomedicine. For instance, when the HPV vaccine, produced in the West, travels to India to be incorporated into its national immunization program on the basis of clinical trials that have been conducted in a number of countries but not in India, what kinds of knowledge about vaccine response or cervical cancer epidemiology are assumed to be portable across territorial and demographic contexts, and by whom? How and when are such assumptions naturalized or challenged? When Gleevec's patent denial is contested in India in spite of it being accepted largely without question in many other countries, what kinds of legal interpretations of invention come to operate in different jurisdictional and legislative contexts? Mobilizations of knowledge are not just transnational, but also operate across domains: of science, law, and policy; of laboratory, clinic, and public health; of experiment, therapy, and epidemiology; of university and industry; of manufacturing and financial capital. During such mobilizations, the representative function of knowledge is not consequent to some absolute truth-value, but rather is a result of its serviceability.[37]

As in my conceptualization of politics, I think here both with and against Michel Foucault, who has provided some of the most important theorizations of the relationship between knowledge and power throughout his work (but most explicitly in essays and interviews collected and published as *Power/Knowledge* [Foucault 1980]).[38] Through an analysis of knowledge, Foucault was able to open up different ways of conceptualizing power. Simply put, Foucault went beyond an analysis that simply read power and politics as ideological corruptions of the truth of science. He recast the question of the influence of power on truth into one that was about the "interweaving effects of power and knowledge" (Foucault 1980, 109). Thus, he was able to ask new questions about the nature of the practice of knowledge production itself, of how such practice was interwoven with the emergence of institutional forms and structures that would regulate social conduct. But Foucault's investment in the conceptualization of knowledge was as truth, especially as he articulated the problematic of Power/Knowledge.[39] How might other concerns with knowledge develop in relation to the situation of highly capitalized biomedicine? Specifically, I am interested in the question of knowledge as being a problem of translation across domains and locales.[40]

A concern with the translations and translocations of knowledge speaks directly to its articulations with value and politics. Which (and whose) representations mobilize knowledge, across which domains, and through what kinds of norms and authority? When (and in what ways) does knowledge come to legitimize or be rendered legitimate by different regimes of value, such as those that promise capital accumulation and appreciation, or mandate ethical clinical practice, or activate foundational constitutional imaginaries, philanthropic ideals, or nationalist sentiments, and through which forms of and spaces for politics? Answering these questions involves attending to the kinds of work that count as valuable knowledge production in contemporary biomedicine—for instance, experimentation, innovation, anticipation, speculation, interpretation, or advocacy—and to the embodied representational forms that knowledge takes as it comes to be mobilized (of the innovator who promises therapies, the industrialist who promises economic growth and national self-sufficiency, the speculator who promises returns on investment, the volunteer who becomes the subject of clinical experimentation, the judge who promises an appropriate interpretation of the law, the activist who fights for social or distributive justice). This speaks both to the labor of biomedicine and to what Michael Fischer (2013) has called its peopling. At stake here is a knowledge-for-itself: all the immediately value-laden, representative political forms that knowledge takes in global biomedicine as it concerns experimentation, innovation, corporate strategy, financial speculation, technocratic expertise, legal interpretation, or civil society advocacy.[41]

This is directly relevant to understanding the ways in which hegemony operates. For Gramsci, understanding representation involved understanding the place of knowledge in culture, society, and politics in deeply situated ways.[42] Gramsci was interested in how the hegemonic organization of coercion and consent was a function of the intellectual authority of dominant groups, and conversely in what kinds of intellectual work were necessary to oppose and transform existing hegemonic orders. The work of knowledge that I trace operates in both directions: toward the consolidation and the contestation of capitalized health. But the kinds of knowledge practices involved in specific forms of hegemonic consolidation or contestation are extremely particular, located within historical, institutional, societal, cultural, and personal investments, and demand empirical attention. Even the question of who counts as a significant intellectual in a given situation becomes deeply fraught and consequential. For instance, I show how it is the financial analyst who disproportionately authorizes what constitutes innovation in the context of the Euro-American pharmaceutical industry (chapter 1), even as high court and Supreme Court judges do so in India (chapter 3); how technocratic clinical research brokers and feminist civil society advocates clash over what constitutes the definitions and priorities of public health, even as those very questions are debated within disciplinary public health journals and forums (chapter 2). What is at stake is not just whose knowledge is right in some absolute, factual sense, but whose knowledge comes to count as valuable and authoritative, where, and through what kinds of mechanisms.

This book thinks through the situated trajectories of global pharmaceutical policy harmonization in India and the cases of HPV and Gleevec while analyzing the conceptual problematics of value, politics, and knowledge. Chapter 1, "Speculative Values: Pharmaceutical Crisis and Financialized Capital," explains the nature of speculative, financialized, multinational pharmaceutical capital. It focuses primarily on the logics that drive the Euro-American, R&D-driven pharmaceutical industry, to argue how an industry that is captured by capital is one that, structurally and constitutively, comes to be in crisis. I show how this crisis extends globally, implicating other national industries as well as consumers and patients in both the First World and the Third. Chapter 2, "Bioethical Values: HPV Vaccines, Public Scandal, and Experimental Subjectivity," elaborates a politics of civil society advocacy as it develops through the public scandal around the HPV vaccine studies. This raises questions not just about relationships between health, value, and politics, but also of the configuration of epidemiological knowledge and technocratic forms of governance within these relationships. Chapter 3, "Constitutional Values: The Trials of Gleevec and Judicialized Politics," illustrates judicialization as it is played out in the Indian courts. It elaborates the legal history of Gleevec in India between 2005 and 2013 to think about the place of the law and judicial governance in articulations of health, value, knowledge, and politics. Chapter 4, "Philanthropic Values: Corporate Social Responsibility and Monopoly in the Pharmocracy," offers a critique of monopoly capital. It describes the incorporation of ethical and normative commitments into the value-generating activities of the multinational R&D-driven pharmaceutical industry through discourses of innovation and materialized through practices of corporate social responsibility. I focus specifically on Novartis's drug donation program, the Gleevec International Patient Assistance Program, and the way in which it was established and run on the ground in India. In addition to imbrications of different registers of value (market and ethical), one sees here complex articulations of experimental and therapeutic biomedical economies. Chapter 5, "Postcolonial Values: Nationalist Industries in Pharmaceutical Empire," identifies Indian free market capitalism as it intersects with global geopolitical configurations and strategies. I provide an account of India's oldest surviving pharmaceutical company, Cipla, which has become a leading player in the opposition to WTO-mandated product patent regimes and hence an ally of global civil society groups fighting for access to medicines. Cipla's history reveals a record of consistent action in its own market interests, and an attempt to define a market terrain in terms of those interests; but it also reflects certain explicit nationalist and (more recently) global humanitarian sentiments, in ways that open up questions about the postcolonial and ethical investments of these market actors. I then think through the global geopolitical landscape that structures these different ethical incorporations in antagonistic and power-laden ways. The conclusion is an attempt to think through the implications of this analysis for considering the future trajectories of politics engaging global biomedicine and global capital.

At the end of each chapter is a postscript that spells out the chapter's concerns to pharmocracy as a politically salient concept. It marks the site of questions concerning the nature of the political as it emerges in and through domains of health that are appropriated by global capital. These postscripts do not provide answers or explanations; they are meant as a reminder that the real challenge here—empirically, conceptually, and politically—is to remain attentive to how pharmocratic regimes put both health and democracy at stake.

Situating Pharmocracy

It is important to locate the analysis of pharmocracy in this book in relation to the specificities of place, history, and event that constitute its empirical substance. The task here is not to provide some sort of comprehensive explanation of what value or politics or knowledge is in some definitive sense as much as it is to multiply the situations from which its various articulations can be seen. Each situated perspective from which this book is written—of speculative, financialized, multinational pharmaceutical capital, of public scandal, of judicialization and the Indian courts, of monopoly capital, of Indian free market capitalism, and of global geopolitics—affords a locus for observing articulations of value, politics, and knowledge.[43]

This book is immediately concerned with a very particular situation in place and time, post-2005 India, in the domain of a specific industrial sector (pharmaceuticals), and with politics concerning health. On the face of it, the story that I am about to tell could be seen as one of a pharmaceutical industry acting and developing in the cause of more innovation and greater ethical consciousness. But it could equally be seen as one of the expanding domain of global capital and of multinational corporate hegemony, resulting in new Third World national regulations that are called upon to facilitate First World corporate interests. Such expansion occurs at the expense of the world's poor, who become guinea pigs in clinical experiments even as they find it harder to access essential medication. The reality involves understanding these hegemonic movements in all their fullness, but also and at the same time the ways in which they are contested. Contemporary India is important in this regard. India occupies a central place in global pharmaceutical politics by virtue of its strong national generic industry, which has been an important source of affordable medication for the Global South over the past two decades. For instance, MSF procures 25 percent of its essential medicines for worldwide distribution and 75 percent of its antiretrovirals from India.[44]

In addition to situating India thus, it is important to situate the period that this book focuses on. Specifically, 2005 serves as an empirical entry point because the legislative events that took place that year signify broader transformations of pharmaceutical political economies. But more generally, the time at stake is the contemporary.[45] How do we situate these legislative moments and the political events that surround them in relation to a broader historical movement in the global pharmaceutical economy and in contemporary India? In order to address this conceptually and methodologically, I turn to Gramsci's notion of the conjuncture, as a conceptual and methodological framework within which to situate my analysis in this book.[46]

Gramsci discusses two kinds of historical movements in relation to one another: the "conjunctural," which "appear as occasional, immediate, almost accidental," and the "organic," which are "relatively permanent" (2000, 201). Conjunctures could most certainly be marked by significant events; indeed, in order for them to be recognized as conjunctures, they probably are. But Gramsci finds them significant not just as historical markers of some kind of epochal shift (as events that radically cause a separation between then and now), but as political ones: the conjuncture provides a terrain upon which politics plays out. This could be a politics that attempts to preserve existing forces and relations, or one that attempts to overturn them. When I say that India's becoming party to the WTO or its attempts to globally harmonize ethical regulatory regimes for clinical trials provides the conjuncture in which this book is written, it does not imply in any simple sense that these events in and of themselves allow for an epochal shift in pharmaceutical economies. What it means is that they are markers of a reconfiguration of the terrain of the political in relation to these economies. Whether we think about the operations of multinational pharmaceutical companies in India, Indian generics companies, or sick Indians who are also citizens and consumers, life (and death), health (and illness), and the nature of markets, production and consumption come to be configured differently in a product patent regime than a process patent one, or in a liberalized clinical trials regime than in a more restrictive one.

The particular events in question, whether in relation to clinical trials or to intellectual property and access to medicines, were themselves contingent events. Nothing was predetermined about India becoming signatory to TRIPS. Indeed, there had been much civil society opposition to India's participation in the Uruguay Round of GATT negotiations in the early 1990s. But trade pressures from the United States, driven by the strength of the multinational pharmaceutical lobby in the U.S. government, coupled with the Indian government's strategic rationalizations that belonging to a multilateral free trade forum would be in the country's economic interests, held sway. Similarly, the political mobilization of CRO interests drove the liberalization of clinical trials regimes, which was hardly an obvious or predetermined movement. Yet elucidating the contingencies that underlie these conjunctural moments alone is insufficient. It remains to be asked at the level of empirical specificity: Why is it that these contingent conjunctures happened together? Why did they happen at a moment of the broader appropriation of various domains of health in India by global capital? And what is the relationship of these multiple, convergent (if contingent) events to the logics of capital and its institutional materialization in corporate strategies and global geopolitics?

For Gramsci, what was most important about the conjuncture was the way in which it always poses the question of its own relationship to the organic. The theoretical task, he suggests, is neither just the elucidation of the conjuncture (which ultimately privileges the contingent as an end in itself or, in Gramsci's terms, leads to "an exaggeration of the voluntarist and individual element" [2000, 202]), nor simply the elucidation of some fundamental organic movement as underlying the conjuncture (which leads to structural determinism). It is rather the determination of the relationship between the conjunctural and the organic.

For this, it is important to locate the conjuncture of pharmaceutical politics in India that I am marking in the context of a broader political economic conjuncture, within a broader trajectory of capitalization of the life sciences and of India. One has seen the progressive privatization of clinical trials since the 1970s alongside the capture of the multinational R&D-driven industry by speculative financial capital, a process I describe in detail in chapter 1. Concomitant to this has been India's transformation into a global market economy, a process initiated in earnest by the 1991 Congress Party–

led government and marked since by various forms of economic liberalization in the interests of global capital. One can see this manifest in relation to changing intellectual property regimes under the guise of free trade and of changing ethical regimes in the cause of good clinical practice. But these are just sectoral instantiations of broader movements of global capitalization in the Indian economy writ large, marked by the opening of markets to foreign investment; intense wealth generation among certain segments of the population in the context of widening inequality and wealth disparity; new kinds of urban-rural divides, along with new forms of sociological mobility (and immobility); the emergence of parallel private infrastructures for essential services such as health, water, and electricity for those who can afford it; and the apparent handing over of the reins of the state to the market.[47]

Yet this period has also been marked by populism of the representative Indian state in relation to the poor. This is different from the feudal populism of political patronage networks, which has existed throughout the history of independent India and which, as Partha Chatterjee (2008) has argued, is important for understanding the functioning of informal economies in India today. It is also different from the state socialist populism of the 1970s, marked by Indira Gandhi's *garibi hatao* (remove poverty) manifesto. Rather, it is deeply coupled to instruments of global capital. An example of this in relation to pharmaceutical economies is the National Rural Health Mission (NRHM), launched in 2005. This initiative has emerged alongside the building of institutional capacity for public health education and research that was previously lacking in India, but also alongside the establishment of global health as a central focus in American medical schools and public health curricula. Programs such as these are closely articulated to institutions of global expertise such as the Gates Foundation, operate with top-down imaginaries of public health, involve public-private partnerships, and are often deeply technocratic in their mind-set.

There are many symptoms of neoliberalism in these formations, but they emerge in the context of representative populism toward the poor as an object and target of state intervention.[48] The NRHM, for instance, happens at precisely the conjuncture that sees India liberalizing its clinical trials regimes and changing its patent regimes to become WTO compliant. But it also happens alongside or anticipates a host of other initiatives launched by the Congress government that was elected in 2004 (and continued in power, albeit with a different set of coalition partners, until 2014) that are similarly populist, and often hitched to rights: for instance, the right to food, right to education, right to employment, and right to information.[49] All of these in various ways represent unfulfilled promises, but they have become important sites of political action. They signify not just the state's acknowledgment of obligations toward its citizens, but also represent modernist promissory notes that emerge out of a conjuncture of economic liberalization. What is at stake here is an understanding of history for the articulation of value and politics, "not the reconstruction of past history but the construction of present and future history" (Gramsci 2000, 202).

This understanding of history, in this book, is grounded in nine years of ethnographic fieldwork with a range of actors involved in various aspects of global biomedicine, pharmaceutical capital, and the politics of health. The research for this project started in early 2006 and involved following the burgeoning CRO industry in India, specifically its attempts to drive regulatory harmonization. This was where, it seemed, all the action was at the time. I was interested in following the intense conversation that was developing within the industry about the importance of developing an ethical infrastructure for the conduct of clinical trials; but the ethics in question was an instrumental and purely procedural one, concerned with good clinical practice and developing the apparatus for informed consent. I became interested in how this conversation around ethics was taking shape, not just for what was being said but also for what was not being said by the actors who were most powerfully involved in substantiating regulatory harmonization on the ground. Specifically, there was no regulatory conversation about whether drugs tested in India would be marketed in India, let alone be made available at affordable prices. The fact that this was happening at a time when actual access to medication could potentially become more difficult under the newly instituted product patent regime exacerbated the stakes of the issue. And so, what seemed as significant as the discourses of ethics that were being articulated were the discursive gaps that were at the heart of this articulation.[50]

I published a piece with this argument fairly early in the game, along with an op-ed in the *Indian Express* (K. Sunder Rajan 2007, 2008). Consequently and unsurprisingly, my access to CRO executives, who were initially very keen to talk to me, started drying up. By this time, my interests were in any case shifting to the question of access to medicines, a shift that followed naturally from attending to the discursive gap at the heart of the conversation on regulatory harmonization. If the CRO actors and clinical trials regulators were not talking about access to medicines, who was? I did not have far to look, since this was the very time when the politics around interpreting the 2005 Patent Act was at its height and becoming heavily judicialized through the Gleevec case. What was a discursive gap in one biomedical and regulatory domain was a site of deep political contestation and thick discourse in another, at exactly the same time. Much of my fieldwork at this point shifted to following the trajectory of the Gleevec case, which involved following its contestation and resolution in the courts, but also tracking the strategies of the multinational, Euro-American pharmaceutical industry in response to this judicial politics, and having conversations with civil society advocates for access to essential medicines and members of the Indian generics industry who had formed alliances with these advocates. I assumed that the clinical trials side of the project was done and dusted, having raised certain questions that I had followed into new research. I thought I had moved on.

But in 2011, I was sucked back into it with a vengeance, as clinical trials became the subject of scandal in India. The specific event that precipitated this was the HPV vaccine study, which became the focal point of political mobilization around unethical clinical trials. At the same time, a slew of other such cases came to light. This included the trials conducted on victims of the Bhopal gas disaster, trials conducted in a hospital in Indore that apparently did not conform to standards of good clinical practice, and trials conducted in Ahmedabad on poor volunteers in the apparent absence of proper informed consent.[51] The specific events in each of these cases was different, but they all suggested that the capacity building undertaken in the mid-2000s to make India a global experimental hub had led to a proliferation of poorly regulated clinical trials. There was no way that the clinical trials issue was a past concern, either politically or for my research.

Hence, part of the structure of this research simply comes from having conducted it in many sites, a process of following significant actors and events around. But more substantially, it comes from thinking about two domains of biomedical politics, concerning clinical trials and intellectual property and access to medicines, together. On the one hand, the specific actors and events that I was tracing in these two domains were different. On the other hand, they were parts of structurally interrelated biomedical and political economies. What I came to be concerned with was the relationship between these two domains, which raised two inverse conceptual problems. The first involves understanding the problem of variance that presents itself here: how it is that similar logics of capital materialize in such different political trajectories, mobilizing different strategies and institutional mechanisms. The second involves understanding norms: how it is that in spite of obviously different and contingent materializations of politics in these different domains, one sees the consistent establishment of certain political economic trajectories and power hierarchies that lead to the progressive capitalization of health.

It is this conjoined relationship between historical variance in the context of structural norms, and conversely of historical normalization of biomedical political economy in the context of contingent variance, that provides the anthropological problem space of this book. It seeks to provoke conceptual and political questions concerning how value, politics, and knowledge come to be related to one another in contemporary global pharmaceutical economies in ways that put both health and democracy at stake.

CHAPTER ONE

Speculative Values

Pharmaceutical Crisis & Financialized Capital

Dialectics of an Industry

This chapter explores how logics of capital grounded in the generation of surplus lead to a structure of crisis in global pharmaceutical industries, leading to trials for the industry itself, for patients and consumers who constitute its markets, and for populations who are excluded from these markets. This is an analysis of the sectoral manifestations of logics of capital. It further explores how these logics operate within a trajectory of the progressive financialization of pharmaceutical corporate capital, especially in the United States. I show how this structure of crisis creates a terrain that allows for situations such as that seen in the conjuncture of the mid-2000s in India, when the country was being conceptualized as a global biomedical experimental hub at the same time that therapeutic access was becoming potentially more difficult under newly instituted product patent regimes (see introduction). This happens at the same time that places like the United States experience prescription maximization and therapeutic saturation among those segments of the population that are included within pharmaceutical markets (Dumit 2012a, 2012b; Petryna 2009).

Antonio Gramsci says of crisis that it "consists precisely in the fact that the old is dying and the new cannot be born; in this interregnum a great variety of morbid symptoms appear" (Hoare and Nowell-Smith 1971, 276). I argue that the pharmaceutical industry is at present defined by a constitutive state of crisis. Crisis is a state that is simultaneously structural (a condition of the present) and exceptional (as being borne of the event).[1] In pharmaceutical politics, crisis manifests in both a humanitarian register and as something that is structurally endemic to capital. This analysis focuses on the latter, analyzing crisis as constitutive to capitalist modes and relations of production.[2]

My concerns in this chapter operate at multiple scales of analysis: first, to general conceptual questions concerning the logics of capital as they are grounded in imperatives to generate surplus; second, to the materialization of these logics in terrains of technoscientific capitalisms that are invested, quite literally, in the ideology of innovation; and third, to the specific sectoral logics of the pharmaceutical industry, as distinct from other kinds of high-technology, research and development (R&D)–focused industries. The most important distinction to note here concerns the specific scales and temporalities of capital investment in R&D-driven pharmaceutical development. The development of a new drug molecule involves enormous initial investment in drug discovery and development. Drug discovery is the process of finding potential target molecules that might have a useful (and marketable) therapeutic effect; this is in the United States largely underwritten by public money, especially through the funding of university-based biomedical research. Drug development involves taking potential therapeutic molecules through preclinical and clinical trials—which is an expensive and risky process, with no guarantee of success. Clinical trials have over the past four decades increasingly moved to the private sector, and this is a capital investment whose risk is largely borne by the R&D-driven pharmaceutical industry. This structure of enormous upfront capital investment into a process that might take over a decade to realize that investment, and whose realization is filled with risk and uncertainty, leads to sectoral specificities in the pharmaceutical industry.

In global pharmaceutical economies, there are at least three sets of actors that are simultaneously in crisis. The first is the multinational pharmaceutical industry, largely Euro-American, which is involved in R&D-based drug development. The second is patients, both in developed-country contexts such as the United States and in developing-country contexts such as India. And the third is national pharmaceutical industries such as the Indian, which is primarily a generic industry with expertise in reverse engineering drugs and selling them at a lower cost than patented medication, and deeply impacted in its business models by patent agreements mandated by the WTO.

Crisis itself, however, is polymorphic—it does not mean the same thing for each of these actors.[3]

Some of the factors that combine to configure the fundamentals of the market terrain that we now recognize in pharmaceutical development include the following: first, the development and growth of the Euro-American pharmaceutical industry, which began to focus on R&D-driven business models in the 1980s, leading to the development of blockbuster drugs that could earn over a billion dollars in annual revenue; second, the elaboration of a regulatory infrastructure in which larger and more complex clinical trials became essential before drugs could be approved for market; and third, the emergent possibilities of biopharmaceutical development (the development of complex biological molecules, as opposed to small organic chemical molecules as drugs), enabled by the growth of the entrepreneurial university, the interest taken in biotech by both private and public speculative markets, and intellectual property regimes that facilitate patenting. All of these were in place as constitutive elements of the drug development process by the end of the 1980s.

In the 1990s, further significant developments occurred. These include, in the United States, first, a restructuring of the regulatory process in ways that recognized the need for facilitating the approval of drugs to market in streamlined fashion;[4] second, the allowance of direct-to-consumer advertising by pharmaceutical companies; third, the release of a study by Tufts University's Center for the Study of Drug Development, which showed that the price of developing a new drug was on the order of $250 million, which made drug development costs a central part of the discussion in business and policy circles on the relationship of drug R&D to drug pricing (exacerbated by the estimation that only one in five drug candidates tends to make it through clinical trials to market; DiMasi et al. 1991);[5] and fourth, the growth of off-label use as a business model, which involves selling a drug for an indication other than that for which it was initially approved.[6] Along with these changes in the business models of pharmaceutical companies, the past thirty years have also seen the progressive movement of clinical trials into the private sector. In the mid- to late 1990s, trials started moving out of the United States to the rest of the world at a rapid rate (Petryna 2009).

By the turn of the twenty-first century, the contours of the pharmaceutical industry were as follows. This was a large industry that was extremely profitable. But these profits were built on the strength of a handful of blockbuster drugs, molecules that made in excess of a billion dollars a year. They offset the high rate of failure of drug candidates to make it through clinical trials (probably four drugs out of every five). Hence, this was an industry whose profits, although huge, depended upon a large amount of money from a small number of compounds. The ability to make so much money from these compounds was secured through strong intellectual property protection. Three historical, institutional factors make this configuration a structure that is potentially ridden with crisis: the place of the pharmaceutical industry in the speculative marketplace, pipeline problems, and the patent cliff. I elaborate.

Most major R&D-driven pharmaceutical companies are publicly traded. This means that value for these companies is determined less by profit (how much money they actually make over the amount expended) than by growth (how much potential there is for future earnings over and above the present rate of earning, which can be translated into shareholder value). The financial community expects a pharmaceutical industry growth rate of 13 percent earnings per share (EPS) annually. The industry growth rate typically operates at 8–10 percent EPS, and between 2002 and 2012 showed an annualized return on equity of −1.2 percent, according to the New York Stock Exchange Arca Pharmaceutical Index.[7]

To reach the kinds of growth the stock market expects purely through the development of new therapeutics requires three to five new chemical entities to be approved each year. This is difficult to achieve. If only one in five drug candidates entering clinical trials makes it to market, then in order to generate three to five new chemical entities a year, the company needs a large pipeline of drugs entering clinical trials. The absence of a robust pipeline in the pharmaceutical industry exacerbates the crisis. The pharmaceutical industry has over the past two decades faced what is referred to as an innovation deficit, a concern that developed in the latter half of the 1990s.[8] This was likely a function of the fact that by this time many of the low-hanging fruit, natural products that could be developed as potential therapeutic molecules, had already been picked, and more sophisticated, targeted forms of drug discovery that could address mechanistic aspects of disease were seen as necessary. The structural relationship between the pharmaceutical industry and the speculative marketplace thus intensified a scientific crisis that had already been in existence.

In this situation, the one thing that has saved pharmaceutical companies is the handful of blockbuster drugs that make billions of dollars a year. The only way these drugs have been able to make so much money is through the monopoly afforded by the patent. Hence, intellectual property becomes the critical factor that allows value generation in this business model. This is where the phenomenon known in industry circles as the patent cliff becomes such a potential source of crisis. Between 2009 and 2012, it was estimated that drugs representing over $74 billion in sales lost patent protection, and hence faced the prospect of competition from generic manufacturers (Deloitte 2009). This means that the pharmaceutical industry has been in crisis from both directions—the looming expiration of patent monopolies on currently profitable drugs; and the lack of an adequate pipeline of new drugs to replace those that start facing generic competition upon patent expiration. This led to the recognition on the part of the pharmaceutical industry of the importance of near-term revenue, and a resulting focus on mergers and acquisitions (M&A) rather than research and development (R&D). Hence, two tendencies are consequent to the structure within which the pharmaceutical industry operates. The first is monopolistic; the second is the tendency to consolidate through acquisitions.

The pressures from the financial markets that R&D-driven pharmaceutical companies inhabit in the context of their current pharmaceutical crises are indicated, for instance, in an article in the pharmaceutical industry newsletter *Pharmalot*. Titled "One More Reason That Lilly Must Do a Deal, Fast" (E. Silverman 2010), it cites figures that point to the crisis faced by the pharmaceutical company Eli Lilly (the makers, most famously, of Prozac), and arrives at the definitive conclusion—acquire or be acquired. Lilly is a big pharmaceutical company that at the time had a particularly anemic pipeline. They had had two major flops, including very poor sales performance of a blood thinner, Effient, and an Alzheimer's medication that was under development and failed to come to market. According to industry analysts, Lilly faced the steepest patent cliff of the big pharmaceutical companies. Another analyst was cited in this article as saying that Lilly's pipeline "still carries considerable risk. In our opinion, management must reconsider its long term strategy and will need to take short term actions."[9]

All the analysts cited in this piece who diagnose the crisis faced by companies like Lilly come from the financial sector—one from Sanford Bernstein, another from Leerink Swann, and a third from Deutsche Bank. In other words, on the one hand, there are actual events and figures—a failed clinical trial, poor sales performances, a certain amount of capital reserves ($5.1 billion in cash and equivalents at the end of the second quarter of 2010, according to the article). But there is also the interpretation of those events and figures through certain kinds of epistemology—in this case, financial risk. It is the financial analyst who assumes the role of the legitimate diagnostician when it comes to identifying the company's problems and its necessary solutions.

In the face of pipeline crises and patent cliffs, the logical response of the speculative marketplace is to push pharmaceutical companies toward M&A. The logic of this step is twofold. First, M&A potentially bolsters pipelines—instead of having to discover a drug candidate from scratch and take it all the way through drug development, companies could either in-license promising late-stage drug candidates from a smaller company that is looking for revenue, or they could acquire the smaller company altogether. This is often the mode of interaction of big pharmaceutical companies with biotech companies, which might have products in the pipeline but do not have the capital reserves or resources to take those products all the way to the market. Second, M&A reduces costs through streamlining, by consolidating projects and workforces in two companies.[10] This leads to the large number of layoffs and redundancies in the industry.

A Deloitte (2009) report on M&A in the life sciences (between pharmaceutical companies, or between pharmaceutical and biotech companies) cites figures that show the increasing trends toward such deals, and the increasing valuation of such deals. For instance, the median value of deals in which a pharmaceutical company acquired a biotech company rose from $80 million in 2000 to $400 million in 2008. There was a similar sort of increase in the median value of out-licensing deals (when a company licenses out a single molecule to a pharmaceutical company, rather than selling the entire company), from $25 million in 2000 to $230 million in 2008. The single largest factor responsible for these trends, it has been suggested, is the patent cliff and the threat of competition from generic manufacturers, which leads to a "laser-like focus on near-term revenue growth and profitability" (Deloitte 2009). What this means is less of a focus on R&D within the companies, especially early stage R&D, since such R&D implies commercial expenditure on projects that have no guarantee of resulting in the successful development of a therapeutic. Therefore, one sees the reinforcement of the very conditions that led to crisis in the first place: there is a pipeline crisis because there are not enough drug candidates coming into the pipeline. Yet the short-term focus on M&A as the way to mitigate that crisis (and as the way that is suggested by the speculative logics of financial markets) leads to a further inattention to R&D within companies, ensuring the continuing lack of an in-house pipeline. Indeed, a 2008 Deloitte survey of 360 senior pharmaceutical industry executives predicted that before 2020, most research and development would be conducted outside large life science companies.

Thus crisis is created by the coming together of a political economic structure of financialized capital that demands growth with an epistemology of risk assessment through which crisis comes to be naturalized. This is a form of diagnosing and understanding crisis that does not question the institutional structure of financialization itself, just the growth and performance of industries operating within the structure. Consequent to this, there is a monopolistic tendency that is enforced through patent protection, which has consequences for drug access, especially (but not just) in the developing world. And there is a tendency toward consolidation through acquisitions, thereby increasingly turning the R&D-driven industry into an M&A-driven one. In the process, one sees a fundamental shift away from the R&D model that has defined the industry for much of the past two decades. Pharmaceutical industries, it could be argued, function less and less as discoverers of new therapy and more like investment banks themselves, controlling, regulating, and betting on the flow of capital.

Ramifications of the Structure of Pharmaceutical Crisis

I argue that the process of the appropriation of the pharmaceutical industry by logics of speculative, financial capital results in the separation of value from considerations of patient needs or good health. Indeed, the very definition of health comes to be at stake and reconfigured in this process. What one is seeing within pharmaceutical industry logics is the implicit understanding of health in terms of surplus health, where health itself becomes a potential source of value for capital (Dumit 2012a, 2012b; see introduction, this volume). Indeed, health has to be thus valuable if one is to even imagine making the kinds of speculative financial bets on it that one sees in this model of pharmaceutical development. This is because the bet that is made here is not one that has anything to do with healthiness or therapeutic efficacy; it is, rather, a bet on market size, market penetration, and the potential for market growth. It is a bet on therapeutic consumption—which, in order to be a source of surplus value, must by definition be potentially greater than the amount of therapeutic consumption required to maintain healthiness. This creates a structure of crisis for patients.

The innovation deficit that puts the pharmaceutical industry in crisis has been compensated for in the American context by a consumption surplus. This is because pharmaceutical companies need to grow their markets in order to create value for their investors. But they have been poor at growing markets by coming up with new drugs for new indications. Hence, American patients get imagined as consumers who can grow markets if they just consume more drugs, leading to Americans consuming more and more drugs and to their becoming, in the language of clinical trials, "therapeutically saturated" (Petryna 2009; Dumit 2012a, 2012b). Given that drugs are fundamentally toxic molecules, this constant growth in drug consumption cannot possibly be harmless, even if it is often invisible (except when it manifests in dramatic crises such as in the case of Merck's blockbuster drug Vioxx, which had to be pulled from the market because of fatal side effects).

If one is considering an industry, such as the Euro-American, R&D-driven pharmaceutical industry, which operates within a value system that is fundamentally dependent on market growth, then one has to consider the various ways in which markets can be potentially grown. One way for a company to grow its market is to come out with a new therapeutic molecule—but this is time consuming, expensive, and risky and has not been as successful over the past decade as capital markets require. A second way is by expanding the indications for medications on the market through off-label use or reframing diseases as chronic or requiring prophylactic and preventive intervention, which is the mechanism of surplus health generation that Dumit has described in his work. This suggests a form of expanding therapeutic consumption that is not necessarily related to expanding the domains of treatment into new arenas, but is rather about expanding the domain of disease itself.[11] A third way in principle is to expand markets spatially, especially into emerging markets. This is harder to do for the pharmaceutical industry because of its concerns with protecting intellectual property (and this is where providing global security to companies' intellectual property through the WTO becomes important) and in maintaining control of their ability to set prices, which itself is limited in ways that I elaborate shortly. Therefore, including developing country populations within a global market calculus, while attractive, is variously constrained. However, value can be increased if the price of drug development is reduced. This is best achieved by reducing the cost of the clinical trials process through outsourcing the trials to the developing world. This does not require the developing world to be constituted as a market—one does not need to sell a drug in a country in which one tests a drug. I elaborate upon this logic with reference to India.

Clinical Trials

India has over the past forty years developed a thriving national pharmaceutical industry, built on the basis of a process patent regime, instituted in 1970, which did not allow patents on drug molecules but only on the process by which they could be manufactured. Unlike many developing (and indeed developed) country contexts, India never instituted a system of nationalized access to medicines, or even a properly functioning system of government-imposed price controls on drugs. Hence, price regulation has largely been a function of the market. This means that the question of what kind of market is operational is critical.

India has become incorporated into the globalization of drug development in two ways since the mid-1990s. As described in the introduction, one concerns the globalization of clinical trials, and the second concerns the globalization of intellectual property regimes under the aegis of the wto. This shift in patent regimes was happening at a time when one was seeing the emergence of a new industry segment in biomedicine—existing solely to conduct clinical trials, and operationalized by companies called clinical research organizations (cros). As clinical trials have moved more and more into the private sector in the United States over the past three decades, these companies have come to constitute an autonomous sector within the drug development industry. Unlike that of the pharmaceutical companies, their locus of value lies not even in the valorized expansion of health but simply in the valorized expansion of pharmaceutical clinical trials. India is a potentially attractive destination for clinical trials because of the presence of low-cost, bioavailable experimental subject populations, combined with good quality medical infrastructure.

And so, logics of capital as they expand globally exclude certain populations from the therapeutic market but include them as experimental subjects in global pharmaceutical clinical trials (K. Sunder Rajan 2007). These are populations that are incorporated as labor in the process of biomedical value generation, but not as consumers. Hence, the very imagination of trial populations in India is merely as risked experimental subjects, without the implicit social contract of therapeutic access at the end of the day. Layered onto these structural logics are the historical conditions that lead to the possibility of the configuration of such merely risked experimental subjectivities in the first place. I have described in earlier work how the kinds of subjects who get recruited into especially early stage clinical trials on healthy volunteers in India are often those who are victims of other kinds of prior dispossession (K. Sunder Rajan 2005, 2007). (Examples include mill workers in Bombay who have lost their jobs because of the evisceration of the textile industry, or, more recently, diamond workers in Surat who are following similar trajectories of de-proletarianization leading to experimental subjectivity).

The clinical trials situation represents a constitutive condition of exclusion from the therapeutic market in order to be enrolled as experimental subjects for drugs that others consume. This reflects the fact that India has cheap, bioavailable bodies.¹² But there is also the fact that India is a country with a burgeoning consumer class and constitutes an emerging market of enormous potential. In this register, there is a desire to include India in a global pharmaceutical market imaginary. Hence, the very same pharmaceutical company logics that make it attractive to outsource clinical trials to developing country locations like India also make it attractive to imagine India as a potential pharmaceutical market. I discuss the manner in which this plays out in terms of impacts on access to medicines.

Access to Medicines

The envisaging of countries like India as a potential therapeutic market by the Western pharmaceutical industry is constrained by one important factor and conditioned by another. The condition is a stringent intellectual property regime, which is what these companies now have post-wTo. This allows companies a monopoly and allows them to set prices as they would in the United States or Europe, which is essential for them in order to protect their high prices in those primary markets. But it is precisely this that limits how much countries like India can be imagined as markets at all, since this necessarily leads to the pricing of many patented therapeutics beyond what many Indian patients can afford. This potentially puts Indian populations into crisis in another register, the denial of access to many essential medicines for large sections that might have been able to afford this medication under a previous process patent regime, not because of market exclusion, but because of the inclusion of India in a global market regime that operates through logics that require the establishment of monopolistic business models at the expense of the free market competition in generic drugs that prevailed earlier.

India's insertion into a surplus health economy also means that it puts the Indian generic industry potentially in crisis, even as it leverages this terrain in strategic ways. Indeed, Indian generics companies use these logics of capital as gestures of public service that are animated both by strategic calculation and often by postcolonial nationalist impulses, even as they thus legitimize their own claim to profits (see chapter 5). Nonetheless, these maneuvers occur on uneven playing fields against powerful competitors. One is already seeing a trend whereby larger Indian companies have emerged as attractive acquisition targets for multinational pharmaceutical companies, not least because of their generic capabilities that are potentially attractive to leverage for revenues by acquiring companies in post–patent cliff scenarios in the West. Hence, there is a movement whereby Indian companies are shifting from being the manufacturers of bulk drugs as commodities for sale in Indian markets to becoming outsourced manufacturing facilities for multinational pharmaceutical companies—that is, if they are not going out of business entirely. Examples of major acquisitions in the past few years include the part sale of Ranbaxy, India's largest pharmaceutical company, to the Japanese company Daiichi Sankyo; of Nicholas Piramal India Limited, India's fourth largest pharmaceutical company, to the American company Abbott Laboratories; and of Shantha Biotechnics, one of India's largest bio-technology companies, to the French company Sanofi-Aventis. These moves suggest the difficulties of surviving as a large Indian generics company in the post-WTO climate, where reverse engineering new drugs becomes legally difficult or impossible and where moving to an R&D-driven business model that involves competing with global pharmaceutical powers is strategically difficult. But they are also consonant with the move of the Euro-American R&D-driven industry to focus increasingly on M&A rather than R&D to build their own capabilities and ensure their own survival.[13]

The progressive acquisition of the Indian industry is consequential not just for Indian patients, but for patients throughout the developing world, especially when it comes to access to essential medications such as antiret-rovirals. This is particularly the case given that drug prices under monopoly regimes are likely to be significantly higher than those under a regime of free market competition, especially if the monopolistic price point is identical to the price point set in the United States. This opens up the broader question of the constraints of drug pricing, which involves understanding the institutional relationships of R&D-driven pharmaceutical companies to the consumer marketplace. I explain the structure of this relationship next.

Consumer Markets and Global Drug Pricing

I have argued that the monopoly provided by the patent to the multinational, R&D-driven Euro-American pharmaceutical industry is fundamental to protecting its market interests. Understanding this involves explaining how this consumer market is constituted globally. The economic rationalization for the patent follows the argument for monopoly capitalism propounded by Joseph Schumpeter (1942), which is that monopoly provides incentives to innovate. The post-1980s history of the R&D-driven pharmaceutical industry—one that sees it driven less and less by R&D—should force us to at least complicate this assumption. What does an "incentive to innovate" mean in the context of an industry that is increasingly speculative rather than innovative? How does the monopoly provide security to speculate rather than or in addition to incentive to innovate? In order to answer this question, I explain some of the complexities faced by pharmaceutical companies as they price drugs globally. But before I do so, it is worth layering this Schumpeterian rationality that justifies monopolistic action on the part of the pharmaceutical industry upon another important rationality from the early twentieth century that is important to understanding the operation of speculative financial markets. This concerns the distinction made by Frank Knight (1921) between risk, as something that is in principle calculable and probabilistic, and uncertainty, which is fundamentally not.

There are three kinds of risk or uncertainty that contemporary R&D-driven pharmaceutical companies potentially face. The first, which intuitively seems the riskiest, is financial speculation. The pressures of the financial marketplace place enormous constraints on the innovative activities of these companies. And yet, from the perspective of pharmaceutical corporate logic, financial speculation is in many ways the safest of the three kinds of risk or uncertainty precisely because it is risky as opposed to uncertain. However speculative financialization might actually be, there remains the constant fiction of calculability.[14] The second is the risk of the clinical trials process. This shades into uncertainty rather than risk, since it is ultimately impossible to predict how a therapeutic molecule will interact with human physiologies, whether those interactions will lead to favorable safety and efficacy profiles, and if those profiles, even if favorable, are attractive enough relative to other drugs for the indication in question to actually garner a market. Reducing the cost of clinical trials by outsourcing them to cheaper locales cannot reduce its biomedical uncertainty, but could in principle reduce financial risk simply by decreasing the amount of capital investment required. But this is also uncertainty that pharmaceutical companies try and convert to risk through innovations in the clinical trials process itself—for instance, by designing procedures that can kill molecules unlikely to come through clinical trials as early in the process as possible (such as through the development of surrogate markers that can provisionally indicate probabilities of safety or efficacy in simulated experimental systems), or by developing adaptive clinical trials that constantly feed results of a particular stage of the process back in ways that allow for a more precise calibration and design of subsequent stages.

It is the third kind of uncertainty that is the least calculable—and that is market uncertainty, especially in different parts of the world. This in part is caused by the prospect of generic competition; but it is also constituted by the fact that drug consumption is mediated by two parties other than the patient—the prescriber and the payer. In some systems, such as the American managed care system, the payer is a private entity such as an insurance company (except in programs such as Medicare and Medicaid, or institutions such as the Veterans Administration, in which the government acts as the payer). In other systems—including most major non-U.S. pharmaceutical markets such as western Europe, Canada, Japan, and Australia—the government is the payer. In a very few countries, India being one, drugs are directly sold (through prescribers) to patients, as commodities in a consumer market. India does not have any system of nationalized dispensation of drugs for the majority of its population (though it does for central government employees through the Central Government Health Scheme), and private insurance, while an emerging market segment, does not structure drug payment the way it does in American managed care environments. Therefore, pharmaceutical companies have to negotiate a different kind of consumer market terrain in different countries, constituted by the willingness of particular kinds of payers to pay for certain drugs. In addition, governments have the ability to control markets not just by deciding (in nationalized health systems) which drugs they will buy, but also by imposing price controls on drugs. In principle therefore, the desire for monopoly is offset (and indeed fueled) by the possibility of monopsony, a market form in which one buyer faces many sellers. Negotiating this uncertain terrain—which is variegated across space and always capable of changing over time because of political pressure or policy modification—is a source of enormous and constant structural and strategic anxiety for the pharmaceutical industry.

Even in primarily free drug consumer markets such as India, the structure of monopsony elsewhere conditions pharmaceutical company pricing decisions.[15] One could imagine a situation in which the vast emerging market that India potentially represents could be tapped by the R&D-driven pharmaceutical industry simply by pricing drugs competitively. While there are certainly examples of such differential pricing strategies in emerging markets or the developing world more generally, it is the exception rather than the norm, which tends toward pricing drugs globally similarly to how they are priced in the United States. This often means setting prices beyond what many developing and emerging markets can bear.[16] One sees this in the case of Gleevec (elaborated in chapter 3), as Novartis's Indian price for the drug was the same as in the United States (at the time of approval, this was approximately $2,700 per patient per month), thereby making it effectively unaffordable even for relatively affluent Indian consumers. At the same time, the company attempted to enforce a monopoly on the drug and prevent generic manufacturers, who were making the drug available for $100–300 per patient per month, from selling it. In other words, it was preventing free market competition in a life-saving drug in a context in which it was not going to make much money on that drug anyway. This intuitively seems perverse, and Novartis indeed garnered enormous bad publicity as a consequence; this was the strategy that epitomized the caricature of the evil pharmaceutical corporation.

Without wishing to defend Novartis's actions, I argue that this reflects the stakes of global drug pricing for the R&D-driven pharmaceutical industry, which are to protect market interests in Euro-American (and Japanese) markets. The two factors that pressure pharmaceutical companies in this regard are monopsonistic government payer systems (especially in Europe) and the threat of arbitrage. Monopsony allows governments to make their own calculations of how much they are willing to pay for a drug, how much they are willing to allow it to be priced on their national market (direct price controls), and what instruments they will use to make these determinations. In some countries—the United Kingdom, most notably—health economics has developed as an elaborate discipline precisely in order to make such cost-benefit calculations, between expense to the government and the quality of life years that would accrue through the use of a particular drug.[17] Other governments (including in the U.K. and most European countries) use systems of international price referencing, by which they will study the prices of the drugs in other markets and determine their own willingness to pay based on those prices. Such interactions with governments—whether through economic instruments of price determination or through more direct political pressures—constrain the willingness of companies to sell drugs far more cheaply in some countries than others. Had Novartis sold Gleevec at $300 per patient per month in India, it might have faced consequences for how much European governments would have been willing to pay for the drug. It would certainly have faced political ramifications in the United States for selling it at a tenfold price differential, given the justifications for high drug prices because of the enormous investment companies put into developing a new molecule.[18]

Largely different prices in different countries also imply the possibility of arbitrage. The homogenization of intellectual property regimes is one form of globalization, an attempt to create a uniformly monopolistic global market. But there is the threat of another kind of globalization, the creation of a diasporic pharmaceutical that crosses borders, especially if drugs in one country are much cheaper than in another. One sees a version of this phenomenon in relation to advanced medical and hospital care through medical tourism, where patients cross borders (usually from affluent nations where care is expensive to developing nations such as India and Thailand that have strong medical infrastructures). Pharmaceutical companies are wary of a similar (though inverse) flow of medication, from cheaper to more expensive markets. Uniform pricing of their drugs is a way to prevent that.

This creates additional incentives for global monopoly, as generic drugs also present a threat of arbitrage. There would not just have been a danger of political ramifications or price referencing had Novartis priced Gleevec competitively in India; there would also have been the danger of patients in Western markets importing the drug from India. And even though Novartis priced Gleevec at U.S. price points, the manufacture of generic versions of the drug in India even as Gleevec was a patented medication in other countries presented the threat of arbitrage and an effective decrease in market monopoly even in markets where Novartis legally had one. Indeed, one saw such arbitrage occurring between India and South Korea: consequent to Novartis's refusal to price the drug competitively in Korean markets, leukemia patient groups arranged to buy the drug from the Hyderabad-based generic company Natco Pharmaceuticals for a fraction of the cost. In addition to such exceptional arrangements that emerged in relation to particular political moments, parallel trading companies have developed in Europe, the Middle East, and parts of Asia as wholesalers that purchase pharmaceuticals in low-priced countries and sell them at cheaper rates in higher-priced countries. The threat of arbitrage, therefore, is not hypothetical.[19]

Speculative Trajectories of Pharmaceutical Development

I have thus far argued that the Euro-American, R&D-driven pharmaceutical industry is shaped and constrained by two kinds of markets, the speculative market and the global consumer market. How might we think about the relationship between these specific sectoral constraints and relationships, logics of capital, and emergent forms of and spaces for politics? Here it is worth remembering two things. First, the particular dynamics of American speculative capital are both specific and differentiated. In other words, the logics of financialization that capture the industry are particularly American materializations of the logics of capital. Many larger Indian pharmaceutical companies, for instance, are also publicly traded, but Indian financial markets do not structure the ways they are valued to the degree and intensity that American financial markets do for the big multinational companies. Hence even as it is important to understand the logics of capital that undergird the structure of crisis that I have outlined, one should stay attentive to the trajectories and dynamics of twentieth-century American corporate capitalism that shape the materializations of this structure.[20] Also, financial capitalism is not singular; it has its own histories and trajectories. The capture of the pharmaceutical industry by speculative financial capitalism speaks on the one hand to certain structural dynamics and constraints in modes and relations of production as they come to be underwritten by logics of capital, as analyzed in the preceding pages. But on the other hand, what this capture means is also shaped by and reflective of evolutions of and transformations within financial capital itself.[21]

How do we think about emergent forms of and spaces for politics in the context of a global biomedicine that is influenced by the capture of the Euro-American pharmaceutical industry by financial capital? Crisis is the structural manifestation of this capture; but crisis by itself does not lead to a destabilization of capital's own impetus toward accumulation and appreciation. On the contrary, as seen in the response across the representative political spectrum in the United States to the 2008 financial crisis, one often sees actions in response to crisis that bail out the entities and structures responsible for the crisis in the first place. This could be because of ideological and pragmatic commitments to institutions of capital accumulation and appreciation, or because of the reality or perception that the consequences of not bailing out those institutions would lead to crisis of even more cataclysmic proportions. It is a function of living in a world where it is not easy to imagine institutional structures that are outside of capital, which in Slavoj Žižek's formulation forms "the concrete universal of our historical epoch" (2004, 294).

What one does see in the case of the pharmaceutical industry is the destabilization of particular processes and actors—the blockbuster model of drug development is widely believed to be unviable; many companies in the United States have gone out of business or have been acquired over the past decade; and those companies that remain are in the process of going through massive reorganization. Both acquisition and reorganization require large-scale retrenchment. There are consequences here both for workers and for patients; for those patients who need drugs, as well as those who are imagined as always already needing drugs; for those who die due to a lack of therapeutic access, and for those who might die due to therapeutic excess. But the power of the speculative terrains upon which the pharmaceutical industry operates and to which it has increasingly come to be beholden continues undiminished. As an example, I discuss an epistemic rationalization for solving the crises I have just described through further intensification of speculative financialization. This speaks to one emergent form of a politics of financialization, which responds to its contradictions and crises by imagining and propounding a horizon of more derivative financialization.

In 2012, Jose-Maria Fernandez, Roger Stein, and Andrew Lo put forward a proposal in *Nature Biotechnology*. Written at the height of the patent cliff, they argued for funding biomedical innovation through financial engineering techniques such as portfolio theory and securitization through the creation of a speculative megafund that would invest solely in biomedical discovery and development.[22] The article provided a rationalization, using economic modeling, for solving a crisis of speculative capitalism in terms of even more speculative financialization.

Fernandez and colleagues recognize the pharmaceutical crisis that I have argued for, most especially the fact that being responsive to shareholders forces the industry to focus on near-term growth, leading to a business model that increasingly moves away from R&D toward M&A. The authors further recognize that a focus on M&A exacerbates the innovation crisis afflicting the industry; they understand that what the industry needs is the freedom to refocus on R&D, which the stock market does not provide. Their solution, however, is not a curtailment of speculation, but its intensification, involving the creation of investment structures that are more willing than public markets to bet broadly and over longer time periods on biomedical innovation. This is a proposal that is based on two ground realities: first, that biomedical innovation is highly capital intensive and requires initial investments that might not see immediate dividends and that are subject to a high risk of failure; and second, that the financial market is itself not a singular entity, but comprises many different kinds of real and possible vehicles for speculative capital investment. Fernandez and colleagues do not diagnose speculation itself as the cause of pharmaceutical crisis; only the particular kinds of speculative vehicles (based either in public equity markets, or, in the case of start-up or private biotechnology firms, often in venture capital) as being insufficient for the kinds of sustainable capital investment that pharmaceutical development requires.

Hence, the problem as diagnosed by Fernandez and colleagues is not that the pharmaceutical industry is beholden to financial markets and the expectations of speculative capital, but that they are to shareholders in public-equity markets, whose speculative horizons are necessarily short term and on the whole more risk averse than what the industry requires. Their solution involves the creation of a special investment vehicle that is capable of bearing greater technoscientific and economic risk, associated respectively with the high probability of failure of any particular drug development venture, and with the high probability of consequent failed capital investment. Precisely because drug development is such a speculative scientific activity—a bet on the promise of a molecule successfully being developed as a safe and efficacious therapeutic that is able to garner enough of a consumer market to recoup the investment of time and capital spent in developing it—the authors argue for a more financially speculative instrument to accommodate it.

The investment vehicle that the authors propose involves creating large diversified portfolios of $5–30 billion called megafunds, consisting of biomedical innovations in different stages of development, and financed by a combination of equity and securitized debt. These are different from traditional investment vehicles for pharmaceuticals, therefore, in the nature of both the portfolio and the financing structure.

In terms of the portfolio, what the authors propose is an investment not in the company, but in particular drug development and biomedical innovation projects. The investors then would not acquire equity in a company, but rather royalties on particular products that might be developed. This allows for capital investment in a wide range of products spanning a large number of companies and is not constrained by the limited pipelines of any individual company. Such a broad range of product investment allows for risk pooling in a manner analogous to, albeit the inverse of, strategies adopted by the insurance industry. The insurance industry hedges its bets on having to make a large payoff on any single event, by offsetting it against many premiums that are collected which might never have to be paid out.[23] Similarly but inversely, the megafund would hedge its bets against a large number of failed drug candidates by hoping that a blockbuster success would offset those failures. This is a portfolio theory that makes use of the structure of the blockbuster model—one that sees a large number of failures, but potential billion-dollar molecules from its rare successes. Investing in a company's equity implies being constrained by the pipelines and growth prospects of each individual company, leading to the kinds of pressures described earlier by financial analysts for a company such as Eli Lilly that might face a patent cliff combined with an anemic pipeline, and the resulting structural push toward M&A. Investing in a broad range of biomedical innovation projects across multiple companies at different stages of development, on the other hand, reduces these near-term, company-specific pressures and would therefore, the authors suggest, allow companies to refocus on long-term R&D projects.

In terms of financing, the authors propose securitization, which they define as "a financing method in which a pool of investment capital is raised by issuing equity as well as several classes of bonds that differ from each other in their risk-reward profile to a diverse population of investors, and in which the funds are used to invest in various assets that serve as collaterals for the bonds" (Fernandez, Stein, and Lo 2012, 965). In other words, rather than just issuing equity—part ownership of a company to a shareholder through stocks in the company—securitization is the creation of a tradable financial instrument (which may include equity in the company, but also other kinds of investments such as bonds). Rather than buying and selling direct ownership in the company, an investor would be trading the instrument itself—in this case, an instrument that is not attached to any single company, but to multiple product pipelines in different stages of development.[24] The classic (and now infamous) example of securitized debt is mortgage-backed securities, which combined mortgages into a large pool that was then divided into smaller pieces that could be sold to investors as a type of bond. As with the megafund proposal, the foundation of mortgage-backed securities was risk pooling—an assumption that if enough mortgages were pooled, then the risk of collective default would be mitigated. Similarly, the assumption of Fernandez and colleagues is that if enough biomedical innovation projects are pooled into the megafund, the risk of collective failure would be mitigated. Hence, the portfolio structure and the financing instruments mutually constitute one another.[25]

Fernandez and colleagues' proposal extends the domain of speculation beyond anything that currently exists. Biopharmaceutical mutual funds, for example, also pool risks by including multiple different companies in the fund, but invest only in publicly traded companies. The megafund proposal calls for investment not just in public companies but also in startups (typically the domain of venture capital), private companies, royalty streams, and intellectual property. However, elements of their proposal do already exist. For instance, there are speculative entities called drug-royalty investment companies that invest in pipelines in exchange for a share in royalties accruing from products that might emerge. But they only invest in product candidates in late-stage clinical trials or acquire royalty interests in products already approved for market. The authors, however, seek to extend financial speculation into the domain of early stage drug discovery, the more upstream components of the process of biopharmaceutical development that have tended to be conducted largely out of universities or smaller entrepreneurial companies (often seeded out of universities). Therefore while the contradictions and crises that emerge from the appropriation of health by capital have led to calls for greater public investment in downstream research, especially in clinical trials (Lewis, Reichman, and So 2007), Fernandez and colleagues, in contrast, call for even greater speculative capitalization of R&D, ever more upstream. The terrain of the political within which pharmaceutical crisis unfolds is constituted by both possible directions in which it could resolve.

There are two problems with the assumptions that underlie the megafund proposal. First, the authors assume that the only thing that prevents pharmaceutical corporations from focusing on R&D is the short-term capital pressures that force them toward M&A. In other words, they assume that given appropriate long-term capital investment and financial security, corporations will innovate and leave it to investors to speculate. This does not account for the radical extent to which the (especially American) corporation has itself become financialized. Pharmaceutical companies do not just respond to investment pressures that are imposed by a financial market that is external to them; they are active speculators in that market themselves. Speculation is no longer just an action undertaken by the (American) corporation; it is increasingly its very raison d'être.

Business historian William Lazonick (2010) identifies the financialization of the American corporation as the major attribute of the post-1970s high-tech corporate economy. Lazonick contrasts many attributes of this "new economy" corporation to that of the older, "managerial" corporation of the early to mid-twentieth century. Most pertinent here is his argument that a speculative and liquid stock market as a defining feature of this financialized economy is an inducement not just to capital (upon which Fernandez an colleagues base their proposal) but also to labor: especially to corporate executives, whose own incentives and compensation have become increasingly tied to speculative instruments such as stock options. In other words, those who run American corporations have over the past two decades been increasingly incentivized to themselves speculate on the financial markets. Lazonick shows that while stock prices were driven in the high-tech economy by innovation in the 1980s, it was speculation that was the major driver in the 1990s. He points to how companies have since 2000 engaged in stock price manipulations through massive stock repurchases.[26] Pharmaceutical companies have been among the largest repurchasers of stock: between 2000 and 2008, Pfizer repurchased $50.6 billion of its own stock, Johnson and Johnson $33.3 billion, Amgen $22.6 billion, and Merck $18.7 billion (Lazonick 2010, 699). Repurchases are an indicator of a move to purer and purer speculation that is not coupled to innovation.[27] Fernandez, Stein, and Lo's assumption that a pharmaceutical corporation is fundamentally an innovative rather than a speculative entity is not borne out by recent history. Add to this Dumit's analysis of how the R&D-driven pharmaceutical industry is now driven also by the fiction of speculative treatments to increase market share, and what one sees is a structure of speculation all the way down.

The second assumption that Fernandez, Stein, and Lo make is a "growing demand for therapeutics from a grateful and price-insensitive clientele" (2012, 964). Undoubtedly, prescription rates for pharmaceuticals in the United States have continued to grow with no signs of abatement. But the idea that this is occurring among a "price-insensitive clientele" is simply wrong. Drug pricing has become an increasingly political issue in the United States and remains a vexed issue globally, as I have described.[28] However, this is elided in the arguments for ever more intense and derivative forms of financialization. Regardless of whether, how, and where such forms are realized, such arguments are a reminder of the sensibilities that have appropriated Euro-American multinational pharmaceutical capital. The global consequence of these appropriations is worth empirically attending to. Indeed, the emergent and constitutive forms of pharmaceutical politics in India are precisely not financialized, and operate through other registers and modalities, as explored in subsequent chapters. But the power of financial capital to structure political economic terrains of global biomedicine remains. It is important to attend to the simultaneous particularity (and hence nonuniversality) of financialized pharmaceutical capitalism and to its hegemony.

In this chapter, I have schematically mapped a political economic structure of crisis, which is also a structure of therapeutic development and value generation. This structure, however, is not singular. It is striated, differentiated, and layered. One can see this in the various kinds of economies that are at stake in this analysis. First, there is an economy of manufacturing and sale, which is an industrial economy and has to do with the making and selling of therapeutic molecules. With the reorganization and downsizing of large R&D-driven pharmaceutical industries and the acquisition of smaller companies and generics companies, this economy is marked by labor insecurity and large-scale retrenchment. But this reflects a more general condition of the crisis of contemporary capitalism, marked by high unemployment and more and more precarious conditions of labor.

Second, there is an economy of research and development, which is a knowledge economy. This operates in the register of innovation, and has to do with intellectual labor. This is a structure of value generation within the pharmaceutical industry that is itself in crisis. This does not mean that R&D

no longer happens; but its nature, contexts, and locations shift. One of the major directions of this shift is toward smaller biotechnology companies and in association with universities that are themselves becoming more entrepreneurial and corporate. There is also a shift toward more rational or translational forms of drug development—the development of drugs that are designed to set right abnormally functioning processes at a cellular or molecular level, developed out of an understanding of basic biological processes.[29]

Third, there is an economy of clinical trials. Institutionally, this has emerged as a more and more autonomous structure, with the development of for-profit CROs as outsourcing service shops to conduct trials for pharmaceutical companies, including especially globally. This creates new forms of labor, especially the labor of experimental subjectivity, a function of the bioavailability of (often previously marginalized and/or dispossessed) subject populations for biomedical research, but also the labor of conducting and monitoring clinical trials, something I do not explore in this book, but which is also usually relatively low-wage, high-intensity work that is often gendered. (Most clinical research monitors tend to be women, since most of this labor pool is drawn from the nursing profession.) This is an economy that maps onto other kinds of globalizing labor that depends upon the bioavailability of (marginal or dispossessed) bodies, such as that of surrogacy and other forms of reproductive labor (Waldby and Cooper 2008; Cooper and Waldby 2014).

And fourth, there is the economy of health itself, which maps onto the various labor economies that are at stake. This concerns the appropriation of health by capital, the way in which health itself becomes the locus of value generation (rather than, as in Marx's analysis of industrial capital, simply the means to reproducing the conditions of production by maintaining a healthy labor force). This is not just about health becoming valuable; it also speaks to all the deeply charged ethical dimensions in play when questions of life and death come to be at stake. It is in part about what Mary-Jo DelVecchio Good and colleagues (1990) have called a political economy of hope but also involves other kinds of affective entanglements, of obligation, commitment, indebtedness, and love.[30] This is an economy in relation to which the development of a critical voice is always fraught and contradictory—how to simultaneously argue for therapeutic access to essential medicines for those who need it while critiquing economies of therapeutic excess and saturation? This is where the turn to the state, and the empirical specificities of political engagement with the state, become important. This is the focus of the chapters 2 and 3, concerning the HPV vaccine and Gleevec cases respectively.

I do not outline the structure of crisis in pharmaceutical economies consequent to their operation under logics of capital simply in order to make a diagnosis. Rather, I develop the idea of contending different relations of production in order to open up questions (tackled in the next two chapters) of the antinomies of the state as it confronts its obligations to fulfill and balance the opposed imperatives of providing for the health of its population (biopolitics) and using biomedicine as an engine of economic and capital expansion (biocapital). For this, understanding the speculative financialized logics under which the multi-national R&D-driven industry operates is important.

The question of market value is a central structural feature of this analysis, speaking as it does to the logics of capital under which pharmaceutical economies operate. This does not mean that all value is reduced to monetary value; quite the contrary. This book as a whole attempts to parse out the multiplicity of value forms at stake in contemporary global pharmaceutical economies (see introduction). But I also want to be attentive to the relations of power between these forms. Logics of capital are never purely internal to capital; they have the ability, indeed the need, to appropriate other kinds of value logics that are seemingly external to capital. This is precisely what happens when health becomes surplus health. This appropriation does not occur seamlessly or similarly across place or time, and these are the differentiations that constitute the terrain of the political. This is where the institutional mediation of the materializations of logics of capital through governance regimes becomes important. The corporation itself is not a singular entity, and different types of corporation are subject to different trajectories of capitalization as they are located in different relations of production. My focus in this chapter has been on the speculative financialization that comes to possess the R&D-driven pharmaceutical corporation; because of the power of such corporations, such financialization has broader structuring effects on global pharmaceutical economies as a whole. But there are other trajectories, such as those followed by Indian generics companies, which speak to different relations of production (see chapter 5).

In other words, even if the logics of corporate capital are based on the generation of surplus, there are still multiple different capitalisms that see the materializations of these logics in different ways, times, and places. At a basic level, two kinds of relations of production I am interested in tracing include that which the Euro-American, R&D-driven pharmaceutical industry operates within and that which the Indian generic industry operates within. There are many intricacies to each of these sectors that I have not explored, but the operational distinction I am making between them concerns different strategies for drug development (based, respectively, on the R&D of novel therapeutic entities and their movement to market after an elaborate process of clinical trials for regulatory approval, and on reverse engineering generic versions of molecules that are already on the market) as well as different market terrains (the former, increasingly, highly speculative and financialized, and dependent upon monopoly protections afforded by the patent; the latter based more in a terrain that sees drugs sold as commodities, competing with each other on price through the free market).

At the start of The Grundrisse, Marx analyzed the banking crisis of 1855 by engaging in a polemic against socialists who attributed the crisis to the malfeasance of the banks. Marx responded by showing that in fact, the so-called malfeasance of the banks was simply a case of banks acting like, well, banks.[31] In other words, what is critical for Marx is an understanding of the crisis in structural terms. But what does structure mean in this case? I suggest that it concerns first an elucidation of the logics of capital, and second an account of the ways in which institutional actors historically came to be captured within those logics, so that it became both sensible and apparently natural for these actors to act in the interests of capital. This does not mean that there is no variance in the particular strategic actions of particular actors. Novartis's refusal to differentially price Gleevec is a different response than GlaxoSmithKline's more aggressive embrace of differential pricing strategies in recent years (Froud and Sukhdev 2006); similarly, the megafund proposal put forth by Fernandez, Stein, and Lo speaks to different modalities, strategies, and intensities of speculative activity and reminds us that financialization is not a singular process but has its own histories and divergences. But it is nonetheless possible to discern certain sectoral trajectories that see the appropriation of health by increasingly financialized capital. This leads to crisis: not just because the interests of capital invariably involve alienation, expropriation, and exploitation, but because, left to itself, capital cannot set itself limits, and hence ends up putting its own institutions in crisis. This is what happened with the banks in 1855; it is what happened with the banks in 2008.

The pharmaceutical industry is an industry that is itself in crisis, and I emphasize the historical tendencies toward privatization, leading to an appropriation of health itself by capital; toward speculation, leading to a move away from research and development toward mergers and acquisitions; and toward globalization, a terrain that is secured through globally harmonized intellectual property and clinical trials regulatory regimes. In the process, the attempts to respond to pharmaceutical crisis lead, on the one hand, to larger, *even more speculative industries, thereby reinforcing the very conditions that led to the crisis in the first place. And on the other hand, the globalization of the crisis impacts people and industries in other parts of the world. What crisis might mean is different for different actors. This difference also precludes the possibility of easy solidarity and makes it difficult to understand the ways in which, for instance, there is a structural relationship between an affluent patient in a therapeutically saturated market who has died because of side effects of Vioxx, which has everything to do with things like off-label use and therapeutic saturation, and a patient who has been excluded from drug markets altogether, perhaps in the so-called Global South, who has died because she could not afford an essential anticancer or antiretroviral medication that could have allowed her to live, and for which manufacturing capacity at an affordable cost exists. Any adequate critical and political response to this crisis has to understand the ways in which health itself has come to be redefined through its appropriation by a globalizing, speculative capital, and has to insist upon an imagination and institutionalization of a form of health that resists such appropriation. Unless we understand the genesis of crisis as residing in the value form itself as it gets appropriated by logics of capital (so that these logics come to define what value means, in all of its material, abstract, symbolic, and agential manifestations), it is impossible to think of transcending the crisis through simply institutional responses.*

CHAPTER TWO

Bioethical Values

HPV Vaccines, Public Scandal & Experimental Subjectivity

From Promise to Scandal

"Bhopal Gas Victims Used as Guinea Pigs," read the June 2010 editorial of the *Monthly Index of Medical Specialties* (*MIMS*), a newsletter edited by the Delhi-based physician Chandra Gulhati (2010). "Chronic Clinical Investigators: New Breed of Body Hunters" was the headline for the May 2011 editorial (Gulhati 2011). Gulhati was the coauthor of an important article in the *New England Journal of Medicine* with Sumiran Nundy, which described clinical trials regimes in India as a "new colonialism" (Nundy and Gulhati 2006). He has been a tireless watchdog and chronicler of unethical clinical trials practices in India, and *MIMS* has been his mouthpiece, through which he has publicized various instances of malpractice over the years. In earlier years, Gulhati's was largely a lone voice. In the period of time between the two editorials cited above, however, the question of unethical clinical trials in India came to the forefront of media attention, not just in India but also internationally, and has been an issue of active political mobilization within India.[1]

Clinical trials in India, in other words, have become the subject of scandal. There are certain recurrent elements to this narrative, for instance: the movement of clinical trials from the West to countries like India because of the lower costs involved; the easy availability in India of poor, illiterate clinical trial subjects; and the virtual absence of ethical or regulatory oversight that allows corners to be cut. It was not supposed to be this way. The harmonization of regulations for the conduct of human biomedical experimentation with guidelines mandated by the International Conference on Harmonization (ICH) in 2005 through a modification of Schedule Y of the Indian Drugs and Cosmetics Act of 1945 was meant to build an ethical infrastructure for the conduct of clinical trials, even as it was geared to consequently attract global clinical trials to India (see introduction). This process was driven by the clinical research organization (CRO) industry, both Indian and multinational. This industry has emerged as outsourcing service providers for pharmaceutical companies, and hence is a component of the complex brokerage economies through which clinical trials operate (see Fisher 2008; Petryna 2009).

The movement of clinical trials to international—non-U.S.—locations started in earnest in the mid-1990s. Adriana Petryna (2005) cites figures that point to a dramatic growth in the number of human subjects recruited into these trials, from 4,000 in 1995 to 400,000 in 1999. A study by the consulting firm A. T. Kearney showed that roughly half of the 1,200 U.S. clinical trials in 2005 made use of an international site (Cruickshank 2009). In the 1990s, as Petryna (2005) notes, most of this growth occurred in countries that had agreed to harmonize standards in commercial drug testing with the guidelines set by the ICH. These primarily included Latin American and Eastern European countries, but not yet India. Since 2005, however, India has undertaken an active effort to build capacity to conduct clinical trials, especially in anticipation of the movement of global trials there.

At that time, a range of actors saw the country as providing an attractive destination for outsourced clinical trials from the West. Contract research in the Indian pharmaceutical industry was estimated by the Chemical Pharmaceutical Generic Association to be worth between $100 and $120 million in 2005, while growing at 20 to 25 percent per year.[2] The most central of these actors were members of the burgeoning CRO industry. These were the most immediate beneficiaries of trials coming to India, and were therefore keen to create conditions for these trials to grow in a sustained and streamlined fashion. The major drivers of the buildup of clinical research infrastructure have been CROs, and they have been particularly influential in building a regulatory framework for the conduct of trials. A few of these have been in existence for over two decades; but more than 80 percent of them were established after 2005.[3]

In the mid-2000s, there was a strong common interest among a number of actors, albeit in different ways and for different reasons, not just in building up a research infrastructure in India, but also in promoting the country as a global destination for clinical trials.[4] But the primary drivers of this promotion were the CROs. These organizations were themselves of different stripes. There were multinational CROs, often American, who set up shop in other parts of the world to facilitate the outsourcing of clinical trials.[5] At the other end of the spectrum were Indian startups sensing a business opportunity in a developing field, some of which were even set up by entrepreneurs with no prior clinical research expertise but with experience in garnering the labor pool to provide various kinds of client-focused services.[6]

But there was also an important history of CROs emerging out of the Indian pharmaceutical industry, which was in the process of retooling its business models as the country was changing its patent regimes to become compliant with the Trade-Related Aspects of Intellectual Property Rights agreement (see introduction). This forced a number of leading Indian drug companies into a research and development–driven business model. Clinical trials became constitutive to this business model, because one cannot develop novel drugs without subjecting them to a regime of safety and efficacy testing. Even more, the attempts of larger Indian companies to expand their generics markets, including to Euro-American markets in post–patent cliff scenarios (see chapter 1), was a spur to their conducting bioequivalence studies, which compare the in vivo biological equivalence of two preparations of a drug, and hence are often used to evaluate the comparative efficacy of different generic medications. Hence while not clinical trials per se, they require similar kinds of capacity building for experimental biomedical interventions in human subjects. In other words, the Indian pharmaceutical industry has itself served as a spur to its CRO industry.

Indeed, India's largest pharmaceutical company, Ranbaxy, was responsible for the growth of the Indian clinical research industry in more ways than one. Its business model over the past two decades or so has been twofold: to aggressively increase its presence in global generics markets (including the United States) and to try to discover its own therapeutic molecules that it might license to multinational pharmaceutical companies in exchange for the payment of various milestone-related royalties. In both cases, developing clinical testing facilities became necessary, and Ranbaxy was one of the first Indian pharmaceutical companies to develop an in-house CRO. It also started outsourcing bioequivalence studies, thereby spurring the development of a CRO industry. Three of Ranbaxy's main clinical researchers left the company in 2000 to create Wellquest in Bombay (itself a CRO seeded by another major Indian pharmaceutical company, Nicholas Piramal India Limited), while two other scientists from Ranbaxy were the cofounders of another major CRO, Lambda, in 1999. In this way, certain sections of the

Indian pharmaceutical industry have generated clinical research work themselves, and have provided the capital and expertise required for this industry to take off. This makes it too simple to suggest that clinical research capacity is being built purely as a consequence of the desire of the West to outsource trials to cheap Indian locations, though Indian actors have certainly bet on such a desire materializing in more research contracts.[7]

Finally, nonprofit entities having clinical research capacity were often set up to provide family planning and contraceptive services in the 1970s, but were acting more and more like CROs in the market climate of the mid-2000s. Major such entities included the North Carolina–based Family Health International (FHI) and the agency that would become a central actor in the human papilloma virus (HPV) vaccine scandal, the Seattle-based Program for Appropriate Technologies in Health (PATH).[8] Regardless of the particular kind of CRO involved, the potential of Indian populations as experimental subjects melded seamlessly with the market potential that CROs perceived from a growth in clinical research.

The infrastructure building occurring in India in anticipation of global trials moving to the country was significant, but it was speculative. This anticipation was based on the expectation that it would serve the interests of Western trial sponsors to outsource these trials to India. A 2002 McKinsey report, for instance, estimated that clinical research in India would be a $1 billion industry by 2010 (NASSCOM 2002). The rationality behind such expectations was based on the various perceived advantages in taking clinical trials to India including that of cost: estimates suggest that lower labor and infrastructure expenses could reduce overall clinical trial expenses for a multinational company by 30 to 50 percent. There was also a perceived recruitment advantage—the assumption being that it would be easier to obtain treatment-naive subjects. A major problem for drug companies conducting trials in the United States is that Americans are therapeutically saturated, already taking so many drugs that it is hard to determine the efficacy of the molecule being tested without having to confront a whole range of interactions that muddy the data obtained. The attempt of the CRO industry was to take advantage of this situation to create Brand India for clinical trials, to establish the country as a primary global destination for clinical experimentation. For instance, CRO leaders in India voiced some of the following expectations at the time:

> So the answer to "Why India?" you must have heard so many times.
> We have a huge treatment-naive population and the cost of getting the

same thing done, with the same quality as you do in U.S. is much lower here. Easily 30 to 40 percent.

The nature of this business is spread across geographies. Therefore you are looking for patients. Your acceleration, your main aim is to accelerate drugs, right? Therefore, you do go globally in search of the right quality patients. Secondly, you also look at the possibility of out-sourcing this. So if you look at—you'll find especially in first five years of 2000s, 2002 onwards, the fact of the matter is that there has been phenomenal growth in the CRO industry, even within the United States. Then they went to east Europe—Europe was anyway a clinical place—and from east Europe they have now started coming to the Asia-Pacific rim. Japan was always there, but countries like, you know, I mean I'm saying like places like Hong Kong, China, India.

I see it very positively. I say that, there's no question about it, that trials are facing east. In my mind, today, trials are facing east in terms of being placed. Tomorrow, after 2010, they will be designing drug devel-opment. I want to see that in my lifetime. Because all the basic sciences are here, the people are here, and this is true largely right across up to China. In this particular case, because you know, I still maintain, it's a people industry, therefore unlike China, we have a slightly greater ad-vantage that we think in English. By *we* I mean industry leaders, and to a large extent—the recruitment strategies, the medical communication, and now with patents being recognized by our country—medical com-munication in all aspects is being important. So in my mind this industry will continue to grow for the next five years, more than 100 percent al-most, year in year growth.

Now India is a nation to reckon with. We've got good practices. We've proven ourselves in GCP [good clinical practice]. We are the brand leaders in generics; we are the brand leaders in bioequivalence. We have practice.

It is getting very big now. All MNCs [multinational corporations] are now setting up their shops in India. You've got all these MNCs, from all over the world. So in one way or another, you will find all MNCs having their presence in India. And that is by itself leading to a simple fact that yes, there is going to be a lot of growth. India, next five years, is going to be a hub of clinical research activity.[9]

How did this promise turn so sour? A typical explanation is cynical: that as clinical trials globalize to places such as India, there is likely to be less stringent ethical regulation compared to advanced liberal centers such as the United States and Western Europe. Petryna (2009) refers to the ways in which such differential ethics emerge in different parts of the world as clinical trials globalize in terms of "ethical variability." But while it might well be the case that cynical manipulation of poorly enforced regulations and genuine malfeasance have contributed to the scandalous situation of clinical trials in India over the past few years, ethical variability is not just a function of bad faith. Petryna's own development of the concept traces its relationship to the political economy of global biomedicine. It is this that I wish to develop by pointing to two complicating factors that render a purely cynical explanation for the scandalous clinical trial insufficient.

First, given that the aim of the CRO industry was to attract global trials, it is worth recognizing that strong regulation and GCP are necessary in order for drugs to be approved for market in the West. The primary concern of GCP is with the collection of informed consent and the apparatus that surrounds it, especially an institutional review board (IRB) infrastructure. This was the focus of the 2005 Schedule Y harmonization exercise. Indeed, members of India's CRO industry would bristle at the suggestion that clinical trials would move to India because it is possible to cut ethical corners there, and were acutely aware of the need to build a positive media image for their industry. One Mumbai-based CRO executive was typically emphatic about the importance of Schedule Y and GCP: "We are new. We don't want to play with the evolution of ethics."[10] Therefore, the public scandal of unethical clinical trials is not a function of an absence of ethics. While it may well be that the inadequate enforcement of existing ethical guidelines contributed to the scandals, it must be recognized that these emerged in the context of active regulatory capacity building for ethical trial conduct (see K. Sunder Rajan 2007).

And therefore, second, it is this broader political economy of global biomedical research that needs elucidation. For instance, most human subject experimentation in India over the past decade has involved bioequivalence studies. Also of relevance are forms of outcomes-based public health research, initiated by the state or by global health nonprofits, which are themselves imbricated in complex relations to global capital flows. The case that would become emblematic of the unethical clinical trial in India, concerning the HPV vaccine studies that I describe in this chapter, is an example of such research. In such situations, a whole set of epistemic questions comes to be intertwined with the ethical and political economic—what one knows from a clinical trial, how one knows it, how one knows when it has gone wrong, or even how an experiment on human subjects comes to be defined as a clinical trial in the first place. The relation between value (as market value and as ethical or normative value) and knowledge itself comes to be rendered political. This is a politics that concerns the conduct of biomedical research; but it is also about constituting and representing the experimental subjects of such research consequent to trajectories whereby bodies and health are made available for knowledge production, value generation, and capital accumulation. It is a politics that has erupted in scandal to mobilize and consolidate civil society advocacy against unethical clinical trials.

HPV Vaccine Studies

The deaths of seven girls in quick succession following the administration of vaccines against HPV in the states of Andhra Pradesh and Gujarat as part of a research study, quickly grew into a scandal and raised a host of questions relating to the lack of regulation and oversight of clinical research conducted in India, especially on marginalized or "vulnerable" subject populations.[11] The scandal turned the clinical trials question into one of general media and political concern in India, something broader than the response of the occasional watchdog such as Gulhati. It put concerned agencies in a situation of having to answer for themselves, aroused indignation, and called forth advocacy. Importantly, it became a political issue not just in the arena of civil society advocacy, but also in that of representative parliamentary politics, as questions of the place of capitalized clinical research in the arena of public health came to be raised.[12]

A brief account of the controversy surrounding the HPV vaccine studies is as follows. In early April 2010, the Indian Council for Medical Research (ICMR) halted a project that involved the experimental administration of Gardasil, a vaccine developed by Merck used to prevent HPV infection, in Bhadrachalam, Andhra Pradesh. The study was shut down because of apparent reports of violations of ethical guidelines. This study had been launched on July 9, 2009, by the Andhra Pradesh Ministry for Health and Family Welfare, along with ICMR and the not-for-profit PATH. PATH itself comes out of histories of global family planning programs, and was founded in the 1970s with a focus on the dissemination of contraceptive technologies to women in the developing world. Initially called PIACT (Program for the Initiation and Adaptation of Contraceptive Technology), the organization was seeded by a small grant from the Ford Foundation. Today, PATH's focus extends to a whole range of health technologies, and its major donor is the Bill and Melinda Gates Foundation.[13]

Therefore, in addition to being not quite a clinical trial, the HPV study operated within a rationale of public health and involved a partnership between the Indian state and a global not-for-profit. The idiom of this collaboration is that quintessentially neoliberal one, the public-private partnership. But PATH has been in the business of public-private partnerships since its very inception, long before that phrase acquired cachet, since its mandate involved taking health (initially contraceptive) technologies from private pipelines and facilitating their introduction into developing country public health programs.[14] The study opens up dimensions of clinical research that operate under the sign of public health or pastoral care. But it does so in a context where public health itself comes into collaboration with private entities and hence does not remain purely a state project.[15] Institutionally, this has implications for thinking about the state's accountability in the appropriation of health by capital, but also for thinking about health itself if even public health cannot be imagined outside private interest. It also has implications for thinking about what a CRO is. Strictly speaking, PATH is not a for-profit CRO, but the functioning within brokerage economies that structure contemporary drug development makes it act as if it is one.

This study was not described as a Phase 3 clinical trial. Indeed, Phase 3 trials had already been conducted for Gardasil, which was approved for marketing by the U.S. Food and Drug Administration in 2006. The vaccine was commercially available in India, and was already being sold in over one hundred other countries. Rather than a clinical trial, the study was referred to as a "postlicensure observational study." While shutting down the trial, the ICMR admitted to lapses in the conduct of the study and said that GCP guidelines had not been adhered to.[16] What this suggests is simply a problem of ethics, compounded by the fact that this was a study conducted on marginal populations, since Bhadrachalam is an area with a predominantly indigenous population (demographically designated as Scheduled Tribes in government classification).[17]

I argue that the emergence of ethics as the dominant problem within structures of public explanation in relation to the scandal of unethical clinical experimentation is necessary but insufficient. On the one hand, ethics provides a useful frame through which problems and violations in the conduct of biomedical research can be pinpointed. But in fact, a focus on ethics potentially black boxes the complex and deeply political imbrications of value (in both its normative and political economic registers) with knowledge that are at stake in such situations. I work through this complex in order to show all the dimensions of knowledge, value, and politics in the HPV scandal that ethics holds in place.

First, the very nature of the experimental comes to be at stake in relation to public health and pastoral care of the population (in this case, when dealing with vaccine delivery to marginal populations). This concerns questions of what Michel Foucault ([1976] 1990) has called biopolitics, but in the context of the appropriation of health by capital through institutional arrangements involving state actors, multinational pharmaceutical companies, global health nongovernmental organizations, and public-private partnerships that operate within brokerage economies. In such situations, the lines between delivery and experiment, the provision of services and the conduct of research, is often blurred. Even establishing what constitutes a clinical trial, as I will show, is anything but straightforward. Second, there is difficulty in establishing causality in case of adverse events. In the HPV case, seven girls who were administered the vaccine died, but none of the deaths could be attributed to the vaccine. In fact, what the controversy highlighted most saliently was the difficulty of retroactively figuring out a causal chain of events from vaccine (or drug) administration to adverse consequence. Third, questions of consent and custodianship emerged in contexts of experimentation on minors, especially minors belonging to marginalized populations. Fourth, one saw the limits and violence of top-down, artifact-driven, technocratic imaginaries of public health that posed solutions to public health problems purely in terms of vaccines, without attending to epidemiological or infrastructural concerns and contexts within which the vaccines would be deployed. In the HPV controversy, this would become a topic of debate and autocritique within the public health community. Fifth, there are materializations of controversy and scandal within domains of representative politics: even as the state was involved in acts of violation within and through biopolitical regimes, it became the institution through which scandal could be publicly highlighted and rendered political. Sixth, in spite of all of these complexities, the one thing that was clear in the HPV controversy—that ethical GCP guidelines had not been adhered to—did not lead to anyone being held accountable, showing that the link between revealing ethical lapse and establishing accountable structures of responsibility to prevent such lapses is a tenuous and nonobvious one, indeed very much a site of politics in and of itself. And seventh, there was the question of how one imagines and represents experimental subjects and what kind of work experimental subjectivity in biomedical research is.

The demonstration study involved the administration of Gardasil to 16,000 girls between the ages of ten and fourteen in the Khammam district of Andhra Pradesh ("Pilot Programme for Vaccination" 2009). PATH was responsible for the mobilization of logistics and project supervision; the Andhra Pradesh government for implementation; and ICMR was officially listed as a facilitator, though it is unclear what that meant. The objective of the study, according to PATH (2009), was that "the demonstration project would help the Ministry of Health and Family Welfare to make recommendations on how to address the problem of cervical cancer in India through vaccination and screening." Therefore, this study was not about the evaluation of safety or efficacy of the vaccine, and no biomedical outcomes were being tested. There was considerable ambiguity in what these observational studies were actually demonstrating, though clearly the study was designed as a via media of sorts toward the integration of HPV vaccines into India's national immunization program.[18]

The study had three phases. The first phase involved assessing the introduction of the HPV vaccine into India. The second phase of the study was the one that was stopped, and involved vaccinating eligible girls between the ages of ten and fourteen in Andhra Pradesh and Gujarat. This was the phase meant to test vaccine delivery in order to incorporate the vaccine into the national immunization program. The focus was to be on strategies for delivering the vaccine, and the acceptance of the vaccine by the population. The third phase was to study coverage, acceptability, feasibility, and cost of vaccine delivery.

The protocol for the HPV study in Khammam district, which emerged as a major focal point of the controversy, involved the administration of three doses of vaccine to girls in three *mandals* (or district subdivisions): Bhadrachalam, Kothagudem, and Thirumalaipalem. These three mandals have diverse demographic profiles. Kothagudem is urban, Thirumalaipalem rural, and Bhadrachalam tribal.[19] Hence, this study had a political economy in terms of its inclusion criteria (regarding the social groups to which the girls belonged who were administered the vaccine); different regional profiles within which the vaccine was administered; and, in the case of Bhadrachalam, a context of war and displacement. This is because many of the tribal girls who had been administered the vaccine in Bhadrachalam belonged to families who had been displaced from the neighboring state of Chattisgarh, which is one of the epicenters of the virtual civil war that is being waged in many tribal regions of India between Maoist insurgents and the Indian state.[20]

The stated rationale for the postlicensure observational study was to generate data about vaccine coverage, feasibility, acceptability, and implementation costs associated with various HPV vaccine delivery strategies. Christopher Elias, the president and CEO of PATH, was quoted as saying about the study, "It was designed, in cooperation with government agencies, to assist India's public health system in identifying the most effective and affordable strategies to help prevent cervical cancer, a disease that kills an estimated 143,000 Indian women every year."[21] The protocols were approved by two ethics committees in India and a private IRB, Western IRB, based in Seattle.[22]

In the aftermath of the study being shut down by ICMR, two separate reports were generated about the study. I use these reports, which needless to say come with their own stakes and biases and also rely upon different methodologies, as a means to read this case. Hence my own reading of the case is mediated, concerning the ways in which catastrophic events around clinical trials get read and become political through emergent structures of public contestation and explanation. One report was produced by an independent commission set up by the Government of India, consisting mainly of physicians and clinical researchers and relying on expert interpretation of available evidence. A second report was written by Sama, a Delhi-based activist group whose focus is on issues of women and health and was based on a fact-finding visit to Bhadrachalam in March 2011 that reconstructed events around the trial through conversations and interviews with involved people, including the parents of one of the girls who died. The Sama report points to the death of four girls, all tribal girls from Bhadrachalam. The government report alludes to the death of seven girls, five from Bhadrachalam and two who were administered Cervarix in Gujarat.

Two issues came to be at stake in the aftermath of these studies. The first concerned the question of ethical violations: was the study conducted properly, in accordance with GCP principles? The second concerned the question of causality: did the girls in fact die because of the vaccines? PATH, in a press release, did acknowledge the death of six girls in Gujarat and Andhra Pradesh (even though the government report cited the death of seven), but denied causality, stating that "none of these deaths was causally associated with the vaccine."[23]

The question of causality is empirical and epistemic: a question of "did this happen because of that?" comes to be closely tied to "how do we know if this happened (or did not happen) because of that?" I am interested in the way in which the empirical, rendered as an epistemic question, gets further imbricated within ethical questions, and how that resolves in terms of structures of accountability. It turned out that the question of whether the deaths were caused by the vaccines did not have a straightforward or already obvious scientific answer, even to the scientific experts who were called upon to adjudicate upon this. Rather, what one saw were specific figurations of causality that came to be naturalized and mobilized by certain individuals and groups at particular moments in time. At stake here is not just the establishment of cause and effect, but a question of what kinds of causal arguments can be made, under which circumstances, and through what kinds of rhetorical devices.

As an example: the HPV immunization card that was prepared as a part of this study made two causal assertions as if they were unproblematic.[24] First, it said that HPV vaccine prevents infection with the HPV virus. Second, it said that HPV virus causes cervical cancer. These statements suggest a straightforward, linear relationship between the administration of HPV vaccine and the prevention of cervical cancer, which gets naturalized and reiterated in statements such as those of Christopher Elias, quoted above. At one level, these are indeed factual statements. But at another, they suggest simple relationships in place of what are in fact highly qualified and contextual ones. This means that Elias's public explanation of why the vaccines might be a tool in prevention ends up short-circuiting a complex terrain of knowledge and value, even if it is not intentional misrepresentation.

For instance, the HPV vaccine only prevents infection from two strains of HPV virus. In fact, more than two hundred strains of the virus exist (though the two strains that are protected against by the vaccines, HPV-16 and 18, are believed to cause approximately 70 percent of cervical cancer cases). Further, the vaccine is not a substitute for cervical cancer screening, which still remains the most effective mechanism for the prevention of cervical cancer, and for which infrastructure hardly exists in places such as Bhadrachalam.[25] And while it is true that this virus can cause cervical cancer, most of the strains do not in fact cause any symptoms in most people. This does not even take into account the possible variations in both cancer etiology and vaccine response among people of different demographics and socioeconomic backgrounds (such as tribal girls in central India), about which next to nothing is known. What one sees in the immunization card is the conversion of something deeply contextual into something technocratic—which dovetails with the very imagination of the vaccine as a technocratic solution to the problem of cervical cancer. At the same time, this shifted the very scientific imaginary embedded in the vaccination procedure, as what counts as "potential risk" and "patient" shifts in accordance with technocratic decisions. I elaborate upon these points at length and return to this question of the technocratic subsequently.

Yet while the immunization card converts a complicated and contextual set of relationships into something linear, straightforward, and factual, the complications of establishing straightforward relationships in the context of whether the vaccines caused the deaths or not would become evident in the various expert opinions that were brought to bear on the case.

PATH's assertion, again almost as a statement of fact, was that there was no causal relation between the vaccines and the deaths. But other renderings of this relationship would come to circulate as well.

While there was absolutely no rendering of the relationship between the HPV vaccine and cervical cancer prevention in sociological or political economic terms (such as, for instance, possible variations in response to the vaccine among tribal girls compared to more affluent populations on whom the vaccine was predominantly tested in clinical trials), the political economic was used as an alternative explanation for some of the deaths. For instance, the official cause of two of the deaths was suicide through the consumption of pesticide. This suggests the larger political economy of indebtedness that provides the context for everyday life in areas such as tribal Andhra Pradesh. It was assumed that this political economy can lead to depression and suicide, but never that it might lead to differential responses to a vaccine. I elaborate upon this and other issues involved in the reconstruction of these studies in the two reports next, through a close reading of each of the reports.

Ethics

Sama is a resource group for women and health, based in Delhi. It was founded in 1999 and has been involved in advocacy around a range of issues having to do with health literacy, health access, and social justice. In recent years, the group has also organized important studies and meetings to consider ethical and regulatory issues emerging around new reproductive technologies and clinical trials. They have been a central actor in the emergent advocacy in India against unethical clinical trials. This engagement with clinical trials has emerged consequent to their involvement in the HPV controversy.

Sama has provided the closest approximation to an on-the-ground report on the HPV study in Andhra Pradesh. The only other report on the HPV trials comes from an expert commission appointed by the Government of India. The government report is a document of considerable interest and importance, and has many worthwhile interventions based on the assessment of study data by biomedical experts. Sama's report is more ethnographic. Members of a Sama team visited two residential schools and a hostel in Bhadrachalam where vaccines were administered, as well as a third residential school called the RBC bridge school, which primarily was for children who had been displaced due to the tribal conflict in Chattisgarh. In this school, most of the girls do not even speak Telugu, the state language of Andhra Pradesh, but rather Koya, the tribal dialect of the Chattisgarhi Koya tribe.

While Sama's report did touch on the question of causality, that is, whether the deaths were due to the vaccine studies, its entry point concerned the various ethical violations that allegedly occurred in the study. It questioned the inclusion criteria in the study, which included girls from various marginalized groups. And it made evident the larger background of tribal conflict in Chattisgarh as an essential context in making these populations particularly vulnerable from the perspective of clinical research.

The HPV vaccines in the study were administered to girls through vaccination camps that were conducted at the schools and hostels mentioned above.[26] In one case, consent for vaccinating 300 girls was given by the teacher in charge of a hostel. In another hostel, it is likely that consent for vaccinating another 300 to 400 girls was provided by the warden. The hostel wardens did not know exactly how many girls had been administered the vaccine, and did not necessarily know who had given consent for the administration. In some cases, the parents of girls who were vaccinated were not even informed about the vaccination (let alone asked for consent). The consent form states that best results are obtained by administering the vaccine to "adolescent" girls. The question of what adolescent means, and how it is translatable across the different contexts in which the vaccine works, was never addressed. Indeed, many of the girls administered vaccine in this case were prepubescent. While the consent form mentions adolescence as an inclusion criterion, primary health center workers involved in vaccine administration that the Sama group interviewed said that they chose girls who were between ten and fourteen years of age because they were not yet sexually active. Since informed consent and proper, clearly defined inclusion criteria for a study are cornerstones of GCP, fundamental questions about GCP, even as enshrined in existing Indian guidelines, get raised in this study.

Before the first dose of the vaccine was administered, the weight and height of the recipient was measured. But the girls were not measured before the administration of subsequent doses. After vaccination, the girls were asked to sit down for ten minutes, and then sent to their classes. (The consent form states that each girl will be "kept under observation for fifteen minutes after she has been injected.") The girls were told that the vaccine would prevent uterine cancer, from which many women die. They were also told that the vaccine would "provide life-long protection, has no side-effects and will not affect future fertility" (Sama 2011).

The entire consent process operated within an imagined context of free choice, that is, the context that is imagined and assumed by the IRBs that approve a study as ethical on the basis, primarily, of viewing the informed consent form. And it is the basis for trial subjects being constructed and referred to as trial volunteers. What is the relationship between such imaginations and assumptions and the actual kinds of experimental subjectivity that were created in Bhadrachalam? Two kinds of subject constitution are operational here: the theoretical constitution of the experimental subject by biomedical ethics, and its practical constitution in the actual conduct of a study in particular places and times, in this case in contexts far removed from the context of liberal voluntarism that informed consent presumes.

This practice of subject constitution is not simply one of coercion. Indeed, some parents actually demanded vaccination for their girls. This was because of the perception of the vaccine studies—which were, in fact, an experimental program—as an immunization program. An experiment about public health delivery was often read as a programmatic public health intervention. This was consequent to the ways in which the studies were framed by those administering it: they were made to seem as if they were about access to the vaccine, not an experiment. The consent form, indeed, was titled "Consent for Participation in Cervical Cancer Vaccination Programme, Khammam Dt Andhra Pradesh." The subheadings in the consent form were "About Prevention of Cervical Cancer" and "Information about the HPV Vaccination Programme." It was mentioned once in the form that this was a "research project." The word "experiment" was never used. The actual consent that was being signed was to the statement "I hereby agree to allow my daughter to take three doses of the HPV vaccine." Given such wording, it is not surprising that this study was often misconstrued as an immunization program and not an experiment.[27]

This opens up the question of how immunization programs relate to the issue of consent. While the norms of ethical experimentation on humans presume that the autonomy of the rights-bearing subject is preserved by asking for consent, in the case of immunization and public health, withholding certain programs from groups may equally constitute a violation of rights. Given that these vaccines are expensive, the fact that they were being administered could actually be considered as providing access to an essential therapeutic intervention. Had this not been an experiment, one could consider the free administration of vaccines in an area of impoverishment as a gift—operating in idioms of gifting similar to those that emerged, for instance, around a drug donation program for Gleevec administered by Novartis (see chapter 4).[28]

The question of consent is tenuous in all medical issues, since patients are divided subjects, caught between being nonexperts and being the owners of (or, in the case of parents, custodians for) the bodies in question.[29] Unlike in (certain kinds of) clinical trials, in an immunization program, the subjects are beneficiaries of the project themselves. If, in this case, the subjects were being experimented upon instead, the question of beneficence also potentially changes. Hence, both autonomy and beneficence, two of the pillars upon which liberal biomedical ethics constructs principles of research protection of human subjects, come to depend upon whether this study was an immunization program or an experimental one.[30] Parents too often thought it was an immunization program. PATH admitted it was an experimental program, but insisted it was not a clinical trial. But among those who either reviewed or mobilized around this issue, some suggested that this was in fact a clinical trial. The distinction between immunization and experimentation marks the line between gifting and violation. Whether a postlicensure demonstration study, by definition, is a clinical trial or not came to be an absolutely crucial scientific and ethical question.

Sama conducted interviews in Bhadrachalam that suggest that misunderstanding about the nature of the study was rife. The report quotes the mother of a vaccinated girl as saying, "Since it was a vaccine being given by the government, we all trusted it blindly and considered it reliable, like any other vaccine that was given as part of the immunization programme" (Sarojini, Anjali, and Ashalata 2010, 8). Another quote states, "We were all told that if your child takes this injection, she will not get uterine cancer and moreover the government is giving it free of cost" (9). This ambiguity was also reflected on the HPV immunization card that was provided to those who were administered the vaccine. Nowhere on the card was it mentioned that this was a research project or an experiment. Rather, it was referred to as the "HPV vaccination campaign" of the Department of Health and Family Welfare, Government of Andhra Pradesh. (Logos of PATH and the National Rural Health Mission were affixed on the top right corner of the card.) The bottom of the card instructed, "Keep this card safely and produce it when you come for next dose of HPV." The card was in English, which opens up questions of language and the translation of information.

It is clear, therefore, that GCP was not adhered to in the HPV study, a fact that was also established by the Government of India commission set up to report on the case. Next I read the government report at length, but want to raise a critical issue at this juncture, which is that, in spite of the evidence of nonadherence to GCP, questions of accountability ended up being impossible to establish. Hence, even though the government report established lacunae in the conduct of the study, it refused to hold anyone responsible for them. This could be seen simply as a whitewash or a cover-up by the government, but in fact important institutional questions arise here concerning who was conducting this study. There was a widespread perception in Bhadrachalam that the vaccine was being administered by the government. But in fact this was Merck's vaccine, and the study was conducted primarily by PATH. How then could it come to be seen as a government vaccine? Some of this elision was seen in the HPV immunization card itself, which suggested that this was primarily a vaccination program conducted by the Government of Andhra Pradesh, as just mentioned. What is articulated explicitly here is the pastoral care dimension of vaccine administration.

What one sees here is a case of ethical malpractice falling through two sets of cracks. One crack concerns the empirical—the difficulty, even impossibility, of establishing whether the deaths were in fact caused by the vaccine, which was the focus of the government report. The second crack is ethical—while it was clearly established that there were ethical lapses, it was difficult, and deemed impossible, to determine who specifically was responsible for these lapses. The end result was a scandal that no one was held accountable for, and that perhaps no one could be held accountable for.

It is worthwhile remembering the lives that were at stake, and that also fell through the cracks. The ethnographic perspective of the Sama report reminds us of this, most especially in a poignant interview with the parents of one of the girls who died. I quote an excerpt from this interview, as cited in the report:

After the first dose of the vaccine, our daughter Sarita did not have any reaction. She fainted upon receiving the second dose in school. This was in the afternoon. Nobody informed us. She was taken to the hospital. That evening, some villagers who had visited the hospital told us what had happened. When we went to see her the next morning, we asked her how she was, and she said she was okay. She said that she had got an injection and after the injection she had felt dizzy and fainted. She was then shown to a doctor. We asked her if she wanted to see another doctor, but she refused saying that she had exams coming up.

When Sarita came home for Sankranti, she complained of constant headaches, stomach pains and mood swings. She used to also tap the top of her head with her hand. On January 21, Sarita did not get out of bed in the morning. Her eyes were red. As we were going to work, we asked her what the matter was and she replied that her head was spinning.

Later that day, she went to her uncle's place in the neighborhood and fell flat at the threshold of his house. She had a fit and began to thrash her arms and legs around. Her cousin sister saw her and came running to the field to get us. She said "Pinni (aunty), chelli (sister) has fallen down and her eyes are not stable. She is not speaking." We rushed her to the PHC (Primary Health Center), where they asked us to take her to the Bhadrachalam hospital. By the time we reached there, she had died. Since we had brought her in a 1-0-8 ambulance, we were informed that a post mortem was required. The hospital in Bhadrachalam kept the body for a day. We brought our daughter back and cremated her the next day.

Our child was active and happy. We lost our child, and we know the pain and the agony of that loss. We don't want any other child to die. We don't want any other parent to suffer. Care should be taken for other children who received the vaccination. We want the government to take immediate action. This is our only appeal. This is why we are speaking out. (Sarojini, Anjali, and Ashalata 2010, 15–16)[31]

Two things emerge from the Sama report. The first are the ethical lapses and nonadherence to GCP, a fact reiterated in the government report. But the second is an ethnographic sensibility that is lacking in the versions that were produced by biomedical experts, and which provides a texture of the suffering and the human stakes when care of the population touches down in technocratic ways in contexts of marginality. Layered onto this are questions of causality that this postlicensure observational study opens up. And it was the inability to establish a clear causal link between the vaccines and the deaths that absolved all those involved in the study of any responsibility for its ethical and practical lapses. I next focus on this question of causality as I read the government report on the study.

The government committee in its investigation was given two terms of reference. The first was to consider the ethics of subjecting marginalized children to these studies, and the second was to consider the links between the deaths and the vaccinations. Hence, the terms of inquiry effected a separation of ethical issues from empirical ones. Accountability ultimately ended up being about the empirical rather than the ethical. The report could not establish a causal link between the vaccines and the deaths, and therefore stated that no one could be held accountable even though it was established that there had clearly been ethical violations in the conduct of the study. That something wrong had occurred was incontrovertible; but who committed the wrong was fuzzy. This could just be because there are too many actors involved in situations such as this, making the apportioning of responsibility difficult if not impossible. But it was also read by actors mobilizing against unethical clinical trials as a symptom of too many actors in collusion: specifically, as the state colluding with multinational corporate interests to cover up a scandal.

The committee did not definitively establish that the deaths were not linked to the vaccine—it just could not be definitively established that they were. The official conclusion of the report, indeed, was that the deaths were unlikely to have been because of the vaccine. The ethical violations were clearly mentioned in the expert opinions that were included in the report, yet the report concluded that there had been "no major violation in ethical norms," but rather only "minor deficiencies in planning and conduct of the study."[32] Further, the questions of ethics here were already preframed in terms of the liberal contract that is the typical framing of biomedical ethics as it materializes in considerations of GCP.

The report was attacked by civil society groups mobilizing against unethical clinical trials as an insufficient indictment of what was to them a scandal.[33] While the conclusion to the report might suggest, if not a cover-up, then at least an absolution of the parties involved in the study, the actual experts' reports that constitute the government report paint a more complicated and nuanced picture. Three leading clinical researchers were asked to evaluate the study. Two of them, A. K. Dutta (head of pediatrics, Kalawati Saran Hospital, New Delhi), and Y. K. Gupta (head of pharmacology, All India Institute of Medical Sciences, New Delhi), considered the link between the vaccines and deaths, and in fact came up with radically different assessments. Gupta's was by far the more detailed and equivocal, yet it was Dutta's assessment that was more or less adopted in its entirety in the conclusion to the report.[34]

Dutta's assessment pointed to problems with the study in terms of poor reporting of adverse events and lack of adequate insurance coverage for the girls in the study (though PATH was insured). But in terms of his primary brief, which was to look at the causes for each of the seven deaths (five in Andhra Pradesh and two in Gujarat), he established no causal relationship to the vaccines.[35] In Andhra Pradesh, two of the deaths were attributed to organophosphate poisoning, which Dutta said were "autopsy proven," and one to drowning in a well.[36] A fourth death was attributed to an "unrelated disease which cannot possibly be linked to vaccine," and a fifth to severe malaria.[37] The two deaths in Gujarat were attributed to snake bite and severe malaria, respectively.

Dutta then elaborated the details of the deaths, based both on doctors' reports and first information reports (FIRs).[38] There are questions here concerning what constitutes data, a record, or an archive of an adverse event, especially since a detailed log of adverse events is necessary to maintain as part of GCP. Causality was being constructed here through two different kinds of reporting mechanisms: biomedical reporting mechanisms (the adverse event forms of clinical trials) and state reporting mechanisms (the FIR). Part of the problem in these studies concerned the fact that adverse events were not properly documented, a point made by Dutta himself in his report. Each of the seven deaths was elaborated upon by him as follows:

1 Sodesai Kumari: the FIR that was filed attributes her death to suicide.[39]

2 Chingiri Alekhya Adeepthi: it was established that she developed severe headache, vomiting, and loss of consciousness ninety-six days after receiving the third dose of the vaccine. In her case, Dutta established cause of death based on the doctor's report, which diagnosed subarachnoid hemorrhage due to the rupture of an aneurysm; an intracranial space–occupying lesion; anaphylactic shock; and dehydration. No detailed hospital records were available for her.[40]

3 Kudumula Sarita: Dutta established the cause of death based on an FIR report, stating "the cause of death was poisoning and hence further investigation was not carried out."[41] It is worth contrasting this conclusion to the interview that Sama conducted with Sarita's parents, quoted above, where they emphatically denied that she had consumed poison. Even if they were wrong and she had, it should be emphasized that Dutta's official conclusion that she died

because of suicide and not because of the vaccine is based entirely on an FIR listing her death as suicide, and not on any biomedical assessment or information.

4 Mudraboyena Suryalaxmi: she died by falling into a well. Dutta concluded, "Since the case was not related to vaccination, hence further investigations were dropped."[42]

5 Kampally Swati: developed fever twenty-three days after receiving vaccination. Dutta stated that "cause of death [was] recorded as viral fever."[43]

The two Gujarat deaths were attributed as follows:

1 Miss Jar [no first name included]: "practitioner had suspected her to be a case of malaria. . . . Medical officer investigated the case and finally opined that the girl died of malaria and severe anemia."[44] No postmortem had been conducted in this case.

2 Vasava Manjula Laxman: had a diagnosis of snakebite. Further investigations were not done because it was assumed that the snakebite caused the death, and hence it was unrelated to the vaccine.

Critical questions of causality are raised by Dutta's conclusions. It may well be possible—indeed, even plausible—that none of the seven deaths were caused by the vaccine, and in each case, an alternative possibility or likelihood was established. But a modality of representation is operational here, involving a twofold set of conjectures. First, there is an interpretation of an event from two very different kinds of data—a doctor's report and a police report. In two of the seven cases, FIRs had been filed, and they alone were read, to the exclusion of any medical reports. Hence, Dutta renders these two very different kinds of reporting equivalent, substituting one for the other without any consideration that they represent entirely nonequivalent forms of medical data. (Indeed, an FIR is not in itself a medical record, but it stood in for medical records in two of the cases here.) Second, even the doctors' reports, when they existed, tended to be partial, provisional, or themselves conjectural, often unaccompanied by proper postmortems or medical histories. Yet the deeply contingent nature of these reports was elided, and one is left with a series of unequivocal arrows: statements that deaths were caused by x, or not caused by y.[45]

Consider, for instance, the kinds of claims that Dutta made in the conclusion to his report:

- Sodesai Kumari: "consumption of poison . . . *proven* by autopsy."[46]
- Chingiri Alekhya Adeepthi: a number of assumptions are made in relation to her death. She died after developing a headache, but there is no detailed medical history relating to her headache. Dutta acknowledges that her medical records state that the headache itself could have been due to a "variety of causes."[47] However, he concluded that the link to the vaccine was unlikely primarily because of the duration (ninety-six days) between the last dose of the vaccine and the onset of Alekhya's symptoms. Of course, what happened in those ninety-six days is precisely relevant to a medical history of the headache, which is lacking. The event that caused the death was the headache, but what caused the headache is entirely unclear. Yet because the death gets linked to the headache, it is automatically assumed that it is not linked to the vaccine.
- Kampally Swati: the recorded cause of death was "viral fever," and it was on the basis of this medical record that Dutta concluded that her death was not due to the vaccine. Yet, in his conclusions, he states, "Diagnosis is uncertain and could be due to malaria."[48] Here, Dutta substitutes one speculative and hypothetical diagnosis, which forms the only record of possible cause of death, with another that is based neither on a medical examination nor a medical record.
- Vasava Manjula Laxman: Dutta concludes that she "was bitten in the leg by a venomous snake and died."[49]

It is worthwhile thinking about the tenuous nature of the evidence here, especially since the entire rationale of a clinical experiment rests on it being evidence-based medicine.[50] Dutta's conclusions definitively ruled out a causal link between vaccine administration and deaths, and these were taken as matters of fact, provided by an expert, as the government report drew its own conclusion regarding the nonrelationship of vaccines to deaths. The hardening of these statements into factual assertions as they traveled from the event of the death of a girl to conclusions in a government report has consequences, especially for establishing responsibility for these deaths (or failing to do so).

I am not suggesting that the deaths were in fact caused by the vaccines—I absolutely have no basis to make a claim about these deaths one way or another. But I do wish to suggest just how contingent and speculative these apparently factual conclusions regarding the nonrelationship of vaccinations to deaths actually were. Part of this contingency is simply a function of the limits of available data, so that Dutta was forced in two cases to read police reports as if they were medical reports, and was often required to draw extrapolative conclusions even from the medical reports that did exist. But part of this contingency is also due to what can only be called extremely creative interpretation of the available data by Dutta himself. Consider for instance two of the more equivocal cases here, concerning the deaths of Kampally Swati and Vasava Manjula Laxman. Swati's death was ultimately a fever of unknown cause—attributed as "viral fever" in the medical report upon her death, and as "could be due to malaria" by Dutta. Manjula's death was unequivocally stated by Dutta as being due to snakebite. But it is worth squaring these conclusions with Dutta's own accounts of these deaths from his report.

Dutta's account of Swati's death is as follows:

> Miss Kampally Swathi 13 years old girl, daughter of Shri Kampally Sreenivas of Ganga Hussain Basti, Kothagudem received the first dose of Gardasil on 7th July, 2009. After 23 days of the vaccination she had developed fever on 1st August, 2009 and was treated by a local registered medical practitioner. She did not improve and was admitted in Kothagudem area hospital on 8th August with breathlessness and went into coma. She was then referred to Khammam civil hospital where she was given Inj Chloroquine, Injection Paracetemol, Injection Ranitidine, Injection Perinorm, Injection Gentamicin, Injection Deriphylline [*sic*], Injection Decadron and Aminophylline drip. High risk consent was taken by the treating doctor. She did not improve with the treatment and expired on 8th August at 9 PM. The cause of death recorded as viral fever.[51]

In other words, what the treating doctor was actually confronted with was a fever of unknown origin. The treatment involved eight different kinds of medication that are used for treating many different kinds of illnesses. Chloroquine is used to treat malaria; paracetemol is used to bring down fever; ranitidine is used to treat heartburn and ulcers; Perinorm is used primarily as an antiemetic, to treat nausea and vomiting; gentamicin is an antibacterial antibiotic; deriphyllin is used to treat lung disease symptoms; Decadron is a corticosteroid (dexamethasone); while aminophylline is a bronchodilator. Some of these must surely have been administered to provide symptomatic relief, while others might have been administered prophylactically; but there was nothing in either the medical records or the treatment records to suggest unequivocally that Swati's fever was a "viral fever," let alone, as Dutta subsequently decided, malaria.

Dutta's account of Manjula's death has even more equivocation, and is as follows:

> Miss Vasava Manjula Laxman, 15 years old daughter of Shri Laxman Lalji Vasava of Nander, Bithli, Shinor of Barodara district received first and second dose of Cervarix on 9th September and 14th October, 2009. The girl complained of mild fever, joint pain and headache on 15th October for which she was treated by a local private practitioner with tablet paracetemol, tablet ranitidine and tablet Liv-52 (herbal medicine for liver). She was asked to come for follow up after two days. She remained well and started working in the field. After 18th day of the second dose she had complained of pain in the leg and some insect bite locally and was not feeling well for which she did not go for work in the afternoon. She was not taken to the doctor for this ailment and rested at home. Her condition became very critical at night and on 2nd November at 7.30 AM 108 no ambulance service was called and shifted to CHC (Community Health Center) Motafolfia. Her condition became very critical during the process of shifting with no recordable vital signs. The ambulance service people started CPR but the girl could not be revived and brought dead to the hospital. CHC doctor advised for postmortem but the family has refused. A diagnosis of snake bite was made *as it is very common in the area and the insect bite which was referred by the family was possibly due to bite by a poisonous snake.* Dr. Shivaji K Kotwal made the FIR and sent the same to District child health officer Dr. RB Patel on 31.12.2009. Dr Patel recorded his signature in the FIR on 02.01.2010. Since the death was not related to vaccine, further investigations were not done.[52]

In Manjula's case, Dutta's own account suggests that no one knows she was bitten by a snake. The medical diagnosis at the time itself was pure conjecture. Yet Dutta's statement that "a diagnosis of snake bite was made as it is very common in the area and the insect bite . . . was possibly due to bite by a poisonous snake" turns into Dutta's conclusion that Manjula "was bitten in the leg by a venomous snake and died."

My point here is not to dispute the conclusions dissociating the vaccinations from the deaths. It is rather to emphasize that this dissociation happened because no unequivocal evidence of an association could be found. Yet other kinds of associations and speculations were made in spite of equally equivocal evidence. And those latter speculations ended up operating as facts and as expert testimony. This opens up questions of the relationship between evidentiary ambiguity and ethical malpractice.

One level at which questions of causality were ambiguous was institutional, as pinpointing accountability in these brokered, multilayered, and multinational structural arrangements of clinical research proved difficult. This was a three-phase, four-nation study, whose protocols were approved for the Indian studies in three IRBS across two countries. It was a public-private partnership, with multinational pharmaceutical companies, global philanthropic public health organizations, state governments, and medical research councils all having a stake. Even some of the most evidently egregious aspects of the study were hard to easily allocate blame and responsibility for.

For instance, the permission to obtain informed consent from hostel wardens to conduct clinical studies on tribal girls was given by a circular distributed by the Andhra Pradesh Ministry for Tribal Welfare. While this absolutely violates any liberal notion of informed consent or parental consent for minors and raises serious questions about research on marginalized populations, who is to be held responsible for this particular practice? Merck, whose vaccine it is, and who stands to gain considerably from its incorporation into a national immunization program, but who was not involved in the study? PATH, who was involved in the logistical aspects of the study, but who was relying on state authorities and institutions to facilitate implementation of the study? ICMR, who as a facilitator, should have been more careful about ensuring GCP, but which also was the organization responsible for stopping the study when violations came to light? The state government, which agreed to conduct the study in Andhra Pradesh, and propagated it as its program? The National Rural Health Mission, which pushed a technocratic vaccine agenda as a stand-in for interventions in improving rural health? The members of IRBS, many of whom serve in voluntary capacities, who approved the study protocol? Or the bureaucrat in the Andhra Pradesh Ministry for Tribal Welfare, who wrote the circular that allowed experimentation on tribal girls based on consent from teachers and hostel wardens?

The other layer of complexity that makes accountability difficult is empirical, and concerns the difficulty of establishing causal relationships between an intervention in a clinical study and an adverse event. The way in which Dutta drew his conclusions was extrapolative, speculative, and irresponsible. But a second expert report to the government commission, by Y. K. Gupta, head of the Department of Pharmacology at the All India Institute of Medical Sciences

(AIIMS), New Delhi, was far more qualified in its conclusions.[53] Gupta stated that the distinction between this observational study and a clinical trial is not clear-cut, since even though the studies were not meant to establish safety and efficacy of the vaccines, they did involve "the study of a pharmaceutical product carried out in humans," and required the observation and maintenance of records of all serious and nonserious adverse events.[54] The definition of a clinical trial under Schedule Y of the Indian Drugs and Cosmetics Act is "a systematic study of pharmaceutical products on human subjects (whether patients or non-patient volunteers) in order to discover or verify the clinical, pharmacological and/or adverse effects, with the object of determining their safety and efficacy."[55] Hence, even though PATH insisted that this was not a clinical trial, Gupta pointed out that under Indian GCP guidelines, it could be considered one.

Gupta's conclusions concerning causality were far more equivocal than Dutta's. For instance, this is Gupta's account of the death of Vasava Manjula Laxman, which had been attributed to snakebite: "The report does not describe the site of bite, the presence or absence of fang marks and local wound condition. It also does not mention the presence of either neurotoxic symptoms (paralysis, head drop, ptosis etc) or hemotoxic symptoms (bleeding from wound/DIC or hematuria etc). In the absence of such signs and symptoms of envenomation, causality assessment is difficult."[56]

Even the death that might appear intuitively to be completely unconnected to the vaccine, Mudraboyeni Suryalaxmi's drowning in a well, received a qualified assessment from Gupta, who merely stated that it is "unlikely" that this happened due to vaccine-induced dizziness. He pointed out that "the case record is incomplete. It just mentions that the subject accidentally fell in well and died. The preceding sequence of events is not mentioned. It is unlikely that the accident happened due to vaccine induced dizziness. *However it is difficult to establish or rule out with absolute certainty association of the event with the vaccine.*"[57]

Gupta was similarly equivocal about virtually all the other deaths. While at no point did he claim a definitive causal link between the vaccine and the deaths, each of his assessments questions the way in which such a link was ruled out in Dutta's assessment. They also point to the inherent epistemic uncertainty in establishing causal relationships to adverse events in the absence of clear statistical clustering or evidence. In this regard, Gupta's conclusions are of a very different order than Dutta's, and raise two important points that never came up in Dutta's analysis—and that were not highlighted in the commission's conclusions to the report.

First, Gupta points out that a clinical trial can never be a sufficient indication of complete safety. For instance, a clinical trial may not pick out a severe adverse event that occurs once in every few thousand patients, since the sample size of a Phase 3 trial tends to be only a few thousand patients.[58] The implications of this in a demographic context that is quite different from the one in which the trials for the vaccines were conducted are obvious: the establishment of the safety of HPV vaccines in clinical trials can indicate the likelihood of, but cannot guarantee, their absolute safety in the context of these studies. Critically, this leads to Gupta's second point, which is that, therefore, this demonstration study must be considered a kind of clinical trial. Gupta returned to the point that he started with, concerning the ambiguous epistemic status of an observational study of this nature.

In the government report, questions of ethics and evidence were uncoupled. This is indicated by the structure of the report, as Dutta's and Gupta's expert assessments were followed by those of Rani Kumar, dean of AIIMS, who looked separately at the question of ethical malpractice and established deficiencies in the processes by which the studies were conducted. The first moment of black boxing occurs here: in the absence of establishing a clear causal relationship between the vaccines and the deaths, the epistemic issues of causality ended up dropping out of the picture, even though equivocations remained and speculations abounded. The ethical remained the only ground upon which adjudication ended up happening. And in spite of establishing ethical malpractice, the institutional complexities by which the studies were structured meant that no one was actually held accountable for them. But the ethical alone does not provide the context for these studies: so too does the technocratic. No amount of ethical regulation or punitive deterrence would entirely ensure the safety of tribal girls in a study that operates within a top-down imaginary of public health that presumes solutions in terms of a linear process of vaccine production → vaccine dissemination → health, without an adequate understanding of social context.

The question I am asking, therefore, is not just, how do we build better regulatory infrastructure for the conduct of clinical research? Indeed, building better ethical and regulatory infrastructure was the cornerstone of the liberalization of clinical trials regimes in India, as driven by the CRO industry in the mid-2000s. The question that must be asked alongside is, how might we construct a biomedical research imaginary that goes beyond the technocratic in order to adequately conceptualize the social that is the target of such research? In the next section, I open up this question by looking at the technocratic dimensions of the HPV studies and considering them alongside the ethical questions that have been explicated.

Technocracy

Ethical violations and the poor adherence to norms of GCP aside, a primary question that must be asked in relation to these studies is, why were they conducted in the first place? This can be asked on two levels. The first, which was posed by Gupta in his assessment, concerns the actual specificities of this particular study. Why did a postlicensure observational study regarding vaccine uptake have to be conducted? What is a postlicensure observational study anyway? Is it or is it not a clinical trial? What led to the study being conducted in the particular states in which it was done? And what were the inclusion and exclusion criteria that led to tribal girls being the subjects of some of these experiments? But the second level has to do with the question of cervical cancer vaccines themselves. Why are they considered an important part, potentially, of a national immunization program in a country like India? What is the place of these vaccines in relation to the broader epidemiology of cervical cancer? And what is their place in relation to the broader imagination that underlies contemporary public and rural health initiatives in India?[59]

At first sight, it would seem as if this latter set of questions would have obvious answers. This is because the safety and efficacy of HPV vaccines has been established in clinical trials, and these vaccines are now a part of immunization programs in at least four major advanced liberal countries (the United States, the United Kingdom, Australia, and Netherlands). The American Academy of Pediatrics (2012) has recommended that the vaccine, which was initially targeted at teenage girls, should be routinely used for boys as well. And in the United States, the defense of the HPV vaccine has been the staunchly liberal-progressive, rational position, which came to light starkly in these terms following Minnesota representative Michele Bachmann's questioning of the vaccine during her candidacy for the 2012 Republican presidential nomination.[60]

And yet, what became evident in the controversy around the vaccine studies is that such questions do not have simple, settled answers. A particular case was being made for these vaccines, most stridently by PATH. But PATH's push for the vaccines and for the studies became the subject of debate within public health scholarship. What is at stake in these disputes is not a pro- versus antiscience position as much as it is a debate between a technocratic imagination of public health and one that is more sociologically embedded.

PATH (2009) made the case for the demonstration studies most strongly in a publication that described the outcome of the initial, formative phase of the studies (what they referred to as Phase 1). This early research, conducted in collaboration with the National AIDS Research Institute, Pune, in 2009, had three objectives: to explore the acceptance of different vaccine delivery strategies; to develop mechanisms for outreach to communities; and to develop an advocacy strategy for outreach to policy makers. The actual work in this phase of research was largely survey, focus group, and interview based, involving conversations with local communities, health workers, and policy makers in order to assess levels of knowledge about cervical cancer and HPV, as well as attitudes toward the vaccine.

In summing up the results of this phase, which effectively served as the platform for the Phase 2 observational studies that were shut down amid controversy, PATH made its epidemiological claims for the vaccine. The claims were ostensibly made in response to the more than 100,000 new cases of cervical cancer that occur each year in India and were as follows: that 270,000 cervical cancer deaths occur each year, of which 85 percent are in developing countries; that based on current global trends, there will be more than a million new cases of cervical cancer each year worldwide by 2050; and that the two vaccines, Gardasil and Cervarix, provide protection against the two strains that cause 70 percent of cervical cancer cases (PATH 2009). What one sees here is a direct correlation that suggests that more vaccine will lead to less cervical cancer. PATH also cited the following figures regarding the cervical cancer burden in India: that in raw numbers, India has the largest burden of cervical cancer of any country in the world; that about one-third of women admitted to hospitals with cancer in India are diagnosed with cervical cancer; that 90 percent of these diagnoses are of late-stage cancer; and that estimates indicate that population-wide prevalence of HPV infection is 7 percent, though that figure has been suggested to be as high as 19 percent in unpublished results (PATH 2009, 5).[61]

PATH did acknowledge that in developed countries, screening constitutes the most effective mechanism to prevent cervical cancer, since it allows for early detection and treatment. Yet in spite of conceding this claim, PATH insisted on the vaccine as the desired mechanism for cervical cancer prevention in developing countries, because "in developing countries ... many women cannot access screening services or do not receive necessary treatment for precancer" (PATH 2009, 3). Of course, in many developing countries, women cannot access the vaccine either, unless the state makes it available to them through immunization programs. What PATH was implicitly suggesting then is that the state can (and should) make the vaccine available to women, but that screening, almost by definition, is inaccessible. In other words, PATH's was a purely technocratic approach focused on vaccine administration.

There are two ways in which that imaginary came to be questioned even from within a public health context. First, questions were raised about whether in fact the vaccine is the best method to prevent cervical cancer, compared to screening, or in the absence of adequate screening facilities. Second and more damningly, questions were raised about the basis of the claims that PATH was making. An argument was made, for instance, that screening outweighs the strengths of HPV vaccines as preventive intervention for cervical cancer (Maine, Hurlburt, and Greeson 2011). This has been argued both in terms of the epidemiology of the disease, and in terms of the feasibility of implementation and cost considerations in developing country contexts (Dunne et al. 2007; see also Miranda 2011). Even if the infrastructure for advanced methods of cervical cancer screening does not exist, it has been suggested that more rudimentary methods could still be inexpensive and cheap interventions (Dunne et al. 2007).[62]

Two PATH researchers responded to Maine, Hurlburt, and Greeson (2011) by claiming that the vaccine is not just a valuable health intervention in and of itself but will be a driver of a more "comprehensive approach" to cervical cancer prevention (Tsu and LaMontagne 2012).[63] They stated that "vaccination and its promotion—including the message that screening must still be provided—are creating a demand for screening and a recognition that a comprehensive approach is essential" (Tsu and LaMontagne 2012, 389). What one sees here is the articulation of a trickle-down public health, where the implementation of a technocratic solution is presumed to drive an overall improvement in public health infrastructure and intervention. A dominant public health imaginary is articulated here that sees health as being driven by the production of artifacts (in this case, the vaccine). Within that imaginary, PATH's claims are entirely consistent and make sense; and the problems for improving health end up being about the gaps that exist between research and manufacture, or (more explicit in this case) between manufacture and dissemination. Regardless of the fact that public health is always already appropriable into logics of surplus value generation, thereby bringing the definition of health itself into question in these situations, the imaginary here is of a health system and infrastructure that is focused on the problem of the artifact, to the exclusion of considerations of policy that might actually facilitate public good in the broadest and most comprehensive sense.[64]

Perhaps the more broad-based indictment of the PATH studies came from an article published by Allyson Pollock and coauthors in the *Journal of the Royal Society of Medicine* (Mattheij, Pollock, and Brhlikova 2012). In this article, the authors question the very basis of PATH's figures, given that national cancer data available for India only cover 7 percent of the population. The data on population prevalence of HPV in India are poor and studies have been highly variable in their findings. There is no cancer registry in Andhra Pradesh, and PATH did not cite any data from the Gujarat registries. The data that do exist, Pollock argues, do not support PATH's claims about cervical cancer burden in India or about the need to roll out a vaccine program. Pollock, therefore, describes the kinds of speculation that have been made by PATH in making their claims, while opening up the question of the relationship of public health claims to data.

Pollock's critique had three focal points: cervical cancer reporting and surveillance systems; epidemiological evidence regarding cervical cancer incidence and prevalence; and the relationship between the epidemiological evidence that exists and the justification for rolling out the study in Andhra Pradesh and Gujarat.

In terms of the first: two agencies are involved with cancer surveillance in India. The first is the National Cancer Registry Programme (NCRP), while the second is the International Agency for Research on Cancer (IARC). The NCRP is a network of population-based and hospital-based registries operating under the aegis of the ICMR. It only covers 7 percent of the Indian population, and rural regions of the country are underrepresented. To the extent that it shows anything, it is a decrease in age-standardized cervical cancer mortality and incidence rates in India, from 42.3 per 100,000 to 22.3 per 100,000 between 1982–1983 and 2004–2005. In addition to these registries, the NCRP draws upon the Cancer Atlas of India, which is a map of cancer incidence using cancer cases registered in pathology departments attached to medical schools as a major source. The atlas covers only 13–21 percent of cancer cases in India, and the hospitals that provide source material are again predominantly urban. The IARC has two different databases, but again the coverage is either limited, overlapping with existing data, or derived through extrapolation from Western data sets. In addition to this generally poor cancer surveillance in relation to India, there exists extremely limited data from Andhra Pradesh and Gujarat, and the data that do exist, as mentioned, was not cited by PATH. Further, the baseline epidemiology of the disease is not properly known, and the surveillance systems that do exist are not capable of assessing the impact of vaccine intervention.

What one has in this case is a knowledge that is based on a very limited information base, but which nonetheless does a lot of work in terms of justifying certain kinds of public health interventions. It concerns itself less with truth or objective validity and more with creating mobility across various domains. This mobility is tied into exchangeability and fungibility of various sorts. Hence, the kinds of comprehensive care for cervical cancer that PATH espouses, driven by the vaccine as a technocratic and value-laden artifact, do not depend on comprehensive knowledge, or at least not on comprehensive information on cervical cancer prevalence and incidence in India. The knowledge that exists, however, is good enough to enable various kinds of movements: of artifacts into rural health programs; vaccines from Merck or GlaxoSmithKline to Indian villages; public health expertise from a Seattle-based nonprofit to the corridors of Indian government and policy making.

At stake here is the creation of multiple regimes of value. This has to do with the value of rural public health, which gets emphasized and which rationalizes and justifies studies whose basis might on closer inspection be deemed questionable. But it also has to do with the market value that multinational pharmaceutical companies accrue from the rollout of their vaccines in national immunization programs. The value of rural public health in this context is that which is legible to capital; it allows vaccines to function as public health artifacts in surplus health economies. The state acts as a facilitator (through, in this case, the ICMR) and as a consumer (through the National Immunization Programme) for these mobile artifacts. The mediation of the movement of these artifacts through these economies is enabled by brokers such as PATH. If the meaning of health comes to be at stake in these movements (as something appropriable into logics of surplus value generation), then so too does the meaning of knowledge (as something that concerns itself with transfigurations and translations of various sorts, rather than with truth). This is knowledge that is articulated to value that can be valorized as capital.

This at one level materializes into profit for companies like Merck and GlaxoSmithKline, should their vaccines be incorporated into national immunization programs. But at a larger conceptual level, at stake are the reconfigurations that become possible when knowledge and health can both be valorized. These questions did not emerge in such terms in the public health discussions around the vaccine, or in media framings of the HPV studies that tended to focus on scandalous ethical malfeasance. But they were central issues in the arena of representative politics in India. Hence if the state through ICMR and the National Rural Health Mission facilitated the capitalization of public health, then it was also the state, especially the Indian Parliament, which provided the arena where such capitalization could be contested and debated on its own terms. In this arena, the scandal of the trial could potentially be reframed as the scandal of the state.[65]

The Science and Politics of the HPV Vaccine Studies

The HPV vaccine studies initially became a political issue through the intervention of the All India Democratic Women's Association (AIDWA), which is the women's wing of the Communist Party of India (Marxist), one of India's two major communist parties. Local branches of AIDWA in Khammam district of Andhra Pradesh got wind of the deaths of the tribal girls who were part of the vaccine studies. They made this issue known to officeholders of the Communist Party as well as to women's groups in Delhi. Brinda Karat, a long-term member of AIDWA and one of the most active political voices in India on women's issues, who was at that time a Member of Parliament in the Rajya Sabha (Upper House of Parliament), raised these issues with Ghulam Nabi Azad, who was at the time union health minister of India, in a letter dated March 22, 2010.[66]

In this first letter, Karat raised the possibility of a connection between the vaccines and the deaths, based on details that were gathered by AIDWA, Andhra Pradesh. Even after such a causal link had been ruled out by the government report, Karat questioned this denial, by pointing, more strongly than Y. K. Gupta had, to the fact that an absence of causality had not been definitively established. In a subsequent letter to Azad, she said of the Government report, "Shockingly even there were no postmortem reports in at least three of the cases, no follow up investigation was ordered. Yet the committee even in the absence of evidence concludes that the vaccinations were *most probably* (emphasis added) not related to the deaths. This can hardly be considered a credible conclusion."[67]

Karat made two further significant moves that are directly related to my interests in the political economic and the epistemic. In terms of the former, she brought the question of corporate interest squarely into the picture by framing the studies as a means for multinational companies to promote their vaccines. How, she asked, could such promotion be allowed within the framework of a public health apparatus? What was global health in the eyes of PATH was reframed by Karat as the interests of multinational corporations acting through foreign nongovernmental organizations. She specifically asked whether the entire project "was designed to promote the interests of the companies."[68]

In terms of the latter, Karat foregrounded the definitional question of whether or not these studies were clinical trials. As already mentioned, PATH had insisted that these were not clinical trials but rather simply "observational studies." Even though they never clearly explicated what an "observational study" was, the point of this rhetorical distinction was obvious: to emphasize that these were not experiments with an untested vaccine, but were rather studies with a vaccine whose safety and efficacy had already been proven in clinical trials. Gupta had, in his expert opinion as part of the government report, already qualified this distinction by pointing out that the context in which the clinical trials had been conducted was quite different from the context of administering vaccines to tribal girls in rural India. This qualification was pushed by Karat, who pointed out that in India, there had been no full-fledged Phase 3 clinical trial, but only what is known as a bridging study.

A bridging study is a clinical study that is designed to ensure that the results of a clinical trial conducted in a certain demographic remain valid when that drug (or vaccine) is used in another demographic. It has become particularly important in discussions around global harmonization of clinical trials, especially in the context of resistance by certain countries, notably Japan, to accept clinical trial results from other countries on the grounds that those results do not necessarily indicate how a drug would work in their populations.[69] Karat's point precisely was that regardless of whether clinical trials had been done elsewhere or not, only bridging studies had been done in India. And hence, her implication was that these observational studies were not merely observation, but still constituted experiment. This was the focal point of active debate in the Indian Parliament between Karat and Azad.

In a calling-attention motion in the Rajya Sabha, Karat made the following claims and asked for clarifications from Azad:

In a latter [*sic*] to me dated 8th April, 2010, the Minister categorically said these vaccines were approved by the DCGI [Drug Controller General of India] in India by following standard procedure and after carrying bridging studies as they were already approved in their country of origin. In other words, from the Minister's letter it is clear that there are no clinical trials because I asked specifically a question about whether there were clinical trials. The Minister in his letter says that there are bridging studies. In his statement today he says that there were clinical trials. I would like to know what is correct, whether letter to me or the statement that is before the House. There is no such thing like bridging studies in any of our protocols for clinical trials or in any other type of study. There is nothing like a bridging study. This is a new terminology which is brought into our system. So, I have looked up all the clinical registry guidelines and I have looked up where the protocols and where the clinical trials are registered. At least, I could not find any Phase-III trial completed with published data. Yes, I could find it in the US Government website where the company says that they have done this or that trial in India. But I could not find it on the ICMR website in India. . . . According to the ICMR guidelines, before you do trial on children, you have to do trial on adult population. What were the trials done? How many women were given this who were screened for HPV that they do not have that virus? Where were these trials conducted? Where has such published material been given?[70]

Azad replied with the following biology lesson:

Now, what is the clinical trial? Let me clarify that. . . . It involves four phases. . . . Number one, trial for establishing safety and tolerability; number two, trial for effectiveness; number three, trial for demonstrating or confirming the clinical and therapeutic benefit; and number four, trials on a large population after post-market approval. The market approval [in India] has been given about two years ago, in 2008, after the third phase was over on a limited number. In one case it was 100 or something like that and in the other case it was 300. In the case of an imported medicine, which has already been cleared by the respective Governments, you are supposed to do a bridging trial, which is called Phase-III, on a very limited number. It is not done on a large number. Then it is given the market approval. So, it is only after market approval is given for two years, the fourth phase starts on a large population. . . . So we are not doing anything wrong. Whether the PATH is there or not, somebody has to carry out this exercise of Phase-IV trial in our country on a large population.

Not only was Azad claiming that a Phase 3 clinical trial is the same as a bridging study, he was also suggesting that PATH's observational studies were a Phase 4 trial. Phase 4 trials are normally conducted by pharmaceutical companies after marketing approval as a follow-up to study safety of the drug in large populations. PATH itself had never, in any of its documents, referred to these observational studies as a Phase 4 trial. Needless to say, Karat did not let Azad off the hook. The debate played out in relation to this thus:

SHRIMATI BRINDA KARAT: I just want to raise . . .

MR. DEPUTY CHAIRMAN: Please be pointed.

SBK: I am being very pointed. The Minister has made a statement in the House that according to him, a bridge study is the same as a Phase III trial. . . .

SHRI GHULAM NABI AZAD: In this case.

SBK: There is no "in this case or that case." . . .

SGNA: In this case because the trial III for the new drugs is totally different. If the drug is already in use, then, this may not hold good.

SBK: Thank you, Ghulamji. You have made my task even easier. There are no exceptions allowed in the present Indian legal framework. . . . How can safety be proved on 110 subjects, and that too by a study done by the company itself? . . . And this has been done by whom? One is Gardasil and the other is Glaxo. They are having a competition amongst themselves as to who is going to capture which market. . . . It was for how many! It was for 354. Sir, only 177 were given the vaccine. The others were given placebos.[71] . . . But these cannot be equated with Phase III trial. And I reiterate today that if you want to change the ICMR guidelines, change them; bring it before the House. But we will not accept tiny population studies to say they are Phase III trials in India. They are not Phase III trials. . . . If you want to change the law and you want to change the guidelines, please change it and bring it to the House. But don't try and say that a trial on 110 people is a Phase III trial. It cannot be accepted.

In response, Azad fell back upon what was known or operational in the American context as justification for their rollout in the Indian context:

SGNA: In America, where it is very difficult to find a large number of subjects for trial for various reasons, this trial has been done on 21000 girls and women. I don't find any clinical trial being done in the United States of America before getting the FDA approval on 21000 individuals. So, it is not that somebody said and somebody started trials here. . . . I don't think the Americans would have done this study on 21000 individuals without any preparation and then allow it into the national immunization programme.

Here, Azad was setting up the trials conducted in America as a gold standard and making the assumption that they could be imported as is, without attentiveness to the very different context into which they were being imported. This difference has to do with epidemiology—how does one know that something will work the same on tribal girls in rural India as it did on urban American women, especially given the paucity of cancer surveillance data and screening facilities in the Indian context? But it equally has to do with the law. Azad was trying to render the "evidence" of evidence-based medicine universal. Karat in response particularized it with her insistence that a bridging study in India could not substitute for a full-fledged Phase 3 trial, but also with her insistence that these studies had to be in accordance with Indian laws and Indian policy. She insisted that in order to produce the bridging study as an epistemically valid entity, it had to be produced simultaneously as a legally valid entity.

Consequences and Trajectories

How did the public scandal surrounding the HPV vaccine studies impact the biomedical terrain of clinical research in India? The answer to this question is complicated and involves the political ways in which logics of capital interact with various arms of the state that are themselves accountable to different interests. I point to two trajectories that emerged after the HPV scandal that raise conceptual questions concerning relationships between knowledge, value, and experimental subjectivity. The first was a parliamentary indictment of these studies that placed the question of multinational corporate power at the center of its concerns, and the second was regulatory changes that were themselves controversial.

In August 2013, a Parliamentary Standing Committee presented a report to the Rajya Sabha concerning the alleged irregularities in the HPV studies.[72] This committee consisted of members of the Upper and Lower Houses of the Indian Parliament from multiple political parties (including Karat), and had been constituted in 2010 in the immediate aftermath of reports of the death of girls in the studies. The report came to unequivocally critical conclusions about the studies, continuing the tone of some of the more pointed lines of questioning in the parliamentary debates on the subject. It only referred to the studies as trials, completely repudiating PATH's insistence that they were not. It stated that these trials had been conducted "against all laws of the land"; that there was an "enormity of wrong-doing/criminality involved"; and that ICMR "lent its platform to PATH in an improper and unlawful manner."[73] But what the report made most explicit was a line of questioning that Karat had initiated in parliamentary debates, which concerned the corporate interests of the vaccine manufacturers. It noted that the four countries in which PATH had conducted these studies, India, Uganda, Peru, and Vietnam, all have national immunization programs which "if expanded to include Gardasil would mean tremendous financial benefit to the then sole manufacturer."[74] It was explicit that the purpose of the study was to exploit the captive market that would be available to the manufacturers through a state-run public immunization program, and questioned the bona fides of PATH's attachments to corporate interests:

> The Committee finds the entire matter very intriguing and fishy. The choice of countries and population groups; the monopolistic nature, at that point of time, of the product being pushed; the unlimited market potential and opportunities in the universal immunization programmes of the respective countries are all pointers to a well planned scheme to commercially exploit a situation. Had PATH been successful in getting the HPV vaccine included in the universal immunization programme of the concerned countries, this would have generated windfall profit for the manufacturer(s) by way of automatic sale, year after year, without any promotional or marketing expenses. It is well known that once introduced into the immunization programme it becomes politically impossible to stop any vaccination. To achieve this end effortlessly without going through the arduous and strictly regulated route of clinical trials, PATH resorted to an element of subterfuge by calling the clinical trials as "Observational Studies" or "Demonstration Project" and various such expressions. Thus, the interest, safety and well being of subjects were completely jeopardized by PATH by using self-determined and self-servicing nomenclature which is not only highly deplorable but a serious breach of the law of the land.[75]

The parliamentary report therefore was as scathing an indictment as one could imagine of these studies, going beyond procedural questions of ethics to condemn the political economy that the institutional configuration of these studies represented. But it is worth qualifying these conclusions in two ways.

The first is to recognize that the appropriation of national public health agendas for monopolistic (or in the case of the HPV vaccines, duopolistic) corporate gain is perhaps as old as the history of vaccines itself. Maurice Cassier (2005) has, for instance, shown how Louis Pasteur commercially exploited the anthrax vaccine in the 1880s and 1890s to develop a monopoly on vaccine production and distribution, in spite of the fact that patents on pharmaceutical products were at that time not allowed in France. Pasteur used contractual strategies such as exclusive operating licenses to restrict technology transfer in ways that would allow his laboratories to retain knowledge and control of reliable vaccine manufacture, even as he had global market ambitions for the vaccine that included the establishment of a company to distribute the vaccine outside France. The corporate agendas underlying the HPV demonstration studies in India were understandably rendered scandalous, but they were hardly new. Perhaps what was new was the complex structure of brokerage that, until the scandal was reiterated through representative parliamentary forums, largely kept the corporate manufacturers of the vaccine out of the picture, focusing attention instead on PATH and ICMR. In other words, what one sees here is an articulation of monopolistic corporate interests through brokerage economies that outsource responsibility as much as they outsource the labor of clinical development or distribution. This is a different strategy of monopoly enforcement than that seen in relation to markets (such as for drugs in India), which are not thus constructed in advance through state biopolitical initiatives (see chapters 3 and 4).

The second is to note that the vociferous criticisms of the HPV studies through parliamentary forums still did not lead to anyone being held accountable for them, even though the Standing Committee Report recommended that action be taken against PATH. Indeed, the most tangible changes after the scandal were regulatory rather than punitive. In January 2013, months before the release of the Parliamentary Standing Committee report, further revisions to Schedule Y were published in almost direct response to the civil society advocacy around unethical clinical trials.[76] Of particular importance was the addition of Rule 122 DAB, which provided for financial compensation of experimental subjects or their families in case of injury or death. This rule made three radical stipulations. The first was that the responsibility for this compensation would lie with study sponsors, not with contractors, service providers, or investigators, thereby placing responsibility for clinical studies upon those at the top of the brokerage chain. The second was that subjects or families would be eligible for financial compensation even in those cases of injury or death that were due to the failure of the investigational product to provide its intended therapeutic effect, hence due to failures in efficacy as well as safety. And third, the sponsor would be responsible for providing free medical management of the experimental subject in case of any injury, whether or not it was trial related. And so, the sponsors were to be responsible not just for adverse events within the study, but for the experimental subjects themselves.

These regulatory changes were not without their own contradictions. Indeed, while their enactment was an understandable response to a situation of proliferating scandal, it also reflected a Catch-22 situation in which failures to implement already existing regulation led to more stringent regulation. This immediately made India a potentially unattractive destination for clinical research, affecting not just corporate-driven trials but also public clinical research. The U.S. National Institutes of Health suspended forty clinical studies that they were conducting in India at the time (Krishnan and Koshy 2013; Carroll 2013); Medicins sans Frontiers became ambivalent about conducting some of its studies in India, preferring countries where the regulatory environment was less unsettled.[77] There were differences of opinion among civil society advocates as well. While many welcomed the regulatory changes, others were concerned about the stultifying impact on research they would have.

The biggest opposition, not surprisingly, came from corporate quarters, including members of the Indian pharmaceutical and CRO industries. This led to an immediate reevaluation of these new rules within months of their passage. The Drug Technical Advisory Board (DTAB), an expert committee of drug regulators that advises the Ministry of Health and Family Welfare on drug regulatory issues, was asked to consider industry objections and provide recommendations.[78] The board recommended modification of the guidelines to restrict the provision of medical management to situations of trial-related injury, and to delete the clause that would allow for financial compensation in case of injury or death due to lack of intended efficacy of the product being tested. The former clause was seen as providing a potentially coercive incentive to participate in a clinical study, while the latter was seen as unreasonable in holding an experimental product to an intended standard of efficacy. But there was also an explicit move to recalibrate regulations back into conformity to international norms, which the January 2013 modifications were seen as exceeding. The DTAB did however suggest retaining the stipulation that study sponsors should bear ultimate responsibility for medical management and compensation.[79]

Politically therefore, the scandal around the HPV vaccines did not resolve in any clear manner. On the one hand, the civil society advocacy around the issue grew into a much larger conversation around unethical clinical trials in India, one that garnered national and global media attention. Other scandals attached themselves to the HPV scandal. The most prominent of these included the scandal of clinical trials conducted on victims of the Bhopal gas disaster and those conducted in MGM Medical College, Indore, that were deemed to be unethical consequent to the accusations of a resident doctor who turned whistleblower, Anand Rai.[80] In the process, one saw legislative intervention and regulatory change. But these changes have been partial and provisional; their consequences for public health and the building of research capacity in India continue to be debated; and questions remain about the ability to implement regulations and enforce accountability in a meaningful way.

Meanwhile, in spite of the advocacy over the preceding four years and the political impacts of public scandal, the Bharatiya Janata Party–led government that was elected to power in May 2014 seemed at the time of writing to be making moves to introduce the HPV vaccine into India's national immunization program.[81]

Knowledge/Value and Experimental Subjectivity

This chapter has explored public scandal and advocacy as emergent forms of and spaces for politics, in the context of the appropriation of public health by corporate capital through highly brokered global economies of clinical research. I wish in this concluding section to reflect upon the issues that arise here for conceptualizations of knowledge, value, and experimental subjectivity.

It is first worth discriminating among various forms of knowledge that come to be at stake in the HPV case. First, there is the question of how something is constructed as an object to be studied and known, and the paradigms or languages one brings to bear on such a study: what might be considered a cognitive structure of knowledge. In this regard, it is worthwhile paying attention to how cervical cancer becomes a problem of knowledge that is an object of intervention. But it is differently structured as a problem from different locations. Second, in relation to this, is the situation that Michel Foucault ([1973] 2003, [1976] 1990, 1980) has described in his explication of the links between knowledge and power—the generation of knowledge of something by subjecting it to study, surveillance, classification, and verification, and thereby constructing it as knowledge. One can see this, for example, in how cervical cancer is constructed through the apparatus of clinical research on a vaccine. This manifestation of a will to knowledge and power acquires particular kinds of salience when it operates in contexts of radical epistemic inequity, as elaborated upon by Edward Said (1976) in his critique of orientalism. In this regard, one can consider the gaze of Western biomedicine upon the Third World, tribal, female, minor body, and analyze how the construction of cervical cancer as an object of knowledge operates through the construction of these girls as subjects of experimentation. The third concerns the forms of anticipatory knowledge involved in rendering certain forms of epidemiological and clinical trial knowledge portable across contexts. Of particular relevance here is what Manjari Mahajan (2008, 585) in discussing policy making around India's AIDS epidemic has called "global foreknowledge": an "already existing, generic template" of a disease that is assumed to operate universally. One sees this in PATH's extrapolations of cervical cancer disease burden in India in the absence of any significant local evidence base, or in Ghulam Nabi Azad's insistence that clinical trials for the safety and efficacy of the vaccine in the United States should be sufficient basis to assume safety and efficacy in poor Indian populations. This leads to a kind of epidemiological harmonization that is purely speculative, but that operates within the normative sanction of evidence-based medicine and enables the rationalization of large-scale, population-level public health interventions. And the fourth is an instrumental knowledge, directed at specific ends—in this case, the efficacy of a vaccine as an instrument of public health via large-scale application, which also sees the fungibility of knowledge as value.

What one sees in the HPV studies is the operation of all four forms, definitions, and registers of knowledge. But there are displacements. Specifically, the goals of public health come to be displaced when it becomes the site of potential valorization. What does it mean when a program that is supposedly about the care of the population, and about the care of marginalized populations, ends up subjecting tribal girls to clinical experimentation, in a situation in which the very definition of what constitutes a clinical trial itself comes to be at stake? What does it mean that this came to light in the context of its failure—that had the studies not been halted, and become scandalous, this site of displacement might never have become visible in the manner that it was? Answering these questions involves reflecting upon the question of experimental subjectivity as it comes to be at stake in such scandalous situations.

If the politics around unethical clinical trials has developed into a complex representative politics, then the experimental subjects are the represented subjects. Whether one is considering PATH's claims about preventing cervical cancer, or Indian regulatory or legislative interventions, or civil society advocates acting on behalf of violated tribal girls or gas victims, one sees a politics that takes shape on behalf of experimental subjects. The experimental subject gets politically represented, but also portrayed in very particular ways.[82] The politics that I have described in India has highlighted dimensions of value, specifically concerning the appropriation of health by corporate capital, which tend to be elided in most biomedical ethics conversations around good clinical practice in Western contexts. But another dimension of value is at stake here concerning the normative figuration of the experimental subject that is worth focusing on.

The entire apparatus of liberal biomedical ethics that has developed around experimentation on human subjects rests on the fundamental fiction that the subject of experimentation is a voluntary subject.[83] This is why the conduct of clinical research on subjects who may not have the capacity for rational, voluntary decision making (children, prisoners, or the mentally ill) is now severely curtailed and regulated. A second fiction operates alongside this first one to rationalize it, which is that the economy of clinical experimentation is a gift economy. This is itself a normative position, a moral repudiation of bodily commodification of the sort that also operates in relation to organ transplantation (Fox and Swayze 1992; Cohen 1999) or sex work (R. Sunder Rajan 2003, 117–146; Kotiswaran 2011). But what happens when the economy itself comes to be significantly commodified and industrialized?

Morenike Folayan and Dan Allman (2011) have argued that given the changing modes of production under which clinical research operates, the fiction of voluntary experimental subjectivity is no longer tenable. Underlying this fiction is a regime of value, that of biomedical ethics.[84] This has been appropriated by surplus value regimes when it comes to the conduct of clinical research, but not correspondingly in relation to the designation of experimental subjectivity. The consequence is not simply a matter of nomenclature, since a denial of wage and contractual rights to experimental subjects ensues. When subjects do get paid, it takes the form of compensation (such as travel reimbursement), since wage is deemed to be coercive while compensation is not. What results is the creation of economic value from the bodily investiture of trial participants without due financial remuneration. The value of volunteerism excludes experimental subjects from economies of surplus value even as they are essential to its creation. Far better, suggest the authors, to call experimental subjectivity what it is: a form of labor.

In their argument, Folayan and Allman mirror Catherine Waldby and Melinda Cooper's diagnosis of experimental subjectivity as one form of clinical labor (alongside new reproductive technologies such as oocyte donation or surrogacy [Waldby and Cooper 2008; Cooper and Waldby 2014]). But if Waldby and Cooper's is more an analytic reconceptualization, Folayan and Allman's was an explicit intervention into bioethical debates as a normative counterprovocation to prevalent liberal norms.[85] Understandably, theirs is a controversial position.[86] But their argument is not that treating experimental subjectivity as labor would somehow be better than pretending it is a voluntary activity; indeed, their constant refrain throughout their piece is that it can be no worse.

Folayan and Allman's refiguration of experimental subjectivity cuts through the pretense that the clinical research economy is still a gift economy, one that the voluntarist fiction protects. Indeed, this pretense is often tenuous in practice. For instance, as the Schedule Y revisions of 2013 explicated the necessity of financial compensation in clinical trials, a critical issue concerned the mechanism by which compensation would be calculated.[87] To this end, the Drug Controller General of India constituted an expert committee to come up with a compensation formula, which was ultimately derived on the basis of the Workers Compensation Act, falling back on labor law as an epistemic basis.[88] Hence in the course of her work, the experimental subject is deemed to be a volunteer; in the case of injury or death, she is imagined as always already having been a laborer.[89]

Additionally, a focus on the laboring experimental subject forces attention upon the differentiated geographies of clinical labor. This opens up important questions concerning relationships between the spatialities and subjectivities of contemporary global biomedicine, and the international divisions and multiplications of labor they engender. This follows Gayatri Spivak's (1998) consistent insistence on the importance of paying attention to international divisions of labor, and Sandro Mezzadra and Brett Neilson's (2013) analysis of the ways in which contemporary global capital sees multiplications of labor. Even though Mezzadra and Neilson trace the concept of international division of labor back to the early political economy of William Petty and Adam Smith and critique its limits for understanding the ways in which contemporary capital expands and intensifies through the proliferation of forms of ever-more precarious labor, it should be recognized that multiplications and divisions of labor are complementary and not antithetical phenomena. The geography of experimental subjectivity that emerges in the context of the increased outsourcing of clinical trials and research over the past two decades on the face of it reflects a colonial cartography, Third World bodies rendered available for First World biomedicine. One sees a discursive reproduction of this cartography in much of the media reportage around unethical clinical trials in India, or in the well-known fictional portrayal of clinical trial geographies in *The Constant Gardener* (le Carré 2001; film version produced in 2005).[90]

None of these are inaccurate portrayals, but they are too simple. What is at stake here is an understanding of the appropriation of bodily potential by global capital (which involves exploitation by both multinational and local capitalist interests) through the production of experimental subjectivity across the "heterogeneity of global space" (Mezzadra and Neilson 2013, 22–23). One axis of this differentiated space is constituted by nation-states occupying unequal positions of global power, but it is not the only one.[91] Alongside the global geographies of clinical research are its knowledge geographies—the ways in which the spaces of the lab and of the clinic come to be reconfigured under new modes and relations of biomedical production and subjection.[92]

The regime of value that is perpetuated by the global regulatory harmonization exercise that India undertook in 2005 therefore allows for surplus value economies to operate within and through institutions of public health, and under ethical fictions that these are gift economies. In the process, I have argued that the hegemonic political economic relations of global biomedicine are obscured (see introduction). More specifically, its transnational and translational dimensions—the ways in which these modes and relations of production operate across territorial geographies and institutional and epistemic domains—get obfuscated. Rather than harmonious, the terrain of global clinical research is deeply striated and structured by various transactional relationships. These transactions could be economic and biomedical— the exchange of money for services rendered in outsourcing arrangements, or of the body for experiment, knowledge, in some cases even therapy—but they become especially political when they occur across fundamentally unequal conditions. The experimental subject, produced in the crucible of capitalist value generation and a normative ethics that serves wittingly or otherwise to naturalize it, becomes a deeply consequential one around which forms of politics get constituted.

Anthropological discussions of subjectivity often focus upon the agential nature of the subject, and recent important concepts such as biosociality or biological citizenship have tended to emphasize the self-molding and creative self-reinvention that occur in response to new biomedical knowledge, even when the subjects of this knowledge are disciplined, exploited, or suffering in various ways.[93] In contrast, what one sees here is subject constitution, the subject whose agency is structured and figured in institutionally and historically specific ways. These subjects may be constituted by many things (the dominant economic order of course, but even by advocates fighting on their behalf) but crucially are represented in a relationship to the state as well as to capital.

A vaccine was administered, and seven girls who received it died. Between these two events, a complex sequence has to be traced. This sequence has a huge number of ethical issues contained within it, and indeed it has been established that ethical violations, as in nonadherence to GCP, occurred. But it remained impossible to hold anyone accountable for these violations. Imbricated with these ethical questions was a sequence of events relating to the empirical and the evidentiary, concerning whether and to what extent the deaths might have been caused by the vaccine. This too ended up being impossible to ascertain and was mired in uncertainty. But these uncertainties ended up being productive in their own right—of regimes of knowledge and value, of instantiations of surplus health economies in public health contexts, and of constitutional moments that played out in arenas of representative politics.[94] This led to various kinds of displacements—of regimes of public health, and of notions of the public, of health, of knowledge, of experiment, of value, of subjectivity. Trajectories of capacity building for clinical trials and clinical research in India have created emergent forms of and spaces for politics that were articulated initially through capitalist interests in global economies, but that have developed through the public scandal and civil society advocacy. This has led to the making of the merely risked, apparently voluntary experimental subject who comes to be at the center of this politics while always being spoken for.

My account of the HPV study has been an attempt to situate the legislative moment of 2005 and the capacity building for global clinical trials that happened at that time in the context of a broader relationship of the conjunctural to the organic that can be traced through a particular critical event. This is a parallel to the story of Gleevec and access to essential medicines traced in chapter 3. If the predominant form of the political in the former case was through the public scandal, then in the latter case it was through judicialization. This mobilized similar (though nonidentical) configurations of institutional actors, but through different trajectories. It is not just the political that gets differentially constituted within these two instances of the globalization of biomedicine; so too does cancer get differently situated.[95]

POSTSCRIPT: PHARMAPUBLICS

The unethical clinical trial lies at the cusp of two normative value systems, the ethical and the scandalous. What kinds of publics are presumed, called upon, and constituted to respond to these systems?

In his essay "Where It Hurts," Lawrence Cohen (1999) considers the problem of organ sales in south India beyond the frameworks of moral adjudication provided by liberal bioethics. The trajectories of Cohen's account are similar to those seen in developments around clinical trials in India over the past decade and involve the layering of formal ethical and legal structures over informal transactional economic activities that are common to many domains of everyday Indian life. The former consists of state attempts to regulate a practice that is viewed with concern; the latter consists of brokerage economies all the way down, with information brokers layered upon organ brokers. Immediately alongside transactions in organs are transactions in narratives and counternarratives, involving the deluge of the usual (often global) suspects—reporters, filmmakers, anthropologists, ethicists, out to document and variously display, adjudicate, and mediate the ethical or scandalous story of the unethical organ sale.

Cohen is interested not just in the content of these narratives, but in the space of publicity that such writing occupies and creates. He diagnoses two conjoined spaces that emerge around such unethical situations, which he calls those of ethical publicity and scandalous publicity. The former is the space of apparently universal moral adjudication, which sees itself as having the capacity and authority to make judgments about the virtues and vices of even geographically and contextually distant transactional activities. Relativist bioethical positions that justify organ sales in contexts that are "not like ours" are every bit as central to such forms of ethical publicity as one-size-fits-all denunciations of the commodification of human parts. What is at stake here is not just the position espoused, but the fact that, as Cohen puts it, "ethics become[s] the dominant mode of public conversation about emergent biosocial situations" (1999, 146). This elides and renders invisible other modes of viewing such situations—such as, in the case of organ trade, political economies of indebtedness that structure organ trade in south India in the first place, and that endure even after the kidney has been sold.[96]

The scandalous is the other of the ethical, but is also contained within it. It is a particular performative and affective mode of describing the lack of ethics, and it is always appropriable to other ends—for instance, as Cohen points out, in rivalries between hospital owners, where the scandal becomes enmeshed not just in normative ordering, but also in business competition, political patronage, and individual feuds. The scandal can never be the pure statement of correct ethical or moral position: it is constantly transacted as it becomes public, and as it constitutes its own publics.

The limits of both ethical and scandalous publicity are that the contours of the ethical and the scandalous are in some sense already known in advance.

I am not arguing for a relativist ethics here, or suggesting that the ethics of a situation is simply and entirely dependent upon the specifics of that situation absent larger normative considerations. Rather, I am suggesting that a discourse limited by the ethical and the scandalous as its normative modalities of inquiry and adjudication does not have space to account for the double binds that emerge in such situations.[97] Cohen points to the nature of this double-bound structure in relation to organ sales. The binary position of ethical publicity there is between coercion (any sale of a kidney is an exploitative act) and volition (but the poor should be free to do with their bodies as they please). Either element of this binary can tip over into scandalous publicity—the scandalous remains here both the opposite of and contained within the structure of ethics that is provided. Cohen's own ethnographic informants provided statements that speak to this volitional aspect: there were those who had sold kidneys in Chennai who told him that they "would do it again" (1999, 147). The ethical position stops here, but Cohen insists on listening further, as he hears: "if I had another [kidney] to give," and further, "I would have to." The ethical short-circuiting of what is in fact a complexly interconnected and interwoven set of determinations, predeterminations, and overdeterminations—such that neither coercion nor volition gets close to the universe within which choices about selling a kidney have to be made—is, Cohen argues, because of the liberal presumption that the ethical moment can be reduced to the moment of primary transaction, when in fact ethical choices are made in the context of ongoing trajectories of lives lived and constraints faced.

There is a difference in the modes of response called to account in scandalous as opposed to ethical publicity. The adjudication that ethical publicity demands is moral; but the scandal, certainly in the Indian context, demands a functional state response to rectify and prevent the scandal, even (perhaps especially) when the state itself is implicated in the scandal through acts of omission and commission. The public of scandalous publicity cannot exclude the state. Civil society response to the unethical clinical trial in India has indeed been directed squarely at the state. There is recognition that the state is both an obligatory point of passage toward any improvement or solution, and is also potentially the most accountable and responsive institution involved in the clinical trials landscape to which demands can be directed.

This was strikingly visible in the months after the HPV scandals broke. At a national consultation on unethical clinical trials organized by civil society groups in 2011, for instance, high-ranking officials of the ICMR were in attendance, both to answer questions and to listen to concerns about the conduct of the studies. The ICMR's own role in the HPV studies was questionable; but the organization's presence in the room was in striking contrast to the absence of anyone from PATH, which not only washed its hands of any accountability for the studies in spite of having conducted them, but also refused any form of conversation or information sharing with civil society groups after the HPV scandal broke. This is not to absolve the state, just to emphasize that there are differential potentials for public accountability here, and the state could be held accountable in a way that PATH could not.

I was about to present a version of this chapter as a talk at the John F. Kennedy School of Government in April 2013. The talk was on a Monday. The Friday before, I received a long e-mail from Vivian Tsu, director of the HPV Vaccines project at PATH. This e-mail was copied to a number of other faculty members at Harvard, including at the School of Public Health and the Law School, none of whom I knew and to none of whom I was introduced in this message. Tsu mentioned that it had come to her attention that I was going to speak about the controversy in India at Harvard and wanted to ensure that there were no misrepresentations in it. I responded that any of the Harvard-based people copied on the e-mail were welcome to attend the talk and directly engage and argue with my interpretation. (To the best of my knowledge, none of them did; certainly none of them introduced themselves to me if they did.) I also said that I would be happy to fully understand PATH's point of view and to that end would come to Seattle to interview Tsu and others involved in the HPV studies if she was amenable. Tsu said she would get back to me about this. That was the last I ever heard from her.

At the start of this correspondence, Tsu sent me a copy of a letter written by PATH to colleagues, explaining what she called the "truth" of the HPV controversies in India. The content of the letter was fairly predictable and covers much of what I have stated in this chapter: that none of the deaths were caused by the vaccines; the studies had gone through proper institutional review; and so on. I asked members of civil society groups whether they had received any similar correspondence or clarification from PATH; they had not. Indeed, they emphasized how PATH had consistently been absent from any kind of dialogue with civil society groups around the HPV issue.

To me, this is the critical pharmocratic question at stake, much beyond whether the studies had been conducted ethically in a narrowly procedural sense or not. PATH was not just pushing a technocratic solution to cervical cancer in India; it was also pushing a technocratic imaginary of the public that it needed to be accountable to. Forget the actual girls in the study or their parents: even representative civil society groups in India did not constitute a relevant public that deserved significant response or dialogue. This is layered on the failure of *scientific accounting in the studies, as extrapolative epidemiological assumptions were made in an Indian tribal context based on data that were obtained largely from (Euro-)American studies. The question of pharmocracy emerges in relation to the different imaginaries of both the public and of adequate epidemiology that were seen in the technocratic public health pushed by* PATH *and the democratic public health demanded by civil society groups raising questions about the study. These are questions of accountability that go beyond the limits of both ethics and scandal to constitute the politics of the situation.*

CHAPTER THREE

Constitutional Values

The Trials of Gleevec & Judicialized Politics

Two Histories of Gleevec

In the past few years, India has come to be seen as a site of deep vulnerability for multinational pharmaceutical interests. This is because of occurrences that suggest a less than favorable climate for intellectual property protection on drugs, in spite of having passed patent legislation in 2005 that is compatible with standards mandated by the World Trade Organization (wto). Ironically, the 2005 Act was passed in order to make patent regimes more stringent, and indeed it does so, having replaced the earlier process patent regime (instituted in 1970) with a product patent one. The 1970 Act was a spur to India's generic drug industry, and led to India's drug prices becoming among the lowest in the world.

In 1995, as India became party to the wto, it was allowed a ten-year transition period to change its patent laws to a product patent regime compliant with the Trade-Related Aspects of Intellectual Property Rights (trips) agreement (see introduction). This meant that as of 2005, any drug developed after 1995 would be subject to a product patent regime; any drug developed before 1995 would still be subject to a process patent regime under the 1970 Act. Hence, the 2005 Act has seen the harmonization of Indian patent laws with Euro-American ones, through multilateral free trade mechanisms, driven in large measure by the interests of the multinational, Euro-American pharmaceutical industry. Yet anxiety pervades the industry around the level and kind of patent protection companies will receive in India. This has to do with the ways in which new patent laws have been interpreted in India through the use of public health flexibilities that allow for a less-than-absolute monopoly under these product patent regimes. These flexibilities have resulted from allowances within TRIPS, especially the Doha Declaration on the TRIPS agreement and public health signed by member nations in 2001, which allowed national governments to use mechanisms that would allow for limitations on or work-arounds of patents in the case of public health emergencies.[1]

The emblematic case that provides precedent for such interpretation is the denial in 2006 of a patent on Novartis's anticancer drug Gleevec. Novartis took the Indian Patent Office to the Madras High Court to dispute the denial, and lost. Novartis then appealed, first to a newly constituted Intellectual Property Appellate Board (IPAB) and then to the Indian Supreme Court. It lost both appeals as well. Gleevec was a landmark case in and of itself, while also serving as a precedent for other cases that have seen the curtailment of intellectual property rights by drawing upon public health flexibilities incorporated into the 2005 Act.[2]

The legal history of Gleevec is vital to understanding contemporary intellectual property regimes and their relationship to pharmaceutical politics in India today. But this is in fact a tale of two histories. The first is the history of Gleevec's own development as a drug, and the place of patents in that history. The second is the history of patent regimes in India. The political is constituted within the relationship between these two otherwise independent histories that have come to be intertwined over the past decade. Gleevec is a drug that received a patent in over forty other jurisdictions before it was denied one in India; yet (perhaps because of this) Novartis felt it important to challenge the denial in India, and even to question the Indian patent regime under which this denial was allowed. Gleevec is just one drug out of thousands for which a product patent has been applied since India's TRIPS-compliant patent regime came into existence. Yet it is the most significant one, because the contestations around its patentability provided the first test case of how flexibilities contained in the new patent regime would be interpreted.

This chapter focuses on the legal history of Gleevec from 2005, when Novartis applied for a product patent on the drug in India, to 2013, when the Indian Supreme Court upheld the initial denial of the patent. First, I focus on the actual dispute around the denial of the Gleevec patent by the Indian Patent Office under the terms of the 2005 Patent Act, followed by Novartis taking the Patent Office to the Madras High Court to litigate against the denial. This played out between 2005 and 2007. I then discuss Novartis's appeal to the Indian Supreme Court, which gave its final verdict in April 2013 upholding the denial of the patent.[3] I do this in order to think through the relationships between value, politics, and knowledge in the context of the judicialization of pharmaceutical politics. After outlining Gleevec's legal history, I consider the nature of the politics of access as it emerges in India in the aftermath of this case. Along with the HPV vaccine case (see chapter 2), this chapter also situates cancer as a disease that emerges within and through particular articulations of value, politics, and global biomedicine.

I provide a timeline of the historical trajectory of Gleevec below, adding certain other events that are relevant to its story in India (table 3.1). Alongside, I outline significant events in the history of Indian patent regimes over the past century, in order to point out that the legal history of Gleevec cannot be understood without reference to the simultaneous history of Indian patent law. Throughout the dispute, Novartis insisted—unsuccessfully—that it could, and that all that mattered was a purely abstract notion of invention, uncoupled from the historical and constitutional contexts within which such a notion would come to be rendered as legal and interpreted thus under national-state jurisdiction.

Alongside this trajectory, it is important to consider two questions. First: what kind of invention is Gleevec? And therefore, second: how does this question come to matter not just as a definitional philosophical question, but in legal and constitutional terms? Simply at the level of the outcome of this legal trajectory, what one sees is a curtailment of the scope of new product patent regimes. This has been celebrated by civil society groups fighting for access to medicines, and attacked by multinational corporate capital and its allies as a lack of proper respect and incentive for innovation. While I believe that the outcomes have been important not just for access to essential medicines, but for bringing into focus the monopolistic practices of the multinational pharmaceutical industry (for which see chapters 1 and 4), what I am interested in here is the mechanisms by which such outcomes are even possible. This involves considering, first, how a question of scientific invention can be rendered as a constitutional one, and therefore concerns the relationship between the technical and the constitutional; and second, how the constitutional itself comes to be rendered through complex and often contradictory forms of state mediation that reflect its own antinomies.

TABLE 3.1. Two Timelines—*Gleevec and Indian Patent Law*

History of Gleevec's Development	History of Indian Patent Law
	1911: Patent Act passed by British colonial regime. Product patents on drugs for 14 years.
	1950: Tek Chand Committee Report submitted to Indian Parliament, reviewing merits and demerits of the 1911 Act. First postcolonial Indian Patent Act passed.
	1959: Ayyangar Committee Report submitted to Indian Parliament, recommending a move from product to process patent regime.
1960: Link established between chromosomal defect and chronic myeloid leukemia (CML) (Nowell and Hungerford 1960).	
	1970: New Patent Act drafted, gets passed in Indian Parliament in 1972, replacing product patent regime with process patents on drugs for seven years.
1973: Mechanisms of chromosomal translocation in genesis of leukemias discovered (Rowley 1973).	
1980s: Screening of growth factor receptors by chemists at Ciba-Geigy leads to identification of compound with possible therapeutic effect for CML.	
	1986: Commencement of Uruguay Round negotiations of the General Agreements on Tariffs and Trade, bringing intellectual property into purview of free trade negotiations for first time.
1993: Ciba-Geigy files U.S. and Canadian patents on imatinib and "pharmaceutically acceptable salts" (Zimmermann patent).	

TABLE 3.1. Two Timelines—*Gleevec and Indian Patent Law* (contd.)

1994: Uruguay Round concludes with signing of Trade-Related Aspects of Intellectual Property Rights (TRIPS) agreement, and the establishment of the World Trade Organization.

Mid-1990s: research to develop pharmaceutically active form of imatinib free base that has therapeutic effect in the treatment of CML (Druker et al. 1996).

1995: "Less developed" countries such as India given ten years to harmonize their patent regimes with requirements of TRIPS. Required to set up a mailbox whereby product patents could be filed in anticipation of a new patent regime in 2005.

1997: Swiss patent application on β-imatinib mesylate, a crystalline salt isoform of imatinib free base that shows potential effect in treatment of CML.

1997–2001: Clinical trials to establish safety and efficacy of β-imatinib mesylate in humans. (None conducted in India.)

1998: "Mailbox" application filed for patent on β-imatinib mesylate in India; to be opened and evaluated in 2005 on passage of TRIPS-compliant Patent Act.

1999: India amends Patent Act to allow for EMR on drugs for which mailbox applications have been filed, until TRIPS-compliant Patent Act passed.

2000: U.S. patent application on β-imatinib mesylate filed.

2001: β-imatinib mesylate approved for marketing in United States as Gleevec. Indian companies start making generic versions of the drug for sale in India.

TABLE 3.1. Two Timelines—*Gleevec and Indian Patent Law* (contd.)

2002: Novartis applies for and receives EMR on Gleevec in India.	**2002:** Further amendments to Patent Act, broadening definition of invention and addition of a chapter "Working of Patents, Compulsory Licenses and Revocation."
2004: Cancer Patients Aid Association (CPAA) files writ petition in Supreme Court opposing the grant of EMR on Gleevec to Novartis, on grounds of right to life and health.	
2005: Novartis applies for product patent on Gleevec. EMR (and writ petition opposing it) null and void because of passage of new Patent Act. Oppositions to Novartis's application, which is denied by Patent Office in Chennai. U.S. patent on β-imatinib mesylate granted.	**2005:** New, fully TRIPS-compliant Patent Act passed in India, granting product patents on pharmaceuticals for twenty-year period. Subsequent to intense debate in Parliament, public health flexibilities incorporated into this act, especially Section 3(d), which prevents pharmaceutical evergreening.
2006: Novartis files case in Madras High Court disputing patent denial and Section 3(d), one of the public health flexibilities based on which the denial was made.	
2007: Novartis loses case in Madras High Court, parts of the case relating to patentability of Gleevec transferred to Intellectual Property Appellate Board (IPAB).	
2009: IPAB upholds denial of patent on Gleevec, but only on grounds in Section 3(d). Novartis appeals IPAB decision to Supreme Court.	
2013: Indian Supreme Court upholds denial of patent on Gleevec.	

Gleevec Patent Denial and the Madras High Court Case, 2005–2007

By the time the new, TRIPS-compliant Indian Patent Act was passed in 2005, the question of the relationship between a product patent regime and access to medicines was already vexed. Gleevec was responsible for this because, before the product patent regime had been instituted, Novartis had been given exclusive marketing rights (EMR) on the drug (see chapter 4). This was in spite of the fact that generic capacity to make the drug existed; indeed, ten Indian companies were making generic forms of imatinib mesylate as soon as Gleevec was approved for sale in the United States. The cost of the generics ranged between 4,000 and 12,000 rupees (Rs.) per patient per month (approximately $100–300 at the time). Novartis's price for its patented medication, on the other hand, was Rs. 120,000 per patient per month (approximately $2,700). In other words, essential, life-saving anticancer medication that was already being sold to patients in a competitive marketplace was now being made potentially less accessible to them through a policy instrument that provided a market monopoly on the drug to a single company. The controversy surrounding the EMR led to active debate in the Indian Parliament about the implications of the new patent regime on drug prices, leading to provisions in the 2005 TRIPS-compliant Patent Act that would temper a product patent regime with public health protections. Thus, the politics around Gleevec were not simply a function of patent legislation that had already been set in place; such politics helped set the context within which the 2005 Act would be passed.

A crucial provision to mention here is Section 3(d). Section 3 of the Indian Patent Act specifies all the things that cannot be held to be an invention. This includes mere discoveries or inventions that might be contrary to the law and public order. But the 1970 Act also excluded, as part (d) of this section:

> The mere discovery of any new property or new use for a known substance or of the mere use of a known process, machine or apparatus unless such known process results in a new product or employs at least one new reactant.

This was amended in the 2005 Act to read as follows:

> The mere discovery of a new form of a known substance which does not result in the enhancement of the known efficacy of that substance or the mere discovery of any new property or new use for a known substance or of the mere use of a known process, machine or apparatus

unless such known process results in a new product or employs at least one new reactant.

Explanation: For purposes of this clause, salts, esters, ethers, polymorphs, metabolites, pure form, particle size, isomers, mixtures of isomers, complexes, combinations and other derivatives of known substance shall be considered to be the same substance, unless they differ significantly in properties with regard to efficacy.

The amended version of Section 3(d) therefore specified a criterion of enhanced efficacy as essential to qualify for the patentability of substances that were modifications of existing substances. This was done to curtail the practice of pharmaceutical evergreening, which is common in product patent regimes and involves the introduction of minor modifications to a drug that is coming off patent so that it can be claimed as a new drug under a new patent. How one might define enhanced efficacy was not, however, made clear in the amended act, and this ambiguity would come to be at the heart of the subsequent controversy around Gleevec.

Once the new Indian Patent Act had been passed, Novartis's EMR on Gleevec was no longer valid, but the company was eligible to file for a product patent, which it did. The Cancer Patients Aid Association (CPAA), a patient advocacy group that had been procuring generic β-imatinib mesylate and making it available to patients, filed a pregrant opposition to the Gleevec product patent application. Pregrant oppositions are another public health provision allowed by the 2005 Indian Patent Act, allowing anybody who feels that a patent application has been wrongly filed to oppose it before it is adjudicated upon. There were three major grounds in CPAA's opposition. The first ground was lack of novelty, based on the fact that a previous patent application had been made on imatinib and all pharmaceutically acceptable salts, including imatinib mesylate, in 1993 in the United States and Canada. Further, CPAA claimed that imatinib mesylate occurs spontaneously as a β-crystalline form. The second ground for opposition concerned the absence of an inventive step; CPAA claimed that for the reasons above showing prior art (a legal term signifying that any part of an invention is already known), imatinib mesylate was obvious to a person skilled in the prior art. The third ground of opposition was on the basis of Section 3(d), which as just mentioned does not allow a patent on a new form of a known substance unless the efficacy of the new form is significantly greater than that of the known substance. The question of significantly enhanced efficacy therefore became a crucial matter of adjudication.

In response to CPAA's pregrant opposition, Novartis claimed that Gleevec was a twofold improvement over prior art: first, because imatinib free base is converted to imatinib mesylate; and second, because the conversion of imatinib mesylate into its β-crystalline form occurs not spontaneously, but through human intervention. Hence, a basic question of molecular production came into being in this dispute—is the β-crystalline form of imatinib mesylate a spontaneous state of being of the salt or the product of human engineering? Novartis also made counterarguments regarding the question of efficacy. They pointed to a study conducted on rats which showed that β-imatinib mesylate is 30 percent more bioavailable than the core imatinib molecule. They therefore claimed that β-imatinib mesylate is more efficacious than imatinib. Hence, Novartis was making a direct claim that increased bioavailability implies increased efficacy. Next CPAA filed a rejoinder, stating that a study on rats is not relevant to a question of efficacy in humans. The organization also claimed that a 30 percent difference in bioavailability is not significant. In this way, CPAA was disputing Novartis's claims of significantly enhanced efficacy by unsettling the definitions of both efficacy and significance.

In January 2006, the Indian Patent Office in Chennai ruled that Gleevec is not patentable. The patent controller effectively accepted all the points in CPAA's opposition. Note that all three grounds on which the patent was opposed and denied are technical, even though Gleevec was already a high-stakes political battle. This in itself is not surprising—after all, the function of the patent office is to make technical determinations, not adjudicate matters of policy. However, the technical, far from providing universal, incontestable solutions, in fact remained entirely unsettled.

The crucial point about this patent application, as earlier noted, is that it was for the β-crystalline form of imatinib mesylate. The opposition claimed that the β-form was simply a polymorphic form of a core molecule that had already been patented in 1993. Since Section 3(d) specifically excludes patents on polymorphs, the contention was that the β-form was hence not patentable, unless it shows significantly enhanced efficacy. So now, the question of adjudicating the ontological nature of a molecule (is the β-isoform of imatinib mesylate created through an inventive step or is its formation an inherent property of the salt?) had to shift to evaluating its efficacy. This, it turns out, meant evaluating what constitutes efficacy in the first place, and what constitutes a significant enhancement of it. It is worth quoting from the patent ruling in this regard:

As regards efficacy, the specification itself states that wherever β-crystals are used the imatinib free base of other salts can be used. . . . As per the affidavit [submitted by Novartis] the *technical expert* has conducted studies to compare the relative bioavailability of the free base with that of the β-crystal form of imatinib mesylate and has said that the difference in bioavailability is *only 30%* and also the difference in bioavailability may be due to the difference in their solubility in water. . . . Even the affidavit submitted on behalf of the Applicant does not prove any *significant enhancement* of known efficacy.[4]

This ruling is made on purely technical grounds, apparently universal and value neutral. And yet there is no clear, universal understanding of what constitutes significantly enhanced efficacy. Further, the assistant patent commissioner inserts the value-laden word *only*. While the establishment of a 30 percent differential in bioavailability (and hence, it is claimed, in efficacy) was framed as a purely technical matter, the rendering of that difference as insignificant was the adjudication of the assistant patent commissioner. This is crucial, because Novartis pointed to the 30 percent difference in bioavailability as precisely being the significant difference. Therefore two moments of black boxing are seen here. First, efficacy was rendered in terms of bioavailability, a correlation that was itself questioned by the opposition and which would remain a significant point of contestation as the legal dispute over Gleevec unfolded in subsequent years. Second, it was deemed that a 30 percent increase is insignificant. A different adjudicator might well have seen that 30 percent in a different light. This verdict rested on such slender threads.

Novartis responded by taking the Indian Patent Office to the Madras High Court in May 2006 to challenge this decision. The company disputed both the denial of the patent and the very constitutional validity of Section 3(d), thereby splitting the case into two dimensions, one technical and the other constitutional. Novartis was not merely disputing the particularities of a single patent decision; it was challenging sovereign legislation of the Indian Parliament in a court of law, suggesting that nation-state sovereignty is not absolute but tempered by and subject to international agreements the state has signed. At this point, the case came to be about much more than the denial of a patent on a single molecule; it came to be about the very grounds upon which other such denials on other molecules could be made in the future. Therefore it also was about the possibilities of and limits to pushing back against trade agreements that constitute unequal relations of exchange and development, the upper hand always going to the advanced industrialized nations of Euro-America and Japan.[5]

The basis of Novartis's opposition to Section 3(d) was twofold. The first claim was that Section 3(d) violated the TRIPS agreement. Novartis asserted that this noncompliance violated the government's constitutional duty to harmonize its national laws with its international obligations, and that the Indian state was constrained in its freedom of legislative action because of the contractual relations of international agreements that it had signed. The second claim was that it violated the Constitution of India. By not properly defining terms like "efficacy," "enhancement of efficacy," and "significant enhancement of efficacy," Novartis said that the provision was vague (though why vagueness should be a constitutional violation as opposed to merely imprecise wording of policy was not made clear). The defense meanwhile claimed that a domestic court does not have the authority to examine TRIPS compatibility. Rather, the exclusive forum for deciding such an issue would be the WTO's Dispute Settlement Board. Corporations cannot take an issue to the board; only member nations of the WTO can, and the Swiss government, which was the relevant member nation in this case, was not doing so. Second, it was claimed that there was no violation of the Constitution of India. Efficacy, the defense claimed, had a clear meaning in the pharmaceutical field. Further, in the field, a one-size-fits-all definition of efficacy could not be held as valid.

In June 2007, Novartis lost the case. The Madras High Court ruled that, on the specific matter of the denial of the Gleevec patent, it did not have the technical expertise to overrule the Patent Office, and it transferred the hearing on the specific merits of the patent denial to the IPAB (which subsequently upheld the original decision of the Patent Office to deny the patent on Gleevec). What the court did rule on was the constitutionality of Section 3(d). And here, the court effectively accepted the arguments of the defense. In doing so, the court further insisted that efficacy had to be understood narrowly, as meaning therapeutic efficacy. And so, while the court did not rule on whether Gleevec itself met the criterion of increased efficacy as required by 3(d), it did provide its interpretation of how that criterion should be defined. This would serve as important precedent for how efficacy would come to be read in the adjudication of subsequent appeals. The court also added a crucial insertion in its verdict. For the first time in the patent dispute, it went beyond technical considerations to bring in considerations of good health care. The judgment, in this regard, says, "We have borne in mind *the object which the Amending Act wanted to achieve*, namely . . . to provide easy access to the citizens of this country to life saving drugs and to discharge their *Constitutional obligation* of providing *good health care* to its citizens."[6]

There are three crucial points to emphasize regarding this verdict. The first concerns the court's willingness to engage in interpretation of legislative objectives in a high-stakes intellectual property case that has become a landmark verdict with implications for the precedents it sets. It is worth contrasting this to another such landmark intellectual property verdict in the life sciences that set a significant precedent allowing the patentability of multiple life forms in the United States, *Diamond v. Chakrabarty*, which allowed for a patent on a microorganism that could break down crude oil spills, in many ways providing the precedent that would open the floodgates to biotechnology patenting in the United States in and since the 1980s.[7] This well-known 1980 U.S. Supreme Court verdict is notable precisely for the majority's extension of plant patents to other living (in this case microbial) forms on the grounds that the U.S. legislature, in specifically coming up with laws that allowed patents on plant varieties, had not specifically excluded the patenting of other life forms. It was thus decided that an implied exclusion could not be assumed. The Madras High Court, however, read the 2005 Patent Act not just in its letter, but in its spirit; and the spirit that is being read concerns not the provisions that provide protection to capital, but those that provide exceptions to patentability in order to protect public health. Therefore, the second crucial point to consider is how the objective of the 2005 Act is read by the court in terms of access—a distributive justice-based interpretation. And the third point to consider is a set of key words—*constitutional obligation* and *good health care*.

What one sees in this case is an example of coproductions between law and the life sciences, a form of what Sheila Jasanoff (2011) has referred to as bioconstitutionalism. It is important to situate such judicial resolutions comparatively. The differences between the Madras High Court verdict on Gleevec and *Diamond* are in part likely to be a function of different kinds of relationships between the judiciary and the legislature in the United States and India, the deep American ambivalence toward perceived judicial activism in contrast to a readier willingness on the part of Indian courts to engage in legislative interpretation from the bench. They are also likely a result of different political imaginaries in relation to property, the deeply protectionist American attitude toward property (which has become almost sacred, especially since Reagan), a contrast to an Indian legal attitude toward property that has generally been much less reverent.[8]

The High Court verdict opened up at least three sets of stakes that would come to matter in significant ways as the legal history of this case subsequently unfolded. The first concerns the purification of technical and constitutional regimes in adjudicating the Gleevec patent. While the technoscientific purports to be universal, it turns out to be contingent, with the means of establishing, defending, and contesting relations of production being actively constructed. While the constitutional always already limits itself to national and civic issues, it does so through the invocation of values that are, if not universal, then at least for the public good. The second concerns the question of comparison. If one looks at the Madras High Court judgment not in isolation but next to landmark judgments in other national contexts, then one can potentially see different relationships to legislation as well as different imaginations of the value of property rights, their sanctity, and their weight relative to the public good. At stake here are comparative questions of judicial cultures, technoscientific imaginaries, and legal histories of property.[9] And the third concerns questions relating to the kinds of social contract that are at stake—between state and citizen on the one hand, and between consumer and corporation on the other—through the imagination of different biomedical economies that presume different definitions of health. In the process, it becomes important to consider how the notion of invention itself is put into question, and how its scientific understanding intercalates with the history and politics of patent law in postcolonial India. These questions emerged as central to the Gleevec case as it further enfolded in the Supreme Court of India.

The Supreme Court Case, 2009–2013

In 2009, Novartis appealed to the Indian Supreme Court. This was not an appeal against the High Court verdict, and hence no longer a questioning of the constitutional validity of Section 3(d), but was rather about its interpretation.[10] Novartis sought to enforce an interpretation that would allow 3(d) to remain on the books, but effectively as a dead letter. First, it disputed the restricted meaning given to the term *efficacy* in terms of therapeutic efficacy by the Madras High Court. Second, Novartis asked that since 3(d) contained no specific guidelines for what constitutes enhanced efficacy, how could bioavailability be rejected as a basis for its evaluation?

This led to a broader disputing of whether or not a 30 percent increase in bioavailability was consequential for the purpose of evaluating efficacy. As mentioned, the Patent Office held that it was not, a point that the IPAB reiterated by making reference to the Madras High Court's insistence that efficacy be narrowly understood as therapeutic efficacy. Novartis claimed that it was impossible to establish therapeutic efficacy in relative terms without clinical studies on humans, since therapeutic efficacy was not an inherent property of a molecule but always dependent on context—the clinical setting, patient population, form of drug, or dosage. Such a context-dependent evaluation of therapeutic efficacy, it argued, was the purpose of a clinical trial for regulatory approval of a drug to market. It could not be a reasonable requirement for a patent claim. Conducting clinical studies as a prerequisite for a patent claim, which is an early-stage claim made long before regulatory preclinical studies, would, according to Novartis's submission, be "highly unethical" (Novartis Supreme Court SLP, 5(F)). Therapeutic efficacy in a clinical setting, it was stated, was only shown for β-imatinib mesylate, and not for any molecular form obtained prior to that. In making this argument, Novartis sought to uncouple the requirements of a patent regime that evaluates invention and a regulatory regime that evaluates the safety and efficacy of a drug. Given that the clinical efficacy of a research compound could not possibly be ethically determined, a proxy was required as a marker of efficacy. Bioavailability constituted such a proxy. Therefore, Novartis moved away from earlier arguments before the High Court that claimed bioavailability as implying increased efficacy, to now suggesting that bioavailability was a necessary surrogate marker for increased efficacy, the best that could exist in the absence of actual clinical studies.

I return to some of these questions in the course of reading the Supreme Court's judgment on this appeal. Before doing so, it is worth considering the modality of adjudication employed thus far in relation to the validity of the Gleevec patent by the Patent Office (and subsequently the IPAB). This concerned asking the question of patentability in relation to the existing legislation, but also in relation to the patent claim itself. These were the two authoritative sources that had to be reconciled. Section 3(d) rendered this reconciliation challenging, because it introduced an additional standard for patentability beyond the establishment of inventiveness and nonobviousness, and therefore legally uncoupled the definition of invention from that of patentability. Nonetheless, what was at stake was the reconciliation of the letter of the law with the letter of the claim. Novartis's appeal sought to effect this reconciliation in a manner that rendered the former effectively worthless as an enhanced standard of patentability beyond invention.

The Supreme Court, however, insisted upon a different kind of reading of the law, one that was hermeneutic as opposed to literal. The court's attempt was not just to reconcile two statements, but to interpret the legislative context within which a patent claim should be evaluated. This meant that the court insisted upon reading legislative intent into Section 3(d).[11] The way in which it arrived at its interpretation of legislative intent was through historical context. In the process, the judgment provided a tour-de-force account of patent history in postcolonial India. The two histories of Gleevec that I set up at the start of the chapter do not just serve analytic purposes; it was precisely by insisting upon the situation of the history of Gleevec's development in the context of the history of Indian patent law that the court arrived at its final denial of a patent on Gleevec.

Writing for the court, Justice Aftab Alam explained the reasons behind such a reading.[12] The patent application for β-imatinib mesylate was filed in India in 1998, when the country was in a transitional period between two patent regimes, and in which the primary change to be enacted was the institution of a product patent regime. This involved important changes in Sections 2 and 3 of the Patent Act (which described the criteria for patentability and specified what does not qualify as a patentable invention respectively). According to the court, "it is necessary to find out the concerns of Parliament, based on the history of the patent law in the country, when it made such changes in the Patent Act. *What were the issues that the legislature was trying to address?*" (Supreme Court verdict, 14, emphasis added). This is a clear statement that the court understood judicial function to involve the reading of legislative intent, thereby setting up the dialogic relationship between different arms of the state as the foundational context for adjudicating a particular patent claim. This understanding was itself based on judicial precedent, from the verdict of *Utkal Contractors and Joinery Pvt Ltd and others v. State of Orissa and others*, which also provided a method for interpreting legislative reasoning:

> A statute is best understood if we know the reason for it. The reason for a statute is the safest guide to its interpretation. How do we discover the reason for a statute? There are external and internal aids. The external aids are statements of Objects and Reasons when the Bill is presented to Parliament, the reports of committees which preceded the Bill and the reports of Parliamentary Committees. Occasional excursions into the debates of Parliament are permitted. Internal aids are the preamble, the scheme and the provisions of the Act. Having discovered the reason for the statute and so having set the sail to the wind, the interpreter may proceed ahead.[13]

Interpretive method was further articulated on the basis of the verdict in *Reserve Bank of India v. Peerless General Finance and Investment Co. Ltd.*

and Others, which stated, "Interpretation must depend on the text and the context. They are the bases of interpretation. One may well say if the text is the texture, context is what gives the colour."[14]

It is again worthwhile comparing this to the U.S. Supreme Court in *Diamond v. Chakrabarty*, cited earlier in reference to the Madras High Court verdict, to suggest the unwillingness of the U.S. court in that instance to similarly speculate upon legislative objectives in relation to a landmark intellectual property decision. Perhaps the most significant decision in American patent law relating to the life sciences was made by purifying the patent claim away from legislative context, rendering it as a separable and separate object that needed to be adjudicated in its own terms.[15] It was precisely such purification that was assumed by Novartis in all its submissions, but that the Indian Court refused at the outset. The comparative question of judicial cultures is in part a question of the way in which the relationship between the technoscientific and the political comes to be differentially interpreted. Both the Madras High Court and the Indian Supreme Court insisted upon the coproduction of the two, such that the question of what constitutes invention could never avoid recourse to the legal definition of invention and the legislative intent behind such definitions. The interpretive formula that was employed could be summarized as follows:

Is Gleevec an invention?
To answer this question, we must ask:
What is invention?

What is invention *in the law*?
↓
What is the *legislative intent* behind such a legal definition of invention?
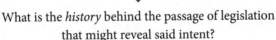
What is the *history* behind the passage of legislation
that might reveal said intent?

It is on the basis of this methodological principle that the court outlined the legislative history of Indian patent law as outlined in table 3.1.[16] This began with the British colonial Patent Act enacted in 1911, which allowed product patents on pharmaceuticals for a fourteen-year period. This was the law of the land at the time of Indian independence in 1947. In 1949, a committee under the chairmanship of Justice Bakshi Tek Chand was constituted to look into the merits and demerits of this act. The committee gave its recommendations the following year and led to the first postcolonial Indian Patent Act passed in

1950, which insisted that inventions needed to be "worked" in India (i.e., the product on which a patent was obtained had to be manufactured in India and could not simply be imported from abroad), and included provisions for the issuance of compulsory licenses (which would allow the government to force the patent holder to license its invention) and revocations of patents in the public interest. The more substantial modification was based on the report of a committee headed by Justice N. Rajagopala Ayyangar, delivered in 1959, which recommended abandoning the product patent regime for a process patent regime. This formed the basis of the 1970 Patent Act. A process patent regime insisted upon the distinction between invention and patentability: even if something might philosophically be considered a technoscientific invention in its own terms, it did not necessarily imply that it was legally an invention that could be granted a patent. The Ayyangar Committee was centrally concerned with pharmaceuticals in its recommendations, both in terms of ensuring affordable access to medicines by preventing monopoly and in terms of stimulating national political economic competitiveness through creating a market terrain that would allow Indian pharmaceutical companies to compete with their multinational counterparts. This was the legislative intent behind the 1970 Act which, the Supreme Court noted, was met in subsequent decades. India's drug prices became among the lowest in the world, and its generic industry became nationally and globally competitive.

The change away from this regime, the court understood, was entirely a function of the demands of the TRIPS agreement. But even this agreement included the subsequent provisions of the 2001 Doha Declaration, which allowed signatory national governments to enact public health flexibilities within their now-mandated product patent regimes. There were three amendments to the Patent Act as India transitioned fully to TRIPS compliance: in 1999, when provisions for exclusive marketing rights were included; in 2002, when the definition of invention was broadened but certain flexibilities relating to public health such as compulsory licensing were included in Chapter XVI, Section 83; and then in 2005, when the law became fully TRIPS compliant with the inclusion of provisions for product patents (which included further flexibilities, including the amended Section 3(d)). The court read the Doha Declaration as entirely constitutive to the formulations and requirements of TRIPS and read the public health flexibilities enacted in 2002 (and 2005) as central to the legislative intent behind the amendments. Section 83 explicitly claimed that patents needed to be in the "public and national interest," and made reference to the importance of affordable pricing in relation to a patent regime.[17]

There was context to the passage of the final 2005 Act that the court paid particular attention to. The initial draft bill introduced in 2004 had not been legislated into an act by the end of the year. Worrying about the possibility of defaulting on its international obligations under TRIPS, the government passed an ordinance at the end of December 2004 that instituted a product patent regime. The ordinance was, however, only valid until March 31, 2005, by which time it needed to be replaced by an act of Parliament. The passage of the act was preceded by spirited parliamentary debates on March 18, 21, and 22, 2005, in which opposition parties voiced concerns about the impacts of a new product patent regime on drug prices. Gleevec was responsible in significant measure for this concern, given the politics that had already developed around the granting of exclusive marketing rights on the drug in 2002, which curtailed the capacity for generic manufacture (see chapter 4), and given that the price at which Novartis was selling its patented medication was up to thirty times higher than what Indian companies were charging for their generic versions. This was echoed by global concerns that were made clear to the Indian government, for instance by the World Health Organization and UNAIDS.[18] Hence, Indian patent legislation was entangled not just in global trade politics but also in a global politics of access to essential medicines. The terrain of globalization here is not simply constituted as an opposition between global free trade and sovereign national interest, but also through challenges between forces of capital and of public interest and public health that play out at both national and global levels of governance and advocacy. The politics around Gleevec was not just a consequence of the legislative history of patents in India; it actively helped shape that history.

The parliamentary debates emerged as a major source for the court to read legislative intent, because of the explicit concerns about product patent regimes in general that were voiced in these debates, specific concerns that were voiced about the extension of monopolies through evergreening, and suggestions that emerged in the course of the debates regarding the various public health flexibilities that could be introduced. The amendments to Section 3(d) were a response to these concerns. The court established a direct relationship between concerns about public health and access to medicines in Parliament, and the incorporation of 3(d) amendments as a response to those concerns. This was fundamental to the court's refusal to read Novartis's arguments about the interpretation of 3(d) simply with reference to the patent claim itself, and its insistence that this technical concern necessarily had to be interpreted constitutionally, with reference to legislative intent.

What one sees in the court's hermeneutic strategy is the coproduction of the technical with the constitutional, but also an interruption of logics of monopoly capital by creating its own interpretive dialogue with other arms of the state. Novartis's assumption in its submissions was that the critical issue in rendering a favorable interpretation of Section 3(d) was to argue for a broader definition of efficacy than therapeutic efficacy, a technical matter. But the court refused to accept it as such. Yet there was a further implicit assumption on Novartis's part, which has largely been unchallenged in the functioning of patent regimes in (especially) the United States (though also in Europe)—which is that the purpose of the patent (certainly in the arena of pharmaceuticals) is the securing of corporate monopoly. That assumption was nipped in the bud by the court through its reading of the parliamentary debates around Section 3(d). One level at which state dialogues operate here is between the judicial and legislative arms as the former reads the intent of the latter. But the voicing of concerns within Parliament, and the accommodation of those concerns by the government, speaks to another level at which they operate, within legislative and representative party politics in a multiparty parliamentary democracy, a point that I return to and detail in the next section.

The actual interpretation of Section 3(d) involved establishing its relationship to Section 2(1)(j), which defined what constitutes invention for the purposes of granting a patent, as the earlier debates in the IPAB about the relationship between molecular production and pharmaceutical efficacy now came to be reframed in terms of the relationship between two sections of an act of Parliament.[19] Counsels for Novartis contended in their arguments that Section 3(d) was not meant to nullify the criteria for invention as stipulated in 2(1)(j). They wished for an interpretation that would render 3(d) a derivative extension of 2(1)(j). Through a reading of legislative intent, the court established that Parliament clearly intended a distinction between invention and patentability. Even if Novartis could show that Gleevec was an invention that satisfied the criteria of Section 2 of the Patent Act, it would have to meet the higher standard of patentability demanded in the act, especially through Section 3(d). Meeting a philosophically intuitive definition of what constitutes invention would not be enough; it would be necessary for Gleevec to meet the legal definition of invention, which required satisfying 2(1)(j) and 3(d) independently. As Justice Alam stated in his verdict, 3(d) could not be read as subordinate to 2(1)(j) because it was "the only provision cited by the Government to allay the fears of the Opposition members concerning the abuses to which a product patent in medicines may be vulnerable" (Supreme Court verdict, 56).

The court used this insistence on a legal definition of invention that required the independent satisfaction of 2(1)(j) and 3(d) as the foundation for its reading of the invention claimed by Novartis for β-imatinib mesylate over that claimed for imatinib and its pharmaceutically acceptable salts in the original 1993 patent application filed in the United States and Canada (this was referred to as "Zimmermann patent" throughout the hearing, after Jurg Zimmermann, the lead author on the 1993 application).[20] But once again, it made a significant departure from the process followed by the Patent Office and the IPAB and from the mode of argument made by Novartis, all of which kept referring to the Zimmermann patent as the original point of reference with respect to which subsequent comparisons could be made, thereby rendering the patent claim the singular material signifier of the invention.[21] Beta-imatinib mesylate had to be established as an inventive, nonobvious modification of the substance claimed in the Zimmermann patent, and further as one that showed significantly increased therapeutic efficacy.

In contrast, the court looked not at the singularity of the patent claim, but at how that patent claim was deployed in the history of Gleevec's development and marketing in order to arrive at its judgment. And it noted a singularly important fact, which was that the U.S. patent for β-imatinib mesylate was filed in 2000 and only given to Novartis in 2005.[22] Yet Gleevec was approved for market in the United States in 2001, and protected in the U.S. market on the basis of the Zimmermann patent itself. The court further looked at the relationship between the patent claim and regulatory approval by studying the New Drug Application (NDA) filed by Novartis with the U.S. Food and Drug Administration (FDA).[23] In the NDA, the active ingredient was stated as imatinib mesylate, and the active ingredient and its composition and formulation were said to be covered by the Zimmermann patent.[24] The court further cited Gleevec's package insert, which describes the drug as follows: "GLEEVEC™ capsules contain imatinib mesylate equivalent to 100 mg of imatinib free base. Imatinib mesylate is designed chemically as 4-[(4-Methyl-1-piperazinyl)methyl]-N-[4-methyl-3-[[4-(3-pyridinyl)-2-pyrimidinyl]amino]-phenyl]benzamind methanesulfonate."[25]

Nowhere was β-imatinib mesylate mentioned in the NDA or the package insert. Furthermore, once the drug was approved for market, Novartis filed for an extension of the patent term of the Zimmermann patent, which was granted, again suggesting that this was the patent that covered the drug. The court also looked at Novartis's own history of enforcing its patent monopoly on Gleevec. Natco Pharmaceuticals had started selling its generic version of the drug, Veenat, in the United Kingdom. This was successfully challenged by Novartis, yet again on the basis of the Zimmermann patent. This history suggested to the court:

> It [is] clear that the drug Gleevec directly emanates from the Zimmermann patent and comes to the market for commercial sale. Since the grant of the Zimmermann patent, the appellant has maintained that Gleevec (that is, Imatinib Mesylate) is part of the Zimmermann patent. It obtained drug approval for Gleevec on that basis. It claimed extension for the term of the Zimmermann patent for the period of regulatory review for Gleevec, and it successfully stopped Natco Pharma Ltd. from marketing its drug in the UK on the basis of the Zimmermann patent. (Supreme Court verdict, 68)

The parenthesis in this statement is particularly important: "Gleevec (that is, Imatinib Mesylate)." Based on Novartis's own claims throughout the social life of the drug, the court decided that Gleevec was, chemically, imatinib mesylate and not β-imatinib mesylate. In addition to its regulatory and patent enforcement history, the court looked at the publication history around the drug, noting a 1996 publication in *Cancer Research* that included Jurg Zimmermann as an author, which discussed the antitumor properties of imatinib and imatinib mesylate; and a 1996 *Nature Medicine* article, also with Zimmermann as author, showing imatinib as the compound that inhibits Abl protein tyrosine kinase (Buchdunger et al. 1996; Druker et al. 1996). And imatinib mesylate, according to the court, was already covered by the Zimmermann patent, which covers all pharmaceutically acceptable salts of imatinib (a conclusion consonant with that arrived at by both the Patent Office in its initial denial of the patent on grounds of lack of inventive step, and by the IPAB). In the court's judgment, the question of whether the conversion of imatinib mesylate to β-imatinib mesylate was inventive or nonobvious or not was irrelevant, because it was imatinib mesylate, not its β-isoform, which was functioning as a drug commercially. Even if chemically, Gleevec was β-imatinib mesylate, legally and from a regulatory standpoint, Gleevec was, simply, imatinib mesylate, based on Novartis's own submissions. Justice Alam made his thoughts on β-imatinib mesylate's legal status clear during the hearing of the case, when he stated that "the β-crystal form is the same person [as imatinib mesylate] in fancy dress."[26]

At stake here are two different modalities of reading the authority that resides within a patent claim. The arguments of Novartis's counsel rested upon the structure of anticipatory knowledge embodied within the claim, as something that covers all potential modifications of the invention that is claimed, but does not disclose any particular one. This allows for a broad scope of coverage (allowing for a broader monopoly from a patent) alongside a narrow scope of disclosure (allowing for subsequent separate patent claims on specific modifications of the initial invention, also thereby allowing for a broader monopoly from a patent).[27] It also presumes broad conceptual and temporal authority of the initial claim, while dissociating it from the specific deployments of that claim in the world.

It is precisely such a presumption that was refused by the court in its reading that rendered the initial claim accountable to its subsequent deployments. This reflected different understandings of the relationship between the monopoly conferred by the patent and public interest. Novartis adopted a Schumpeterian perception of the monopolistic function of the patent, which is that providing the inventor with an absolute monopoly as an end in itself serves public interest by providing incentives to innovate (Schumpeter 1942). In the case of Gleevec, Novartis would maintain that these incentives were repaid to the public through the company's charitable drug donation program, the Gleevec International Patient Assistance Program (GIPAP), which provided the drug free to eligible patients unable to pay for it.[28] In contrast, the court read the patent as an instrumental monopoly in the public interest. In such an understanding of a patent regime, the boundary between the scope of coverage and disclosure that Novartis was arguing for was rendered untenable, because it would allow the initial patent to function as a blocking patent.[29]

By refusing this distinction, the court restricted the authority of the patent claim as an instrument to secure future monopoly as an end in itself. The implications of this go beyond the specifics of the Gleevec case, even beyond the specifics of the interpretation of Section 3(d), to providing judicial precedent for the rationale of the patent system itself. The court made this clear as it stated, "We certainly do not wish the law of patent in this country to develop on lines . . . where the scope of the patent is determined not on the intrinsic worth of the invention but by the artful drafting of its *claims* by skillful lawyers, and where patents are traded as a commodity not for production and marketing of the patented products but to search for someone who may be sued for infringement of the patent" (Supreme Court verdict, 81, emphasis in original).

By situating Section 3(d) within the broader history of patent law in India, the court had determined that it was a criterion that had to be satisfied in its own right, and not simply as derivative of Section 2(1)(j). By reading the Zimmermann patent not just as a discrete claim with its own authority but as a strategic instrument that was deployed in the world toward particular ends, the court questioned whether the patent on β-imatinib mesylate would even matter given Gleevec's legal and regulatory history as imatinib mesylate in the United States and elsewhere. And by refusing to accept the distinction between scope of coverage and disclosure, the court made clear that it saw imatinib mesylate as already covered by the Zimmermann patent, which was not enforceable in India, while also clarifying that it saw the patent as an instrument of public interest that had to be interpreted and enforced as such. Through these lines of reasoning, the court established that Gleevec did not meet the criteria for legal invention established in Section 2(1)(j).

This still left the question of the specific applicability of Section 3(d): was β-imatinib mesylate a modification that conferred significantly enhanced therapeutic efficacy over the known substance? And what was the known substance, imatinib free base or imatinib mesylate? Recall that this was the primary question in Novartis's appeal to the Supreme Court. It therefore was a question that still needed to be adjudicated. However, the hermeneutics employed by the court rendered it a tertiary question as far as the Gleevec patent itself was concerned: whatever its verdict on 3(d), Gleevec could not be granted a patent because it did not satisfy 2(1)(j). Nonetheless, the stakes of the court's interpretation of 3(d) were high in terms of the precedent it would set in the long term regarding how efficacy would be interpreted. Novartis was attempting in its appeal to force the issue of defining significantly enhanced efficacy by revisiting the question of the relationship between bioavailability and efficacy, with the hope that this would lead to a broader interpretation of efficacy than that allowed by the Madras High Court and upheld by the IPAB.

In the Supreme Court, Novartis's case was supplemented by an independent brief submitted by legal expert Shamnad Basheer, who argued against the narrow definition of efficacy as therapeutic efficacy granted by the High Court.[30] Basheer's brief was an attempt to lend legal and regulatory clarity to Section 3(d), by establishing a consistent definition on the basis of which it could be enforced, which he felt was important for "the robust development of sound patent jurisprudence for India" (Basheer intervention, 8).

Basheer argued that the U.S. Orphan Drug Act (ODA) should provide the basis for a definition of efficacy in terms of "therapeutic advantage."[31] This would be a broader criterion than therapeutic efficacy, and would explicitly allow physical properties of a molecule such as bioavailability to be taken into account while evaluating enhanced efficacy. This was a peculiar line of argument. For one thing, Basheer was arguing for an interpretive guideline for 3(d) that did not even include the word *efficacy*, which appears not once but twice in the section. For another, the ODA is not even patent legislation, and its intent is to incentivize research into rare or neglected diseases for which there might not be a sufficient market incentive; the intent of 3(d) is to prevent pharmaceutical evergreening. This means that 3(d) is specifically an instrument to reduce monopoly, whereas the ODA provides extra market exclusivity and monopoly to companies as reward for developing orphan drugs. Rather than clarifying the legislation, Basheer seemed to be rewriting it in terms of categories that existed in neither the wording nor the intent of 3(d).

The ODA provides complete market exclusivity of seven years to the originators of orphan drugs. But it does allow a competitor to market a structurally similar drug that is "clinically superior." The question of what constitutes clinical superiority then becomes a crucial interpretive question, which Basheer suggested was a problem similar to that confronted in the evaluation of efficacy with respect to 3(d). Clinical superiority is defined under the ODA as showing "a significant therapeutic advantage over and above that provided by an approved orphan drug" (as cited in Basheer intervention, 13). The grounds upon which therapeutic advantage can be established include not only greater therapeutic effectiveness of the competitor drug, but also superior safety. Basheer argued that in principle, increased bioavailability could lead to increased therapeutic advantage by leading to lower dose requirements and thereby reduced toxicity, which could lead to improved safety. He was not claiming increased therapeutic advantage in the specific case of Gleevec by virtue of the 30 percent increase in bioavailability of the crystalline isoform over free base, which he said needed to be independently established. But he was arguing for a lower threshold for establishing efficacy than the establishment of therapeutic efficacy.

Basheer's intervention did not turn out to be significant to the verdict in the case (except ironically, as indicated below, to Novartis's detriment), though it did cause anxiety among Novartis's opponents given that it was providing a persuasive alternative to therapeutic efficacy as the definition of efficacy. But it is important to point to the conceit behind it. If Novartis sought to enforce a narrowly technical definition of invention purely with respect to the patent claim, then Basheer's attempt was to enforce a narrowly legal one, in which the letter of the law would transparently and without reference to history or context provide a clear definition of efficacy that could be uniformly enforced. Both Novartis and Basheer were pushing technocratic interpretations of patent law that could consistently isolate and purify inventive criteria in ways that did not allow for the interpretive license taken by patent adjudicators and the courts as they attempted to establish the applicability of 3(d) to Gleevec. For the court, however, such license was essential to allowing the kinds of thick interpretation necessary to situate a molecule's patentability not just along a linear imaginary of romantic invention that materializes through a patent claim, but also in relation to the legislative intent to prevent monopolistic corporate practices at the expense of public health and access to affordable medicines.

The court established that β-imatinib mesylate needed to meet the test of Section 3(d) since it was derived from a "known substance" that had already been patented. To this end, it referred to the Indian patent application for β-imatinib mesylate, which states that "all of [its] indicated inhibitory and pharmaceutical effects are also found with the free base . . . or other cells thereof" (cited in Supreme Court verdict, 84). This statement alone, according to the court, made it clear that β-imatinib mesylate could not qualify for a patent under 3(d), since "when all the pharmacological properties of beta crystalline form of Imatinib Mesylate are equally possessed by Imatinib in free base form or its salt, where is the question of the subject product having any enhanced efficacy over the known substance of which it is a new form?" (85).

However, what was the known substance? The court pointed to the ambiguities of Novartis's own position in the matter. Its patent application pointed to imatinib free base as the original molecule from which β-imatinib mesylate had been derived. Yet its claims for the inventive nature of the crystalline form claimed that it was two steps removed from the free base, suggesting that the known substance preceding it was not the free base but imatinib mesylate. The court had already established that both freebase and imatinib mesylate were disclosed in the Zimmermann patent and therefore not eligible for a product patent in India; but the question was which one of the two would serve as the reference with respect to which the efficacy of the β-crystalline isoform would have to be established?

To answer this, the court referenced two affidavits submitted on behalf of Novartis before the controller of patents at the Chennai Patent Office in 2005, by the chemists Paul Manley and Giorgio Massimini, in order to show that Gleevec met the requirements of Section 3(d). Manley's affidavit pointed to the greater stability, flow, solubility, and hygroscopicity of β-imatinib mesylate, while Massimini's described the rat study showing 30 percent increase in bioavailability—in both cases, the point of comparison was to the free base. The court could not find any submission that showed the efficacy of β-imatinib mesylate over noncrystalline imatinib mesylate. It wanted to know: does noncrystalline imatinib mesylate have equivalently higher solubility relative to free base as the β-crystal? The assumption was that it probably did, given that "one does not have to be an expert in chemistry to know that salts normally have much better solubility than compounds in free base form" (Supreme Court verdict, 88). And if so, then how could the β-form be an improvement over its immediately preceding substance, imatinib mesylate?

The relationship between chemical ontology and legal reasoning is worth unpacking here. The reason that imatinib mesylate does not appear as an entity in any of Novartis's submissions is likely because it is chemically a transitional or interstitial entity. The patent claim on the β-crystalline isoform suggests that methanesulfonic acid salts of imatinib tend to crystallize. A common crystal form is the α-crystal form, which is less thermodynamically stable, needle-shaped (and therefore less easy to absorb), and difficult to reproduce. The β-form is more thermodynamically stable, non–needle shaped, and can be reproduced. Yet legally, imatinib mesylate was an entity that needed to exist in order for Novartis to claim a two-step improvement over imatinib free base, and did exist in its regulatory submissions and package insert. For β-imatinib mesylate to satisfy Section 3(d) legally, the court demanded a comparison with imatinib mesylate, a comparison that was chemically untenable. Imatinib mesylate was deemed to be a known substance for the purposes of comparing efficacy because it was anticipated by the Zimmermann patent claim, which included "all pharmaceutically acceptable salts" of imatinib, rendering it legally a real substance and a relevant standard of comparison.

The final question concerned efficacy—how was it to be defined for the purpose of interpreting Section 3(d)? The court concurred with the Madras High Court that it had to be in terms of therapeutic efficacy, using as its basis the linguistic definition of efficacy as stated in the *New Oxford Dictionary of English* (1998 edition), which describes it as "the ability to produce a desired or intended result" (cited in Supreme Court verdict, 90). The court deemed that, in the case of medicines, this had to imply the ability to cure a disease, and hence necessarily suggested therapeutic efficacy.[32] What then would be the parameters by which therapeutic efficacy could be defined?

The arguments for Novartis's counsel echoed Basheer's interventions, suggesting that these parameters had to be broad enough to include attributes such as bioavailability, which could confer therapeutic advantage by leading to reduced dosage requirements and hence decreased drug toxicity. In opposition to this position, Anand Grover, lead counsel for CPAA, insisted on the basis of pharmacological textbooks that therapeutic efficacy had a clear meaning in the field and was established in terms of pharmacodynamics (what the drug does to the body), not pharmacokinetics (what the body does to the drug, which is relevant for considering attributes such as bioavailability).

The court accepted the fact that bioavailability of a drug is necessary for its effectiveness, but cannot in itself be regarded as an indicator of therapeutic efficacy. Ironically, it drew upon Basheer's intervention to disregard bioavailability as a criterion for therapeutic efficacy, since he had stated (citing another commentator) that "a determination that a drug product is bio-available is not in itself a determination of effectiveness."[33] On this basis, the patent was denied on the basis of 3(d) as well, and precedent was set for the interpretation of the section on narrow grounds of therapeutic efficacy.

The Science and Politics of Gleevec

The Supreme Court verdict led to predictably polarized responses from those supporting and opposed to Novartis's position. For instance, a *Wall Street Journal* article cited Novartis's executives and representatives of the multinational pharmaceutical industry making straightforward and oft-cited correlations between a favorable patent environment, innovation, and public health. Ranjit Shahani, vice chairman and managing director of Novartis India, said, "This ruling is a setback for patients that will hinder medical progress for diseases without effective treatment options." A Novartis spokesman linked this to the threat of reduced investment in India as a market: "If innovation is rewarded, there is a clear business case to move forward [in India]. If it isn't rewarded and protected, there isn't." The Pharmaceutical Research and Manufacturers of America, the major U.S.-based lobbying group for the multinational pharmaceutical industry, stated that the ruling "marks yet another example of the deteriorating innovation environment in India" (Krishna and Whalen 2013).

In contrast, those involved in advocacy for access to medicines celebrated the ruling as an important victory. A collection of essays in the *Economic and Political Weekly* provides various legal and civil society perspectives and contexts on the case, and the stakes and consequences of the verdict, from this oppositional position.[34] Particularly important in this collection is an essay by K. M. Gopakumar (2013), who argues that while important, this was nonetheless a limited victory, and that what was needed was legislation that would prevent patenting on all known substances, regardless of improvements in efficacy, as existed in the 1970 Act. Such positions are also taken in the interests of innovation but more stringently defined, with an insistence that practices such as evergreening in fact reflect the lack of innovation in an industry that often protects its monopoly through minor modifications to existing drugs.

It is perhaps ironic that such an argument could effectively be made against Gleevec, widely regarded as one of the most innovative and revolutionary anticancer medications ever developed. Indeed, much has been written about Gleevec as a magic bullet in the treatment of cancer, and as an exemplar of translational research that sees basic research into mechanisms of disease translate into medically available treatments. Some of these accounts, such as the one written by Novartis CEO Daniel Vasella (2003), provide a linear and romanticized model of scientific invention. More reflexive and sociologically intricate accounts of Gleevec's development have been provided by Siddhartha Mukherjee (2011), and by Peter Keating and Alberto Cambrosio (2012). It is worth constructing some of the complexities of Gleevec's story from these accounts; but even they are not attentive to how the political gets constituted if one recognizes that Gleevec's is a global story, not just one that plays out in Euro-American research laboratories, clinics, and corporate boardrooms.

Mukherjee's account of Gleevec's development is part of his magisterial account of the history of cancer research and treatment (what he refers to as a "biography of cancer"), *The Emperor of All Maladies*. It is exemplary of a move that began in the 1980s toward targeted cancer therapy, which developed out of a mechanistic understanding of cellular and molecular triggers for particular cancers that then serve as therapeutic targets. The breast cancer drug Herceptin (trastuzumab, developed by Genentech) and Gleevec are the two early success stories of targeted cancer therapy. The histories of both drugs indicate the importance of corporate involvement in biotechnology research toward therapy. This involvement is not politically straightforward. On the one hand, it is unlikely to imagine the translation of basic research on molecular mechanisms involved in cancer into therapeutic development without the pull of corporate investment in capital and human resources. On the other hand, these investments are always predicated on strategic market calculations, which means that the developmental trajectory of a drug is always dependent upon how potentially valuable that investment seems in terms of financial rather than therapeutic benefit. Both the Herceptin and Gleevec stories involved particular researchers (Dennis Slamon at UCLA in the case of Herceptin; Brian Druker at the Oregon Health and Science University and Nicholas Lydon at Novartis in the case of Gleevec) having to fight against corporate market calculations to push ahead with their research programs.

A second common thread in the two histories concerns the importance of cancer patient activism for access to medicines and putting pressure on researchers and regulatory agencies to speed up clinical trials. In the case of Herceptin, Mukherjee traces the history of breast cancer activism that led to an expanded access program to the experimental drug even before it was approved for market.[35] Therefore, access politics was imbricated in the politics of clinical trials, in ways radically different from a context such as India's where clinical trials for these drugs did not take place, and where the political resonances of experimental subjectivity emerge quite differently. Questions of such differential constitutions and resonances of the political across different locales are precisely what concern me here, as I will elaborate.

Any account of the scientific developmental trajectory of Gleevec must be located in these two contexts, of corporate involvement and of a politics that was about speedier access through greater investment in novel drug development and quicker approval to market. But the purely scientific trajectory is itself complex and involves the serendipitous intersection of two independent histories—of basic research and of corporate screening for potential drug targets—that merge and continue into a third: of clinical trials. I briefly describe this trajectory for Gleevec, by summarizing accounts from Mukherjee and from Keating and Cambrosio's account of the history of cancer clinical trials, *Cancer on Trial*.

The basic research trajectory did not begin with the search for a drug. It was, rather, perhaps like all basic research in biology, full of moments of discovery that could retrospectively be reconstructed into a linear trajectory toward a drug. Some elements of this include the discovery of a particular chromosomal abnormality (the Philadelphia chromosome) in patients with chronic myeloid leukemia (CML) in 1960 (Nowell and Hungerford 1960); the discovery of translocation between fragments of chromosomes 9 and 22 as the mechanism causing this abnormality (Rowley 1973); the identification of genes involved in these translocations, *abl* (on chromosome 9) and *Bcr* (on chromosome 22), whose fusion was found to result in the *Bcr-abl* oncogene; the engineering of a mouse containing *Bcr-abl*, which proved the relationship between this oncogene and the development of CML; and functional studies of *Bcr-abl* that identified it as a tyrosine kinase.[36]

The trajectory of research at Ciba-Geigy was on a quite different problem, a search for molecules that could inhibit the family of enzymes called kinases (which are involved in regulating cellular activity through phosphorylation, that is, adding phosphate groups to molecules to cause their activation, inactivation, stimulation, or inhibition), but selectively (since kinases are essential enzymes that are involved in the regulation of all manner of biochemical pathways, and a nonselective kinase inhibitor would be impossibly toxic). This was a team led by the chemist Nicholas Lydon, who found a molecule with potential selective kinase inhibitory properties. Jurg Zimmermann, who became the lead author on the 1993 patent claim for imatinib, created thousands of variants of this molecule, while Elisabeth Buchdunger tested these molecules on cells. In the process, Ciba-Geigy scientists were coming up with kinase inhibitors without a specific disease target, while basic research on CML had led to an understanding of disease mechanism that involved a tyrosine kinase, *Bcr-abl*.

One of the researchers studying *Bcr-abl* kinase was Brian Druker at the Dana-Farber Cancer Institute of Harvard Medical School, who heard of Lydon's collection of potential kinase inhibitors and approached him to collaborate. In spite of the enthusiasm of the individuals concerned, the collaboration could not proceed institutionally because of legal objections from Harvard's side (see Keating and Cambrosio 2012). Ironically, this was because of an exclusive agreement between Dana-Farber and Ciba-Geigy's competitor Sandoz (which would subsequently merge with Ciba-Geigy to form Novartis). It was only after Druker left Harvard to join the Oregon Health and Sciences University (OHSU) that the collaboration could proceed, as OHSU's lawyers allowed a collaboration that Dana-Farber's did not. Druker conducted a series of studies on Lydon's molecule—first, in vitro studies on CML cells in a petri dish; then experiments in mice implanted with CML cells; and finally, experiments on human bone marrow from CML patients. These were the results published in *Nature Medicine* that would subsequently come to be central to establishing the trajectory of the drug in the Supreme Court case, albeit in the specific matter of the name of the molecule disclosed in the article, which had no mention of the β-crystalline isoform of imatinib mesylate.[37]

This history suggests a trajectory of invention very different from that implied in a patent claim, which implies simply that the pharmaceutical company is the innovator of a new drug. But it also suggests a trajectory different from that claimed by opponents to Novartis, in whose eyes the real inventor of Gleevec was Druker.[38] Both of these are based in romantic imaginaries of invention, whether by the innovative company or by the genius scientist. In fact, what was critical was the collaboration between Druker and Lydon that allowed two independent research trajectories to find each other and merge. This set the stage for the clinical trials of Gleevec, which required further collaborations with physicians and clinical researchers.[39]

The Gleevec trials can be seen as revolutionary, both because of their outcome (showing significantly better results than the current standard of care, which was interferon and/or bone marrow transplantation) and their speed (the entire process from the start of Phase 1 trials to market approval took less than four years, unlike the typical ten-to-fifteen-year process that most drug trials involve). The Phase 1 results on eighty-three patients were published in the *New England Journal of Medicine* in 2001 (Druker et al. 2001), but Novartis had activated Phase 2 and 3 trials even before this publication. Keating and Cambrosio point to the unusual nature of these trials, not just in terms of their speed, but also in terms of the relatively large number of Phase 1 enrollees, since Phase 1 studies are toxicity studies that typically enroll only about ten volunteers. Most enrollees in early-stage oncology trials tend to be patients in the terminal stages of the disease: given the high toxicity of most anticancer drugs, they cannot be tested on healthy volunteers, and are often tested only on people for whom other avenues have been largely exhausted. Yet the Gleevec trials included patients in less terminal stages. This meant that the Phase 1 trial was not simply a test of the drug's toxicity, but already was an initial test of its potential curative effects. Because those effects were so substantial, many Phase 1 enrollees were still receiving the drug at the time of the *NEJM* publication, making for an unusually long experimental duration of a Phase 1 trial. Keating and Cambrosio draw upon Vasella's account of the development of Gleevec to suggest the pressures the company felt from patients who had heard of the promising early results from the Phase 1 trials, leading to their fast-tracking of Phase 2 and 3 trials even before Phase 1 was completed. This is an example of what they refer to as oncopolitics.

Ironically, Novartis was reluctant to initiate clinical trials even after Druker's promising early results, mirroring similar reluctance on Genentech's part to invest in the R&D of Herceptin. Druker and Lydon's collaboration was throughout conditional on institutional enthusiasms, and was nearly scuttled by both the academic and corporate institutions involved. Mukherjee emphasizes this in his account as he describes the Gleevec story in terms of "an inverted world in which an academic researcher had to beg a pharmaceutical company to push its own products into clinical trials" (2011, 436). Druker assembled his own team to run the trials, and managed to persuade Novartis to give him a few grams of the drug to use for the Phase 1 studies. In Mukherjee's words, "Druker would have a shot—but only one shot. To Novartis, CGP57148 [the name given to Gleevec when it was still a research molecule], the product of its most ambitious drug-discovery program to date, was already a failure" (436).[40]

The imbrication of science and technology in the political is explicit in Mukherjee's and Keating and Cambrosio's accounts of Gleevec, but they are focused on the United States and Europe. I argue that understanding politics involves a situated perspective from beyond Euro-American centers of R&D in the life sciences, and requires a comparative attentiveness to the differentiations and striations that such perspectives provide. While India is not considered a part of the scientific story of Gleevec to the extent that R&D and clinical trials for the drug did not take place there, the legal trajectory that emerged around the drug there put into question particular authoritative narratives of invention. As Gleevec's history gets situated out of India, interruptions of logics of capital and of romantic ideologies of innovation as underwritten by the decontextualized authority of a patent claim come to be at stake. This has consequences for understanding politics, but also for understanding science.

There are two elements to the oncopolitics that Keating and Cambrosio describe. One concerns the politics of institutional collaboration, especially between academe and industry, and the second concerns the politics of especially American patient advocacy in accelerating R&D into anticancer therapies. The second element of oncopolitics is most certainly present in the Indian story, since the initial pregrant opposition to the Gleevec patent in India was initiated by CPAA, a cancer patients' advocacy group. But how politics is constituted and what it means is very different in a context where patient advocacy around access is not coupled to R&D the way it usually is in western Europe and North America. I wish to add to and complicate Mukherjee's and Keating and Cambrosio's accounts with a simple observation: the fact that R&D into anticancer therapeutics is almost exclusively a Euro-American enterprise, yet people get cancer in other parts of the world as well. What kind of an oncopolitics might emerge in such situations where questions of access are dislocated from those of experiment?[41]

I have thus far emphasized the active interpretation of legislative intent by the judiciary in India. But how did legislative intent itself come to be what it was? In other words, what were the pulls toward the enactment of legislation such as Section 3(d)? Answering this involves understanding the dialogues between executive and legislative branches of the Indian state in the context of coalitional parliamentary party politics, especially the involvement of leftist political parties in intellectual property–related policy debates. It should be emphasized that there is a long political history of Left-progressive mobilization against multilateral trade and intellectual property regimes in India, dating back to opposition to the Uruguay Round of GATT negotiations in the late 1980s and early 1990s (Sengupta 2010, 2013). Understanding what happened with Gleevec involves situating it within a longer trajectory of activism that rendered questions of intellectual property and access to medicines in India already deeply politicized.[42]

Leftist political parties became aware of intellectual property–related issues because of the concerns of their powerful trade union of pharmaceutical medical representatives, the Federation of Medical Representatives Association of India.[43] Their involvement was "part of a policy movement to have aspects of public health enshrined in our policy regime"; "the question of having a proper, people oriented drug policy, where main emphasis was to have generic drugs."[44] This involved not just taking an oppositional political position with respect to TRIPS, but also intervening in the process by which its provisions would come to be enshrined in policy. The Indian Constitution contains an omnibus provision whereby international treaties, whether bilateral or multilateral, do not have to be legislatively ratified by Parliament. According to Nilotpal Basu, CPI-M Member of Parliament, this was intended as an interim arrangement at the time of the drafting of the Constitution to allow executive flexibility, but was never changed. It was also based on the assumption that governments would be single-party majorities in Parliament, and therefore that "the ruling party, or the prime minister, who represents the majority of the ruling party . . . can be deemed to be the representative of the Parliament as a whole, or at the least the majority of the Parliament as a whole" (Basu interview). Between 1996 and 2014, India was ruled exclusively by coalition governments, which means that the ruling party did not even necessarily represent the majority will of the ruling government, let alone of Parliament as a whole.

Because of this provision, TRIPS was passed without any of the underlying issues being debated in Parliament. This is important to emphasize, because the parliamentary debates before the passage of the 2005 Patent Act in March 2005, which proved so crucial to the Supreme Court verdict against Novartis, were the only time the institutionalization of TRIPS into pharmaceutical patent policy was extensively debated legislatively. This was a function of the fact that while TRIPS itself was ratified through purely executive means, its implementation required legislative changes—such as in the Patent Act—that could not be ratified through the omnibus provision covering international agreements. This led to a series of legislative events prior to the parliamentary debates that Basu describes as follows:[45]

The NDA [National Democratic Alliance, the BJP-led ruling coalition from 1998–2004] initiated moves to legislate the Third Amendment, and we had forced the government to have a, what you call a Select Committee. . . . On very very serious issues of public concern, where there was a major public debate and discourse, we have what you call Select Committees, [which] . . . can come up with its own version of a draft legislation, which is quite distinct and different from the initial draft legislation that the executive is obliged to move in the House. So there was a Select Committee, where of course we in the Left were in a minority. But we fought gamely. I mean, while there was [a] campaign outside—we had run a very good campaign on this GATT process, Dunkel Draft, so on and so forth. And we had at that time evolved also very well defined amendments. On that Select Committee, there was a great degree of convergence between the Congress and the BJP. . . . The entire set of amendments that we had was ultimately registered by the Left members in the committee was [a] note of dissent. And it is very interesting that subsequently when the UPA [United Progressive Alliance, the Congress-led coalition] government came [in May 2004], since they were depending on our critical support—at that time, there was a lot of political speculation as to how the absolutely conflicting approaches of the Left and the Congress could be reconciled in terms of legislation-making process. And it was specifically mentioned that what happens to the patent amendment? [This was a] pending thing, the legacy that the new government had to bear. So we made it clear that the Third Amendment that was moved by the NDA regime led by BJP, that is not acceptable to us. So no way that the government can push *that* legislation. But at the same time, these people also had a problem, because you see there was continuous pressure that while India has signed this WTO agreement, but they are not changing their patent regime. (Basu interview)

It was in this context that the Left decided that the pragmatic mode of dealing with this issue could not involve an outright rejection of TRIPS, but required critical engagement. This involved drawing upon the principles of the 2001 Doha Declaration, which would allow for the enactment of public health flexibilities in any TRIPS-compliant patent legislation. The Left pushed for various such flexibilities to be introduced in the draft legislation, one of which was the amendment to Section 3(d). According to Basu, the Congress was open to incorporating flexibilities, but was resistant to the specific changes sought to 3(d). While the extent of distance between the positions of the two parties was not made public at the time, the Left made clear in closed-door negotiations that their continued support for the government would depend upon 3(d) being incorporated into the legislation along with other proposed flexibilities.[46] Hence, the letter and spirit of 3(d) was upheld by the state, through a judicial act that read legislative intent. But this was in spite of executive ambivalence that continued to be on display years after the passage of the amendments in the 2005 Act.[47]

I have described the intricacies of Gleevec's legal trajectory in India in part because it is so central to the interpretation of TRIPS-mandated product patent regimes in India. But it is also important in showing how the logics of capital interact with, and can potentially be tempered by, the dialogic ways in which the state is constituted, which is itself in part a function of civil society organization. The clinical trials situation was driven in contrast by logics of capital that were unfettered for a significantly longer period of time, until the trials became the subject of scandal (see chapter 2). At stake here are questions of relationships between technoscience and representative politics. The state functions as a critical transacting agent that both serves the interests of capital and can potentially be held accountable to public interest.

This is perhaps more generally true of the southern world.[48] For instance, access to Gleevec was a contentious issue in South Korea even before it had become politicized in India.[49] A Korean professor of mechanical engineering contracted CML in 2000, and found out about the clinical trials being conducted on Gleevec in the United States. He was able to organize other leukemia patients in Korea to petition the government to allow Novartis to expand its experimental access program for the drug in Korea. Thus, Korean patients became enrolled as trial subjects even as they started to politically organize to ensure broader access to Gleevec in Korea after its market approval. This was particularly important because, as in India, Novartis priced Gleevec in Korea at the same price point as in the United States and Europe.

The first salvo in the postmarket politics around Gleevec was an attempt by leukemia patient groups to get the Korean government to issue a compulsory license on the drug in 2002. This failed, leading to two other fronts being opened. The first involved approaching generics companies in India for the drug. This was facilitated by meetings with activists for Indian patients and access to medicines at the World Social Forum in Bombay in 2004, who connected Korean activists with companies that were manufacturing generic versions such as Cipla and Natco. The second involved a longer-term engagement with both Novartis and the Korean government regarding the pricing of the drug in Korea.

In contrast to India, drug prices in Korea are regulated through price control mechanisms rather than intellectual property laws. Korea had harmonized its patent regime to a product patent regime in 1986, but has a monopsonistic system of national health insurance, with the state as the major buyer for drugs it deems essential to public health.[50] The locus of contestation therefore concerned whether the Korean government could impose price controls on the drug. The government attempted to set a ceiling price on the drug of U.S. $15 per 100 mg capsule, but Novartis refused to accept the price and demanded a 34 percent increase. The basis for Novartis's price point was that this was set in seven advanced industrial nations (the so-called A-7 group of countries)—the United States, United Kingdom, Canada, France, Germany, Switzerland, and Italy. Bilateral trade agreements between the United States and Korea stipulated that Korea would adhere to A-7 pricing of pharmaceutical products, even though it was not formally part of the group of A-7 countries. Eventually, a negotiated settlement was reached between Novartis and the Korean government, whereby the government agreed not to restrict the price of Gleevec, while Novartis donated toward the cost of the drug. In this way, the amount that patients themselves had to pay was only 10 percent of the price of the drug (the rest being paid for by national health insurance and Novartis together), but the price of the drug remained the same as it was in the United States.

The pricing of Gleevec was a contentious issue in other developing country contexts as well. For instance, the Brazilian government was able to negotiate with Novartis and brought the price down from U.S. $19 to $13 per 100 mg capsule. Hence, the politics surrounding Gleevec in India reflect a much broader constellation of southern politics around access to medicines that call into question the assumptions and paradigms of innovation in relation to drug development as they operate in Euro-America. These are histories that play out through law and advocacy that are differently coupled (or not coupled at all) to R&D than is the case in Europe and the United States. They are also histories with their own comparative intricacies, for instance around different structures of health care access (nationalized health insurance in Korea as opposed to free market competition in generics in India); different loci around which drug prices come to be internationally contentious (the patent in India, price controls in Korea); different global relationships around which this contention materializes (bilateral trade agreements with the United States in Korea's case; conformity with TRIPS in India's); different industrial and market capacities (India as largely a Third World market but with globally competitive generic manufacturing capacity; Korea as a more developed market that nonetheless depended upon Indian generic capacity to make the drug accessible until price negotiations with Novartis could be concluded); and different configurations and articulations of patient advocacy with other forms of civil society and political advocacy (in India's case, a Left-progressive civil society that came to be highly politicized around intellectual property matters in the late 1980s and early 1990s as concerted opposition to the GATT negotiations was mounted; in Korea's case, a civil society that traced its politicization to the prodemocracy student movements of 1986).[51] Finally, there are South-South articulations to be attentive to, such as those between Korean patient groups and Indian generics companies. A more striated, differentiated, and multiply located notion of the political than the Euro-American "oncopolitics" that Keating and Cambrosio (2012) describe is necessary to understand the global manifestations of the politics of access to medicines.

In this chapter, I have focused on the importance of legal reasoning and its alternative paths to global pharmaceutical politics. This is not just about ideological positions around innovation and access to essential medicines (of which there are plenty, on the sides both of the multinational pharmaceutical industry and of activists who oppose it), but about the technical virtuosity of the lawyers and judges involved. Indeed, I suspect that one of the reasons Novartis kept losing its cases in India was that it employed some of the most famous lawyers in the country, who were big names but did not necessarily have that virtuosity when it came to the strategic interpretation of patent law and its relationship to scientific development, something that lawyers for Novartis's opposition seemed to possess in ample measure.[52] Therefore, the courts and legal reasoning itself are important sites for ethnographic attention to the articulations of value, politics, and knowledge.

Judicial Ethics and the Spirit of Constitutionalism

This chapter has explored judicialization as an emergent form of and space for politics, in the context of an economy that sees the expansion of multinational corporate monopoly, underwritten by ideologies of innovation and presumptions of romantic invention, and inscribed in a patent claim. The Gleevec case as it has played out in the Indian courts potentially interrupts these monopolistic logics in at least two ways. First, by providing other interpretive modalities for trajectories of invention, the verdict holds the authority of patent claims accountable to existing national-state laws. And second, it thereby denaturalizes the ideologies of innovation that allow patents to function in the cause of increasingly unfettered corporate monopoly. I wish in this concluding section to think about the value systems that animate the kinds of judicial impulses that have been seen in the legal trajectory of Gleevec, which has continued in subsequent curtailments of intellectual property rights in India in the cause of public interest (see note 2).

The stakes of the Gleevec verdict are obviously high in terms of allowing access to a potentially life-saving anticancer drug for larger segments of people who need it. Activists fighting against the Gleevec patent have pointed to the stark (up to thirty-fold) differentials in price between Novartis's patented drug and generic versions on the Indian market. The multinational pharmaceutical lobby has meanwhile itself argued that verdicts such as those seen in India will have adverse consequences for drug access in the long term by removing incentives for innovator companies to market their drugs in countries that do not provide stable monopoly protections. One sees here a structure of polarization similar to that described in chapter 2, between Euro-American biomedical interests demanding a harmonious playing field that facilitates global movements (whether of patented medications or of clinical experimentation) underwritten by norms of spreading the health (and logics that demand growing it as surplus value), and opponents railing against multinational corporate hegemony.

Without trivializing the stakes of accessing essential medication, I wish to thicken them. The question of access in practice is more complicated than just establishing the price of the drug. Mechanisms of enabling and constraining access within particular pricing environments are a function of other kinds of infrastructural development (for drug manufacture and distribution, for instance) and themselves come to be a site of strategic maneuver and politics.[53] Similarly, indeed, the question of health goes beyond one of access to biomedical artifacts such as drugs or vaccines. The story of the HPV vaccine scandal discussed in chapter 2 is, after all, one that saw provision of a vaccine through a national immunization program, but led to concerns about pharmaceuticalization in the absence of adequate epidemiology or screening in order to expand multinational corporate markets. While Gleevec is a historic anticancer drug and the moral imperative to ensure that it is as widely available as possible to those who need it is obvious, I believe the true stakes of the long battle around its patentability in India lie elsewhere. After all, the Gleevec patent itself expired in July 2015. Even if Novartis had won the Supreme Court case, it would have enjoyed patent protection on its drug for just a couple of years. Such a lengthy judicial battle could surely not have been undertaken for such trivial gain.

I suggest that the stakes of the Gleevec case include but go beyond access to an anticancer drug. For the multinational pharmaceutical industry, there are the stakes of establishing monopoly regimes globally (including at the expense of prevalent free market systems such as those seen in India, for which see chapters 4 and 5). It is also about the establishment of a narrow idea of invention that furthers romantic ideologies of corporate-driven innovation and which provides a normative justification for monopolistic regimes. But there are also stakes here for conceptualizing the ways in which judicialization operates as a strategy of politics. There has clearly been a Global Southern turn to judicialization over the past two decades. This has specific inflections in different situations; can both interrupt and instantiate global capital flows; and operates in complex relationships to informal and illicit economies depending on prevalent structures of representative and regulatory government.

Understanding judicialization as a form of and space for politics involves being attentive to its own spatialities and to the subjectivities it engenders. Jean and John Comaroff have posed an important series of provocations about judicialization as a condition of contemporary postcolonial politics (Comaroff and Comaroff 2006). Following their lead, I suggest that cases such as Gleevec's pose a number of conceptual and immediately political questions concerning the citizen as legal subject. How does this articulate with biomedical subject constitutions, such as those of patient-consumer-experimental subject? In what ways does the law imagine biomedical subjectivity in particular contexts of governance and representative politics? What kinds of accountability do these legal subject constitutions demand, and of whom? How is responsibility configured for those in positions of institutional power? These are some of the pharmocratic issues that emerge from intellectual property and access politics in India.

I argue that answering some of these questions requires attention to the ways in which the judicialization of pharmaceutical politics in India activates and is animated by constitutionalism (see introduction). This has often taken recourse to a discourse of rights, especially Article 21, which guarantees the right to life and suggests a liberal normative template that derives from Western legal frameworks.[54] But when I interviewed Justice Prabha Sridevan, who wrote the Madras High Court verdict on Gleevec, I heard something more. She insisted that as a judge, what was at stake for her in such cases was "the upholding of the spirit of the Constitution."[55] This is not a strict foundationalist constitutionalism, but rather an interpretive, hermeneutic, dynamic one.

It also goes beyond what Comaroff and Comaroff have called the "fetishism of constitutionality" (2006, 24), in that it is not a theological reification of the authority of a foundational national text. It is rather a strategic political deployment of both constitutional authority and rights-based norms in ways that serve to realize the "promise of justice."[56]

But where does this spirit of the Constitution come from? One of the most powerful functions of national-state constitutions is their ability to perform their own mythos, to call into being a people and their values (Ackerman 1991). Constitutions represent value-laden origin stories. Postcolonial constitutions such as India's have an obviously Euro-American, liberal inheritance, but their origin stories render them political in very particular ways.[57] The question of constitutional authority therefore is at least in part a comparative question, whose answer involves attention to the foundational myths that nations tell themselves; to the judicial cultures of constitutional interpretation that emerge in particular places and times; and to the conjuncture of their actual origination.[58] Therefore, constitutions are themselves conjunctural documents that reflect the ethos of a time and a place, even as they provide occasions for what Spivak (1990), following Jean-François Lyotard (1984), calls "paralogical legitimation"—a legitimation that operates through movement against an established way of reasoning, and thereby opens up the possibility of its own innovation and thus also of justice.[59] Constitutions must be situated if some sense of their spirit is to be understood.

First, they must be historically situated. Upendra Baxi has argued that the Indian Constitution is not simply an abstract normative document, but an "inaugural postcolonial form" (Baxi 2010; see also Austin 1967). Baxi (2010) describes how the Indian Constitution performs a creative modification of the ideas of constitutionalism by combining the (sometimes contradictory) concerns of governance, social development, rights, and justice. The contradictions of the Indian Constitution, however, are not just a function of different normative impulses that might not easily coexist. (For instance, concerns with governance often justify egregious human rights violence by Indian police and security forces fighting insurgent or terrorist movements.) They are also a function of the multiplicity of constitutionalisms that Baxi argues come to inhabit the Indian Constitution over time. Baxi suggests that, since the drafting and adoption of the Indian Constitution, there have in fact been seven kinds of constitution, replacing or coexisting with one another.[60] Critically, Baxi suggests that the seventh incarnation, which defines India entirely in terms of global market interests, is "fully at odds" with previous ones. What one sees in the Gleevec case is not just a dialogue between different arms of the state, but also between different generational impulses and constitutional moments.

And second, constitutions must also be spatially situated. The very idea of the spirit of the Constitution demands a spatial attentiveness. When Justice Sridevan speaks of the Constitution whose spirit she wishes to uphold, she is speaking of a specific thing, of this Constitution, one which operates in this nation of India in order to provide a governing rationale and a set of directive obligations to the state. This is reflected in the critical line that she wrote in the Madras High Court verdict quoted earlier, which I reiterate here with a different set of emphases than before: "We have borne in mind the object which the Amending Act wanted to achieve, namely . . . to provide easy access to the citizens of *this country* to life saving drugs and to discharge their Constitutional obligation of providing good health care to *its citizens*."[61]

Just as a particular set of obligations is emphasized, and a particular idea and ideal of health assumed (one that is about healthiness, and not about generating surplus value for capital), so too is the nation-state as a jurisdictional and representative body of governance invoked;[62] and further, a specific nation-state, with its values and normative commitments, which in the case of the Indian Constitution have been enshrined most explicitly in its directive principles. Granville Austin (1967) has described the importance of these principles. He has argued that while "negative obligations," providing domains of protection for citizens from the power of the state and usually articulated in terms of rights, are inherent to most liberal democratic constitutions, the uniqueness of the Indian Constitution lies in its further attention to the state's "positive obligations" toward its citizens. These were written into the constitution as directive principles, which are not legally enforceable, but nonetheless provide an idealistic roadmap for the state to follow.

In discussing judicialization as a form of and space for politics in this chapter, I have described the ways in which the Gleevec case initially resolved, in an apparent purification, into technical and constitutional components; how the technical components remained unsettled and in some sense could not be settled without taking recourse to the constitutional; and how the constitutional components open up questions regarding what Sheila Jasanoff (2011) has called bioconstitutionalism, moments of resolution and adjudication that put both law and health/life at stake. While I have focused on judicial problematizations and resolutions of the technical and the constitutional—and in the process, upon the coproduction of the patent as something that is legally and scientifically determined—broader trajectories are at stake in this story.

First, there is the question of the movements of a product patent to India through the dictates of multilateral forums such as the WTO. This speaks to the nature of relationships between different scales and forms of governance, and more specifically the question of how global governance dictates or impacts national-state governance, or fails to do so. It might seem like the export of patent regimes is a purely technical matter, but in the Indian context it came to be rendered a constitutional one: not just in the narrow textual sense of homogenizing global agreements with the letter of the Indian law, but in the broader sense of forging and defining the contours and the terrain of the technical and the political in relation to which the product patent can operate in a given national-state context.[63] Second, this rendering of the apparently technical as constitutional has to do in part with the specific judicial and political cultures in India, and the ways in which these render and animate constitutional histories. But it also has to do with historical contexts of pharmaceutical development in India, the building of generic manufacturing capacity under an earlier process patent regime, and the particular ways in which that has more recently come to be inscribed within a global politics of access to essential medicines (see chapter 5). And third, there is a broader ideology that provides political traction and sanction to monopolistic product patent regimes through a valorization of innovation (but that also defines innovation in the rather narrow terms of making new drugs).[64] The trajectory of Indian judicialization interrupts these arguments, even as it opens up possibilities of interpretive legal innovation.

One way to ground a conceptualization of constitutionalism and judicialization is to specify it in terms of national histories and locations. Another way to do so is by asking how science comes to be lodged in the court (Jasanoff 1997). This question is not merely an institutional one, but is a broader conceptual question concerning epistemic authority. When the spirit of a constitution that emphasizes a right to health and distributive justice is deemed to have more authority than a patent claim, one is seeing the consolidation of certain modes of public reason over others.[65] Who has the institutional authority to make such determinations is a deeply political question, one that has fundamental stakes for democracy.

Within the structure of pharmaceutical crisis described in chapter 1, bioconstitutional moments play out in ways that constitute the state as a site for political struggle. Financialized, multinational pharmaceutical capital attempts to capture the state, but is opposed by (national and global) civil society, which itself forms strategic alliances with certain (in this case, Indian generic) corporate interests to keep the state accountable. The constitution of the political in relation to the Gleevec case is thus coproduced with the situating of cancer in India (or Korea, or Brazil) in different ways than those seen in Euro-America. Chapters 4 and 5 elaborate upon such politics by situating it in terms of the materialization of logics of capital in/as different capitalisms, resulting in a competition between the monopoly capitalism of the Euro-American R&D-driven pharmaceutical industry and the postcolonial nationalist free market capitalism of the Indian generic industry that itself comes to be less and less viable in post-TRIPS global market environments.

POSTSCRIPT: PHARMACO(LAW)GIC

The Indian Supreme Court verdict on Gleevec has provided a significant precedent for limiting the practice of pharmaceutical evergreening, one that certainly establishes interpretive room for maneuver within India's product patent regime, which could also have implications that extend beyond India.[66] But there is more at stake in this verdict than simply policy precedent. It is worth thinking about the court itself as an institutional site of democratic articulation. The particular mechanisms of such articulation—the very texture of legal argumentation that was employed, and the modes of interpretation of the patent (literal versus hermeneutic) that brought the different assumptions underlying invention to the fore—are worth paying attention to. And institutions such as the Supreme Court have their own aura, lending a certain kind of authority to verdicts, a gravitas borne of a self-conscious sense of justice being dispensed. It was clear for instance that the judges hearing the Gleevec case were aware of the precedential power that was vested within them. The length, detail, and explanatory reasoning of the verdict, and the insistence on wiping the slate clean and adjudicating all aspects of the issue (concerning both Sections 2(1)(j) and 3(d)) suggest that the justices knew that they were hearing a landmark case whose consequences would be felt over the long term and well beyond access to a single drug.

Is this form of judicialization, one that orients pharmaceutical politics toward socially just possibilities, in principle democratic? It is easy to be swept away by romanticism while considering a judicial intervention such as this. The emergence of the Indian Supreme Court as a bulwark against corporate capital is in stark contrast to recent decisions of the American Supreme Court such as Citizens United, which provide corporations with First Amendment rights to free speech as if they were people.[67] More generally, the Indian Supreme Court has taken on an activist role on a host of social justice issues, ranging from corruption to food distribution to women's rights, demanding that the state act to fulfill its representative obligations to its citizens. It is important to acknowledge the radical potential of such judicial intervention.

But it is equally important to think through its limits. At one level, these are the conceptual limits of the law itself, as the question of justice always exceeds formal legal adjudication and can never be entirely contained within it (Derrida 1992). But at another level, there are pragmatic, institutional, and political limits. Scholars have recognized that judicialization constitutes a complex terrain and site for politics and does not necessarily result in socially progressive outcomes. João Biehl and Adriana Petryna (2011) have shown, for instance, how the judicialization of pharmaceutical politics in Brazil serves as an instrument of pharmaceuticalization, whereby individual citizens make demands upon the state (in the context of nationalized health care) for drugs as a matter of entitlement. This puts burdens on the health system even as it often bypasses the authority of evidence-based medicine; the right to health operates as consumer demand upon the state, which then becomes the broker in procuring drugs for an ever more demanding citizenry that also emerges as a market for pharmaceutical companies. Jean and John Comaroff have pointed to the hyperlegal sphere of postcolonial politics that comes to operate in the judicialized context of South Africa, with consequences not just for promises of justice but also for state conceptions of crime and policing (Comaroff and Comaroff 2006). And Gautam Bhan (2009) has shown how the public interest litigation has served as an instrument to enforce evictions in Delhi, thereby serving simultaneously to uphold tenancy as a right even as it has acted in certain situations to displace people from their homes.[68]

Hence if the emancipatory potential of judicialized pharmaceutical politics comes to be obvious in situations such as the Gleevec case, then its democratic potential is more tenuous. At an empirical historical level, the story of the Indian judiciary is marked by failures as much as by stunning successes. The structure of judicial politics in India today sees the operation of activist higher courts that intervene substantially in the making of policy alongside virtually nonfunctional middle and lower courts that are often mired in corruption and inefficiency. In terms of political horizons, it is possible to imagine a judiciary that is not invested in the ideals of social justice, as witnessed in rulings such as the criminalization of homosexuality through the upholding of Section 377 of the Indian Penal Code, an article of the law that traces back to a colonial British statute enacted in 1860 that defines homosexuality as an "unnatural offense."[69]

The judiciary as an instrument of social justice is also a historically and generationally specific institution, reflective of a turn in this direction that occurred after the lifting of Indira Gandhi's state-imposed Emergency in the late 1970s

(Baxi 2010). There is no guarantee that it will always remain thus. Indeed, in the domain of access to essential medicines, one has seen moves to sensitize the Indian judiciary through programs that have involved teaching Indian judges the principles of intellectual property law. This has included programs facilitated by the U.S. embassy in Delhi in concert with industry lobby groups in India and the United States.[70] Judicial common sense is not static, and one could envision the pedagogical indoctrination of a new generation of Indian judges who are far more sympathetic to multinational corporate ideas and ideals of intellectual property than the current generation has been.[71]

The law itself, the courts themselves, cannot therefore be deemed just or unjust, democratic or not, in any absolute sense. What is significant is the particular way in which the Constitution came to be activated in the Gleevec case. An image that endures in my mind from the Supreme Court hearings is that of Anand Grover, representing the CPAA, arguing in court and walking around its halls during recess with a copy of the Indian Constitution tucked under his arm, his inseparable companion, resource, and recourse. A spirit of constitutionalism that depends upon an interpretive, nontechnocratic hermeneutics has emerged as a democratic counterweight to logics of multinational pharmaceutical capital.

CHAPTER FOUR

Philanthropic Values

Corporate Social Responsibility & Monopoly in the Pharmocracy

Monopoly and GIPAP

This chapter describes Novartis's philanthropic drug donation program for Gleevec, the Gleevec International Patient Assistance Program (GIPAP). Established in 2002, GIPAP is a mechanism to make Gleevec accessible to patients who cannot afford the drug. Since its inception, it has come to be operational in over eighty countries, and Novartis claims that it has helped over 60,000 patients through the program. I show how this ethical program is imbricated with Novartis's insistence on monopolistic protection for its drugs, which drove its extensive legal battles around Gleevec in India. I further argue that corporate philanthropy provides the justification for monopoly even as monopoly provides the conditions of possibility for philanthropy. This is a case of the multinational pharmaceutical industry projecting itself as an agent of humanitarian redemption while emphasizing the necessity of monopoly protections in order to do so. This articulates not just to politics of access to medicines but also to that of clinical trials and therapeutic care.

At the very start of the Supreme Court hearings on the Gleevec case, and periodically throughout, Justice Aftab Alam asked Novartis counsel a simple question that was never answered: why not just price the drug on the free market so that Indian patients could afford it, thereby avoiding extensive patent litigation altogether?[1] On the face of it, Novartis's insistence in fighting for its patent on Gleevec over an eight-year period while pricing the drug higher than the Indian market could bear indicates two things. First, the end game from the perspective of the multinational pharmaceutical industry is not the patent but monopoly. India's patent regime now affords the full protection of a product patent as mandated by TRIPS. What it does not allow as readily as especially the American patent regime is the unfettered expression of that patent as corporate monopoly. There is an insistence instead that patents should not operate in ways antithetical to the public interest. Second, the stakes for Novartis in this case are not so much the penetration of Indian markets as the protection of Western markets.[2]

Novartis's actions came to be seen as egregiously opposed to the public interest and manifested in advocacy against the company at the national and global levels throughout the duration of its legal entanglements in India. Much of this was initiated in 2006 and 2007, when Novartis was disputing the Gleevec patent denial in the Madras High Court. Such struggles involved patient advocacy and civil society groups involved in battles for access to essential medicines, but garnered a broader spectrum of civic and political attention because of Novartis's challenge at the time to the constitutionality of Section 3(d), which was seen as an attack on national legislative sovereignty by multinational corporate interests. The broadest oppositional advocacy was orchestrated by the Access to Medicines and Treatment Group of Médecins sans Frontières (MSF), which organized a Drop the Case campaign against Novartis (Access Campaign 2014). Opposition to Novartis was voiced from a range of quarters, including the South African Treatment Action Campaign, Archbishop Desmond Tutu, U.S. Congressman Henry Waxman, German Members of Parliament, and the Berne Declaration.[3] In India, a group of doctors called the All India Drug Action Network organized a boycott of Novartis and its products.

Perhaps the most telling critique came from Brian Druker of the Oregon Health and Science University, who was arguably the researcher most central to the discovery of imatinib's therapeutic properties against chronic myeloid leukemia (CML), and therefore one of the most important figures in the history of Gleevec's development as a drug (see chapter 3). Druker published an article in which he clearly expressed his concerns at Novartis's strategy, emphasizing the important role of the public sector in drug development and insisting that patents should not simply serve as tools of corporate monopoly. It is worth quoting extensively from Druker's piece:

Many scientists . . . are engaged in research primarily motivated by the pursuit of knowledge as a means to help patients. . . . It is therefore a matter of great concern that the results of these efforts can't reach patients and save lives because of pricing strategies and patent policies such as "patent evergreening" (minor changes to existing molecules designed to extend patent monopolies) used by partners further down the drug development process. . . . Imatinib has radically improved the success of treatment for [chronic myeloid leukemia] and patients treated with the medication can retain a high quality of life. The development of this drug is a journey in scientific discovery that highlights the collaborative and open process of innovation, where both the private and public sectors play an indispensable role. . . . In the late 1980s, I began collaborating with industry scientists at Ciba-Geigy (now Novartis Pharmaceuticals) who were developing inhibitors for the class of enzymes to which Bcr-abl belongs. Both the scientific community and the pharma industry were highly skeptical of the utility and selectivity of these enzyme inhibitors. Despite this, I suggested that the CML enzyme (Bcr-abl) would be an ideal target of therapy.

In 1993, I moved to Oregon Health and Science University in Portland and had a single goal of finding a company that had the best inhibitor of Bcr-abl and to bring it into clinical trials. My work in Oregon for CML was primarily funded by public sources. . . . My persistence with scientists at Ciba-Geigy (now Novartis) helped to keep the development of imatinib on their agenda despite uncertainty from product managers. . . . The approval of imatinib in May 2001 was the culmination of a 10-year project for me, something I had dreamed of since medical school.

However, the price at which imatinib has been offered for sale by Novartis around the world has caused me considerable discomfort. Pharmaceutical companies that have invested in the development of medicines should achieve a return on their investments. But that does not mean the abuse of these rights by excessive prices and seeking patents over minor changes to extend monopoly prices. This goes against the spirit of the patent system and is not justified given the vital investments made by the public sector over decades that make the discovery of these medicines possible. (Druker 2007a)

Purely from a public relations perspective then, Novartis's actions in India garnered it a reputation not that different from the one Monsanto had developed in the politics of agricultural biotechnology in the 1990s. My interest in this chapter lies in how Novartis in contrast aggressively defended its monopolistic practices as ethical. Conceptually, theirs followed a typical Schumpeterian line of argument: that monopoly leads to incentives to innovate, leading to public interest (Schumpeter 1942). But specifically, this ethical position was articulated through the company's charitable drug donation program for Gleevec, GIPAP, which was referenced throughout the drug's legal history in India.

To be eligible for GIPAP, a patient must meet medical and financial criteria. She must be diagnosed with CML or gastrointestinal stromal tumor (a rare stomach cancer for which Gleevec is also indicated); not be part of a reimbursement or insurance scheme; and be unable to afford the drug out of pocket. The Max Foundation, which is a U.S.-based nonprofit with offices around the world that is "dedicated to improving the lives of people with blood cancer and rare cancers," manages and administers GIPAP.[4] In India, the program is administered through relationships with key physicians who recommend patients (their own, as well as those recommended to them by other physicians in their region) to the foundation for enrollment in the program. The foundation manages the paperwork to ensure that the patient meets the criteria for enrollment, while Novartis provides the drug. Drug donation programs instituted by multinational pharmaceutical companies are not new, and Novartis itself has much larger drug donation programs for malaria and (through its generic arm Sandoz) tuberculosis. But GIPAP is probably the world's largest operational drug donation program for an anticancer drug.

I consider GIPAP at three registers. First, I trace its emergence as an important justification for monopoly as ethical in the legal history of Gleevec in India. This involves focusing not on the period from 2005 to 2013 that I have already discussed, but looking earlier, from 2002 to 2005. At this time, India did not have a functioning product patent regime, but did have provisions mandated under TRIPS for exclusive marketing rights (EMR) on drugs for which mailbox patent applications (i.e., patent applications made in anticipation of a product patent regime, which would be opened and considered subsequent to the institution of that new regime in 2005) had been filed. Novartis had filed for and obtained EMR on Gleevec in India in 2002, which itself led to legal and political controversy, as I describe below. Second, I consider the intricacies of GIPAP as it was instituted and practiced in India. This involves considering interactions between Novartis, the Max Foundation, physicians involved in administering the program, and generic manufacturers of imatinib mesylate. I do so by quoting extensively the perspective of one of the physicians involved with the program. And third, I describe some of the controversies that emerged around GIPAP in India and elsewhere. This elaborates the ways in which a political debate set up around the specific issue of access to essential medicines bleeds into broader questions of pharmaceutical politics, including around the relationship between experiment, diagnosis, and therapy.

I wish thus to consider the relationship between legal and political statements made in opposition to and in defense of monopoly, and the intricacies of practicing corporate philanthropic drug donation on the ground. What are the stakes of instituting policy positions regarding the extent and scope of monopoly allowed in pharmaceuticals (which is ultimately what the battle around Section 3(d) as it extended all the way to the Indian Supreme Court was about), given the necessarily more flexible ways in which these policy positions play out in terms of actually getting essential anticancer medications to patients who need them?

The Gleevec EMR Controversy

I begin with a discussion of issues that had already come up around Gleevec prior to the patent dispute, but which remained unresolved once India adopted its product patent regime in January 2005. In the period between 1995 and 2005, India still formally had a process patent regime, but, due to its obligations under TRIPS, needed to institute provisions that would facilitate a transition to a product patent regime. Two such provisions included the provision of mailbox facilities for filing patent applications and a provision for EMR, which would allow for market exclusivity on a drug even before a product patent regime could be instituted. Provisions for mailbox facility and EMR were provided through an amendment to the Patent Act in 1999.

Soon after Novartis developed Gleevec, ten Indian generic companies started manufacturing reverse-engineered versions of the drug. Novartis responded by applying for EMR on the drug and filing injunctions against these companies in the Madras and Bombay High Courts. While the Bombay High Court refused to grant an injunction against three companies, the Madras High Court did grant an injunction preventing seven companies from making the generic drug. Novartis itself was selling the drug at Rs. 120,000 per patient per month, which was up to thirty times more expensive than the price at which generic companies were selling their versions. Therefore, the Cancer Patients' Aid Association (CPAA), a patient group that procured the drug to distribute to patients at a subsidy, filed a writ petition in the Supreme Court of India in 2004. This writ petition challenged both the granting of EMR to Novartis for Gleevec and the very provisions of the 1999 amendment to the Patent Act that allowed for the granting of EMR. While the challenge was never adjudicated upon, since the 2005 Patent Act was passed in the meantime rendering the EMR null and void, the issues raised in CPAA's writ petition are worth outlining and analyzing. Equally worthwhile is an analysis of Novartis's counterpetition to the court, arguing against CPAA's petition.

The grounds of CPAA's petition were the right to health and equality enshrined in the Constitution of India. The basis of this framing was that if Novartis had the exclusive right to market Gleevec, then at its prohibitive price of Rs. 120,000 per patient per month, "the overwhelming majority of 24,000 patients that suffer from CML every year in India will die." A direct correlation was made by CPAA between unaffordable medicines and dying "a premature death."[5] The case had certain aspects that made the granting of EMR particularly pernicious from the perspective of the petitioners. Most important was that an EMR grantee could sue for infringement of its EMR, even if the drug for which EMR was granted was not valid for a patent and the patent was later denied. Gleevec, it was argued, was not a drug that was valid for a patent, since it was not novel but simply the modification of an existing substance (an assertion that was later proven correct). Yet it was granted EMR. This implied that EMR was purely monopolistic, without any basis in patent rights, and its purpose was purely for profit. According to CPAA, this monopoly was a constitutional violation of Article 21 of the Indian Constitution, which protects the right to life.

It is worth noting how CPAA foregrounded the question of rights as the basis of a politics of access to medicines, raising a tension between different kinds of rights, the right to life and intellectual property rights. The group was claiming that the right to life is an absolute right, and therefore trumps property rights, and was further claiming a subsumption of the right to health as automatically implied in an article of the Constitution that protects the right to life. It is precisely such an embodied idea of health, as healthiness, that I have argued gets abstracted when health gets appropriated by capital. What is at stake here is not just a contest between different kinds of rights, but the very definition of health that is implied depending on which right gets prioritized.

In order to prove that the high price of Gleevec affected the right to life, CPAA argued that 25,000 new CML cases per year in India are projected, of which about 18,000 die per year because they cannot even afford to pay Rs.

1,000 per month for the drug, which is the price at which CPAA was selling the drug to patients after procuring it from generic companies for Rs. 4,000. Hence, CPAA was suggesting that even if Gleevec was being sold by generics companies on the market at a competitive price, and even if that price was being further subsidized for patients by CPAA, still nearly three-fourths of patients suffering from the disease every year would die because the drug was too expensive for them. In a situation of monopoly pricing, the implications were obvious. Under these circumstances, CPAA argued that the Government of India was obliged to do one of two things—either invoke a compulsory license, or set the price for the drug. This is the point in its argument when CPAA turned to the state. At this point, it moved the battle beyond Novartis to the Indian state's duty to deliver on its constitutional obligations.[6]

Also, CPAA was making a more fundamental argument about intellectual property rights. It was suggesting that an EMR is an example of a pure monopoly, which goes far beyond the potentially monopolistic tendencies involved in upholding a patent regime. This forces us to consider the constitutive tension that exists between the public interest and monopolistic functions of patents. But it also forces us to think conceptually about both public interest and monopoly on their own terms. It is important to think about how monopoly is at odds with the free market and yet works as its exception. Monopolies, after all, are abjured by industries themselves, not just by opposition groups like CPAA or consumers. It is also a site where the state, in this case, aids the corporation through its active legal intervention, almost as a form of corporate protectionism. (In other instances, the state might well intervene to prevent a monopoly in the cause of the free market.) Further, in the logic of a monopolistic corporation, a monopoly need not be antithetical to the public interest.

Two kinds of legal provisions provided the basis for CPAA's arguments regarding the public interest. One was in terms of patents themselves. The CPAA petition highlighted the inherent dual character of the patent, as simultaneously existing in the cause of public interest and acting antithetically to it. This duality of the patent was both a crutch and a target for CPAA, simultaneously allowing for a contrast between a patent regime, which does have a kernel of public interest animating it at its heart, and EMR, which is purely monopolistic, while emphasizing the patent's own potentially monopolistic nature. And hence, the second kind of legal provision that the CPAA petition draws upon is in terms of public interest as opposed to the interests enshrined in intellectual property rights. Public interest therefore was argued for both in terms of, and against, patents.

The antinomy, of whether the patent is in the public interest or monopolistic, exists within the Indian Patent Act itself. Here, Chapter XVI, Section 83 of the act, which specifically brings in the notion of public interest, and points to public health as an exemplary case of public interest that should not be violated by a patent regime, was a crucial point of reference.[7] This section reflects the inherent tension of patent law. It is the user, here, who has to be given protection from the patentee (though the animating rationale for the patent is to protect the patentee from the user copying and disseminating an invention, thereby indirectly promoting public interest through providing an incentive for disclosure through such protection). It is the protection of the user, as a necessary condition for such disclosure to serve public interest, which is protected in these clauses. Once recognized and acceded to, however, the patentee's rights are in some sense absolute. It is the trimming of this absolute right that the law has to undertake through imposing limits, conditions, and cautions of different kinds.

It is in this context that arguments about the cost and availability of Gleevec compared to generic versions of the drug need to be situated, and in which the apparently simple opposition between public interest and monopoly has to be rendered in terms of the imperatives to be balanced and the double binds at stake. In its petition, CPAA pointed out that (at the time, in 2004) it had managed to procure generic imatinib mesylate and make it available to thirty CML patients. Even then, they had to turn away approximately 300 patients who had come to them for the medication. In other words, even the generic drug did not address the problem of affordability for many people who needed it. The CPAA petition pointed to some relevant figures in this regard. The generic drugs CPAA procured cost Rs. 90 per 100 mg capsule. Typically, the dosage of the drug involved taking four capsules a day, leading to a cost of about Rs. 360 per day.[8] Gleevec's cost was Rs. 1,000 per 100 mg capsule, which meant that what a patient who received a drug through CPAA would pay in an entire month for the generic drug would have to be paid for a single capsule of the patented medication (since CPAA was selling the procured generic drug to patients at a discounted price of Rs. 1,000 per month). With monopoly rights for Gleevec in place, CPAA's calculation was that 24,000 CML patients would die per year, leading to approximately 120,000 "preventable premature deaths" over the five-year period of EMR. This is the scale of the potential impact of a monopolistic legal regime on drug access, and the stakes from the perspective of patient activists.

In such a framing, one sees a particular resolution of a tension between public interest and monopoly rights resolving into matters of life and death.

The state acts as a biopolitical mediator, in Michel Foucault's words, "making live and letting die" ([1976] 1990, 135–161). But when left to itself, the monopolistic functions of intellectual property lead to what the CPAA petition refers to as "the relative deprivation of access to health between those *who can afford to live* and those *who cannot afford and die.*"[9] There is a stark poignancy to the fact that, in India today, *affordability* refers not just to consumer goods or luxuries, but to life itself.[10] One sees a set of stakes more severe than the technical ones that were at the heart of the patent adjudication as described in chapter 3. The framing of the issue in terms of public interest directs the argument explicitly toward the state. The CPAA petition showed that the state was violating its citizens' right to life in a twofold manner—by incorporating amendments that grant EMR on drugs to corporations and by then allowing those rights to be granted and exercised, and by not invoking compulsory licensing or price protection as a means to prevent the violations that could be perpetuated through an exercise of monopoly rights. In the process, battle lines were drawn not only between Indian pharmaceutical companies and Novartis, or patient groups and the multinationals endowed with EMR, but between Indian citizens and the Indian state.

It is instructive to look in contrast at Novartis's counterpetition, which was submitted on April 28, 2005. By this time, India had passed its new, WTO-compliant patent laws under the amended Patent Act of 2005. Hence, effectively, the EMR had become null and void. Novartis's counterpetition therefore is not a document that was adjudicated upon. But it is interesting for its arguments, which point both to the value logics that multinational pharmaceutical companies operate within, and to the strategic and tactical maneuvers that they adopt in order to counter civil society attempts to dispute their monopolies. In the process, the relationship between public interest and monopoly gets reframed, away from the opposition between the two depicted by CPAA, and toward a suggestion that monopoly might actually operate in the public interest.

At the heart of Novartis's response was the insistence that the suffering of cancer patients was "addressed proactively and on a larger scale" than anything CPAA has done through Novartis's drug donation program, GIPAP. The program opens up the question of corporate social responsibility as the idiom in which pharmaceutical companies think about drug access, thereby suggesting how the conceptual terrain of access to medicines is marked by an opposition between public interest–based demands and corporate social responsibility. It was claimed that GIPAP covered 98 percent of the patients who were given the drug.[11] In the process, Novartis claimed that 3,638 patients

TABLE 4.1. Comparison of Gleevec Sales versus GIPAP

	Sales	GIPAP
May–December 2002	Rs. 9.67 crore (Rs. 96.773 million)	Rs. 11.85 crore (Rs. 118.55 million)
January–December 2003	Rs. 11.98 crore (Rs. 118.87 million)	Rs. 72 crore (Rs. 720.04 million)
January–December 2004	Rs. 6.2 crore (Rs. 62 million)	Rs. 257.10 crore (Rs. 2,571.09 million)

had been helped by GIPAP in India, and more than 9,000 worldwide. In India alone, it was claimed that more than $76 million worth of Gleevec had been distributed for free. Novartis cited the following figures to justify its claims, comparing sales of Gleevec from 2002 to 2004 to the amount of drug distributed under GIPAP, thereby showing that in fact Novartis distributed more drug free than it sold (see table 4.1).

These figures suggest how complicated questions of drug access actually are even if one goes by numbers. It is worth paying attention here to Novartis's own wording: "The argument that the grant of the EMR has made the anti-cancer drug out of reach of the cancer patient would hold no ground at all. In India, under the GIPAP programme, 98% of the patients are given the drug free of cost and only 2% pay for the drug."[12]

This is a carefully worded, even somewhat disingenuous, statement because who the patients are is not specified. At first glance, it might appear that "the patients" refers to all patients with CML. In fact, however, it refers to all patients who are on Gleevec. Indeed, if 3,638 patients in India were being helped, then by Novartis's own figures, this could not constitute 98 percent of CML patients in the country, given that approximately 25,000 new CML cases are estimated to occur every year. On the one hand, therefore, Novartis appears to counter CPAA's claim about the lack of drug accessibility by stating that 98 percent of "the patients" are covered under GIPAP. But CPAA's claim is based on their estimated numbers of 25,000 new CML patients per year; Novartis's response is based on the much smaller percentage of patients who actually get prescribed Gleevec. On the other hand, assuming the veracity of Novartis's figures, the fact remains that the 3,638 patients that they had helped as of April 2005 was considerably larger than the 30 patients for whom CPAA had been able to afford to procure generic imatinib mesylate.

This is a basic facet of the complex terrain of drug access. If one is simply looking at how many patients are able to get access to the drug, then it is very likely that Novartis was able to make the drug as accessible (or more) to people in India as any other entity. This is partly because Novartis was not seeing India as a primary market for the drug; its stakes were in maintaining the price of the drug in India, so that it could protect that price in its more lucrative Western markets. In other words, logics of selling dictate against Novartis making Gleevec affordable in India. But logics of giving make it reasonable for the company to donate the drug free. In that sense, Novartis could afford to give away free drugs, because it was not going to make money off those patients anyway. Purely from the point of view of the accessibility of a single drug, for a single disease, a monopoly need not therefore deprive people of a drug, as long as the holder of the monopoly is well enough disposed to donate the drug to those who need it. Indeed, it is monopoly that allows Novartis to switch Gleevec out of a market economy, where differential pricing does not make sense, to a gift economy, where philanthropic donation does.

However, CPAA was not simply looking at the Gleevec question from the perspective of how many people get access to the drug. They were concerned about how many people could potentially access the drug relative to those who have the disease. By that count, even GIPAP only reaches a relatively small proportion of people who are actually suffering from the disease. Given the large number of people who are not reached either by GIPAP or by their own procuring mechanisms, CPAA's contention was that free market competition that ensures lower prices is a better mechanism to ensure wider access than a monopolistic regime. The crucial point to note here is that logically and empirically, a question of how one evaluates drug access comes to be at stake. If one evaluates drug access in terms of the number of people who received a drug free or at affordable cost for a given disease and under given sets of contingent conditions, then Novartis's claims are justifiable. If one evaluates drug access in terms either of the number of people who received a drug free or at an affordable cost relative to the number of people who have the disease, or in terms of the structural and policy conditions under which, in principle, drugs can be accessible to as wide a section of the population as possible, then CPAA's positions make sense.

While grounded in the specifics of the Gleevec issue, CPAA's arguments went beyond it. This is because they were arguing for general principles of policy against monopolistic regimes. In other words, Novartis in its counterpetition chose to respond to a broad claim about the principle of granting monopolies on essential drugs as if it were a specific argument about the accessibility of Gleevec alone. By doing so, the company managed an aggressive ethical position, contrasting its own philanthropic ventures to the actions of generic companies, which it claimed "helped very few patients on a philanthropic basis."[13]

I argue therefore that a certain kind of structural terrain gets set up through these debates, where free market competition on the one hand is opposed to a combination of monopoly and philanthropy on the other. Monopoly provides the conditions of possibility for philanthropy; yet at the same time, philanthropy is invoked as the ethical justification of a monopolistic regime. In the process, it might seem in either case that the market might come to look like an angel, the only question being which kind of market serves patient interests better. And yet, when we go back to CPAA's figures, we recognize that, regardless of whether we are talking about free market competition through generic companies or monopoly through Novartis, most patients who needed the drug could not afford it. In fact, therefore, the market, in either guise, does a very poor job of ensuring treatment in absolute terms. This is where CPAA's turn to the state becomes crucial.[14]

The GIPAP program was also used as a counter to CPAA's arguments that EMR violated the right to life as enshrined in Article 21 of the Indian Constitution. Novartis stated that EMR did not violate the right to life because "while maintaining a uniform international price to prevent movement of the drug out of India, the drug is available in plenty and free of cost to eligible patients."[15] However, Novartis ignored the fact that even if GIPAP allowed access to free drugs, it was not a part of EMR provisions, but external to it. It was Novartis's own provision, and not something that was required of an EMR holder. Further, though projected as a response to right-to-life arguments, GIPAP itself was not a right; it was a gift. It was not enforceable, and was only continued at Novartis's will and privilege. Hence, in considering questions of access, it is essential also to consider the questions of power that go with different modalities of access. Undoubtedly, GIPAP was generous; but it was also arbitrary. Indeed, Novartis threatened to stop enrolling new patients in GIPAP in countries that allowed generic manufacture of imatinib mesylate, a threat that was directed strongly against India. Suffice to say that the very condition of philanthropy such as GIPAP is the power to arbitrarily withdraw such philanthropy.

By opposing EMR through recourse to Article 21, CPAA had effectively set up a binary between (monopolistic) commodification and rights. Through Novartis's response, corporate social responsibility becomes a third leg, as an alternative to rights and as a public interest response that does not have to be opposed to commodification. In this way, corporate social responsibility functions as a neoliberal articulation of public good that can be entirely consonant with monopolistic commodification. What one sees in the EMR dispute, then, is the polarization of the debate into two different kinds of CSR—corporate social responsibility on the one hand, invoked by Novartis, and constitutional social responsibility on the other, invoked by CPAA. The former has emerged as central to the apparatus of neoliberal capital. The latter harkens back to the kind of social contract that was embedded in the welfare state ideal, but which has been thoroughly discredited, leaving the field open for corporate philanthropy. What this results in, then, is another kind of polarization—not just between monopoly and rights, but between a response to needs and demands for rights.[16]

Perspectives on GIPAP in Practice

In this section, I provide a physician's perspective on the operation of GIPAP. My attempt is not to set up an opposition between legal fictions as they emerged in the EMR dispute and the reality of practice. Rather, it is to shift the ethnographic scale of analysis. The issues that came up in the dispute, and in public positions taken around GIPAP, point to certain important policy and political stakes having to do with access to essential medicines. However, the physicians involved with GIPAP were the actual transacting agents involved in ensuring access to this particular essential medicine for their patients. This involved the articulation of institutional and personal relationships not just with Novartis, but also with the Max Foundation and with Indian companies making generic versions of the drug. And, as I will show, it opened up aspects of health care that go beyond the provision of a pharmaceutical product for the treatment of disease, articulating broader questions of cancer epidemiology, public health, and clinical experimentation.

I preface this account with three points. The first is a simple contradiction— which is that GIPAP continues to exist in India at all. As described, GIPAP was instituted in India in 2002, at the same time as it was globally; but Novartis threatened to stop further enrollment in the program if India allowed the marketing of generic versions of Gleevec. The publicly stated position on eligibility criteria for GIPAP is clear: "Patients must be in developing countries that have minimal reimbursement capabilities where regulatory approval or at least an import license for Glivec for CML/GIST has been obtained; and *where no generic versions of imatinib are available*."[17] Indeed, in the period between 2002 and 2005, when the controversy around the grant of EMR was ongoing, it had seemed as if GIPAP would be discontinued in India; but since then, the program has continued.

The second concerns the implications of having access to the drug, whether Gleevec or the generic versions. The political debate around access to Gleevec, as already mentioned, has been framed in the stark terms of life and death—and to those CML patients who might have been able to access the drug but for its cost, those are indeed the stakes of the matter. Once the patient is on the drug however, the cancer becomes a chronic disease that can be pharmaceutically managed—a transition similar to that seen in the case of HIV-AIDS once antiretroviral therapy made it a manageable disease. This potentially raises a host of subsequent issues that are different from those that emerge in the initial framings of access politics. For instance, Julie Livingston (2012) has discussed the cancer epidemic in southern Africa that is consequent to the success of antiretrovirals, which has led to people living with AIDS rather than dying from it, but also living long enough to manifest cancer as a secondary or subsequent disease. The subsequent issues having to do with living on Gleevec involve providing the infrastructure for long-term, proper therapeutic compliance; dealing with the development of resistance to the drug, which has been seen in an increasing number of cases; and doing research that can provide a better understanding of both epidemiological outcomes of patients on the drug and the underlying biology of response (and resistance) to the drug. Physicians are not just brokers involved in making the drug accessible to patients; they are also crucial actors involved in the long-term care of (and occasionally research upon) patients. A politics that seems restricted to questions of access in its legal and policy framing in fact concerns multiple other dimensions of research, experimentation, infrastructure, logistics, and care.

And therefore third—my own stakes in this account are not to get to the bottom of how GIPAP operates, but rather to provide a situated perspective of how the politics of access and care looks to physicians involved in the program. The reality of GIPAP is complicated—as already suggested, the publicly available information on the program is not necessarily reflective of the complexities of its practical implementation. Also, GIPAP has had its own share of controversy, including in India, as I describe in the next section. And it has been difficult for me to get access to the institutions most directly involved in the administration of GIPAP, the Max Foundation and Novartis. I did write to Viji Venkatesh, who is in charge of coordinating GIPAP for the Max Foundation in India. I got a response, not from her but from the Corporate Communications division of Novartis India, enquiring after my interest in GIPAP. I responded indicating my desire to learn more about it from the company's perspective, but never heard back. I also contacted the Corporate Communications division of Novartis at its global headquarters in Basel regarding my interest in GIPAP, but did not receive a response there either. I talked to a few of the physicians involved with GIPAP in India, and the general sentiment about the program was positive.

The interview that I quote extensively here is with Raghunada Rao, a hematologist at the Nizam Institute of Medical Sciences, Hyderabad. Rao was willing to discuss GIPAP with me in a taped interview. He was one of the physicians involved in GIPAP from the beginning of its rollout in India. Rao was involved not just with recommending his own patients for enrollment in the program, but also with responding to and medically evaluating requests from other physicians in the region who might have eligible patients. He was involved with the Max Foundation even before Gleevec was approved for market in the United States, and had positive experiences with GIPAP. But he has also worked closely with generic manufacturers of imatinib mesylate. I provide some of his perspectives at length. It is worth remembering that this is a conversation from 2010—hence long after the initial battles between CPAA and Novartis over EMR, but before the final Supreme Court verdict on the patentability of Gleevec. His perspectives therefore speak to a nearly decade-long involvement with both Gleevec and generic imatinib mesylate, and a similarly long association with GIPAP.[18]

Rao's background in the treatment of CML:

I started treating CML way back in 1990. I joined Tata Memorial Hospital, and at that time what we had for treatment of CML was purely hydroxyurea. In 1992, interferon became a craze. Interferon was established as the treatment of choice because it did make a difference in . . . the first drug to show that you can probably in a small percentage of patients achieve a molecular remission, although in a larger percentage you can achieve a cytogenetic remission. So we used interferon extensively and then I did lots of interferon studies here, both with the normal interferon and the pegylated interferon.

Rao's early involvement with Gleevec:

The imatinib trial was not done in India. The nearest trial center for us was Singapore. So some of my patients went to Singapore, some went straight to M.D. Anderson Cancer Center. They participated there—those who could buy a ticket. And very peculiarly for that trial, in those countries, only the citizens of those countries were eligible for full reimbursement of the investigative workup and the stay. So all other foreign, I mean, entrants into this study were denied that. But they were given the drug free. So in about [a] couple of years the drug got approval and so I did continue, I made an argument and plea to Novartis at that time that all patients who were on that trial should be given lifetime free drug. So I still have patients from the original trial taking the drug with me. And when imatinib itself was launched in India by several, by Novartis for a long time, [a] majority of my patients went on the GIPAP program.

Rao's dealings with Novartis, however, must be situated alongside his encounter with generics, which is imbricated within a politics of access to essential medicines, but also in relation to a postcolonial nationalist position:

India as you know had both a process patent as well as a product patent initially. So [a] very good number of generics were launched with minor tweaking of the process, and you could file a patent and market the drug. So that was not a problem. At about the same time, what was a major concern amongst politicians, social groups, and patient activists as well as the medical world was the nonavailability of antiretroviral drugs. India became aware that it is at the epicenter of the AIDS epidemic. My state, Andhra Pradesh state, as you know, has the dubious distinction of having been one of the first, highest reported state[s] for AIDS. So the AIDS activists wanted selective permission to manufacture antiretroviral therapy in India, and they were highly successful in convincing the politicians that yes, this is possible.

At about the same time, I became aware that Shantha Biotechnics had manufactured hepatitis B vaccine for 25 cents and wanted to market it for $1 a dose in the world market for WHO-sponsored vaccination programs in the Third World countries. I supported that move very well. So, I became associated with Mr. Varaprasad Reddy, who was the chairman and managing director of Shantha Biotechnic, to lead the campaign of educating doctors that, yes indeed, this is a good vaccine. So we did a very successful campaign for hepatitis B. I used to go for lots of camps along with the gastroenterologists who lead Shantha Biotechnic camp. At that time of course, Bharat Biotechnic launched its own biotech kit, launched its own hepatitis B. So that was my interest in getting drugs into the country, which were absolutely essential for the health of its millions. And I felt, yes, it was justifiable to probably infringe, to tweak the agreement to provide drugs for our own people.

This was a politics that bled into Rao's early interactions with Novartis as well, especially in relation to their early strategies to combat generic versions of imatinib mesylate:

RR: So imatinib as you know was launched in India as a generic. There was a lot of campaign against it by the multinational[s]. The typical campaign is usually in that it's poor quality or its ineffectiveness. Then storage, transportation, things like that, lack of clinical trials and all that. So the same campaign was launched by Novartis in India. So I used to vehemently oppose them when they met me, that this is not the way to campaign for your drug. We should talk about your drug and you promote your drug, not decry other drugs. Because, that is, under the Monopolies and Restrictive Trade Practices Act, this is an unfair trade practice. You cannot talk about another drug. It is like Election Commission declaration or diktat, which says that you can promote your own party, [but] you can't talk ill of the next party. So I brought this to the notice of the Drug Controller [General of India, the authority that regulates drug approval and marketing in the country].

KSR: What was the basis of the Novartis argument against the generic?

RR: That it is a copy of its own drug and that they have infringed the copyright [*sic*: patent] law.

KSR: Were they making quality arguments also?

RR: They did make quality arguments, but they stopped the quality arguments within about six months. They didn't make any printed material, but they did tell their field force to argue against the generics. Fortunately for me, I did know all the Novartis field force, and did counsel them that it is not right on your part to talk about the generic. You might be working for a multinational company but you are still an Indian, and you should look at the scope of a drug being made available. Of course, they countered it by saying there is a GIPAP program available, and hence the GIPAP program is in place, and so you should not promote any generic drug at all.

Novartis's strategy and tactics also involved getting Gleevec into the Public Distribution System for drugs. While India does not have a nationalized health scheme for therapeutic access for the larger population, it does have a substantial scheme (the Central Government Health Scheme) for employees of the government:

> So the argument was countered by the fact that you are not promoting, just giving the drug free, but you are politically lobbying at the level of the central and the state government to buy only your drug for its distribution. That means for hospital distribution, for dispensary distribution, they persuaded the Central Government Health Services, and the Defense and whatnot to make huge purchases. Which I said is counterproductive. That means you are asking the taxpayers' money to be used for purchasing one dose of a drug where you can benefit ten people if you buy a local brand. So I used to counter it like that. So it is not correct on your part. And finally, the Central Government did see reason. So, a couple of years later, it did promote the generic brands, and now only the generic brand is permitted in the Central Government Health Services dispensaries. It's no longer promoting the Novartis brand.

Meanwhile, Novartis was working on refining its criteria for GIPAP in order to make it optimally functional to serve its stated goals:

> It modified the GIPAP program. There were several patients enrolled onto the program who came in Rolls Royce, very expensive cars in metropolitan cities. Not in Hyderabad, but perhaps in Delhi, as has been reported by their own dispensing agents. That these patients are probably filthy rich and they can afford the drug, to buy the drug, and they should not be provided [it]. So two years back, the financial assessment and recommendation became split. The recommendation is now being made by the physician, but the financial assessment for eligibility is made by an independent financial assessment group which Novartis has employed all over the country. So that is where it stands. So I still have a large number of patients on both generic and the innovator molecule. Both are equally effective.

The procedure for enrollment in GIPAP was as follows:

> I will enroll them online. The financial aspect has to be taken care of; that's not my job. It's an independent organization. Then the patient gets a phone call after his credentials are verified from a person who speaks the patient's own language, all of whom are volunteers from the Max station. They may be anywhere in the country, but they will evalu-

ate using the web. Some of them are former patients. Some of them are physicians' sons. So they will approve, and they ask the patient to come and visit the center three days after the phone call. Because the drug has to be physically lifted from Bombay to the local area. And we can transfer patients between centers anywhere in the country. We can also get the delivery to be done to the nearest Novartis depot. All of them need not come to Hyderabad. If they want to collect from Cuttack, Berhampur, Vishakapatnam, Vijayawada—wherever this is a Novartis depot, yes they can collect the drug from there. If there's another physician caring for the patient, that physician will continue caring; I won't take away his patient. I will only continue approval based upon the report submitted by that physician. So it's an online, instantaneous approval for renewal. Renewing the prescription is a physician's prerogative.

Once there is a death, we report the death. We have to report two causalities, drug or disease. Ninety-eight percent of the time it is disease related, there is a progressive disease. So we sign them off, saying they died because of progressive disease.[19]

Therefore, Rao's position with respect to GIPAP is more pragmatic than the polar positions adopted by Novartis or its opponents, whether in the EMR controversy or in Gleevec's subsequent legal history. He expressed ambivalence toward some of Novartis's marketing tactics, and unequivocally supported the importance of generic competition as a means of providing access to essential medications to the Indian population. But he also had a relatively smooth experience with GIPAP per se, in terms of the mechanics of its operation; and with Novartis, who for the most part responded positively and without excessive reluctance or bureaucracy whenever Rao recommended patients for the program to them: "One good thing about Novartis is, Novartis knows where I work. So, I work in a place where people can't have one square meal a day. So they don't trouble me for prescriptions or . . . they don't trouble me. They know I don't see patients who can afford the drug. Simple. I live at the foothill, not at the top of the hill."

Not everyone's experience with GIPAP has been so positive. Purvish Parikh, another GIPAP physician based at the Tata Memorial Hospital in Mumbai, filed an affidavit in the Madras High Court as the patent case was being heard, pointing to some of the difficulties he had with GIPAP in its early years, especially as Novartis reevaluated its decision to continue enrolling patients in the program given the existence of generic competition.[20] Parikh's affidavit was not central to the legal trajectory of Gleevec as I described it in chapter 3, since it did not concern the patentability of the drug. But it is an important document in providing an equivocal physician experience of GIPAP. Parikh pointed out that until the time of his affidavit (2006), the Max Foundation had rejected eleven of the patients that he had referred to the GIPAP program even though all of them were too poor to afford the drug, a contrast to Rao's more positive experience. But the real uncertainty around the program was in 2003, when doubts existed about its continuation. It is worth quoting the trajectory of events at this time, as recounted by Parikh in his submission to the court:

> Apparently in May 2003, Novartis had modified GIPAP and had stopped accepting new patients. On 24.12.2003 I received an e-mail from Novartis India . . . informing me that Novartis had been granted the Exclusive Marketing Right for Glivec and that they were now changing their program and were restarting to accept new patients, including those enrolled in other generic imatinib patient assistance programs. The letter also confirmed that pursuant to the launch of generic imatinib mesylate brands in the Indian market, the scope of GIPAP had been modified in May 2003 to stop accepting new patients. However, they changed that after getting the EMR on the drug.[21]

I asked Rao about this, and his response was more positive. In addition to providing the drug, the company also provided infrastructural support to ensure that the program was functional in ensuring the drug would reach intended patients:

> KSR: So did Novartis . . . what happened around 2003? Did they actually stop enrolling patients in GIPAP?
>
> RR: They said, as long as the drug is not within the reach of [the] common man, we will support [it]. So we had a meeting in Madras. The big man who saw imatinib through its launch, who has now moved on from being vice president, international vice president, to become one of their board of directors, he flew in by a private jet from Geneva to Madras, and he promised that he will continue providing the drug. We requested for three more forms of assistance. One was with the investigative work-up and response evaluation. Second one was to make the drug available at the doorstep. That means, could you ensure delivery to the home? Then the patient doesn't have to come here. Third was transportation assistance. So we requested three forms of assistance. So he agreed for all three forms.

As you know, Novartis [actually Sandoz, Novartis's generic division] has a program in antitubercular drugs which is ten times the size of GIPAP. Because there are ten times more tuberculosis patients in India. In that, they use a courier system to deliver the drug home. They use . . . I forgot—they are called barefoot representatives. They locally employ youth, give them a bicycle and a mobile phone sim card. And for each delivery they make, if I remember right, they pay 90 rupees or something like that. So it's an income generation for the village youth, unemployed youth, and at the same time the compliance of the patient is assured. They can't come to the center to collect the drug; the drug is delivered to their home. So they promised that they will use the same schema for the Gleevec patients also. So that was readily agreed, since they already have something in place. But I'm not so sure about the investigative part because that's pretty expensive compared to the transportation cost, which may not be very expensive.

KSR: So even when the generics came into . . .

RR: They did not withdraw any support.

KSR: Didn't withdraw any support and didn't stop enrolling any patients?

RR: Initially we thought it might happen, but Max Foundation as well as Novartis have agreed that they would not. So we were hearing about these budgeting plans. He did say that the global demand on the free drug assistance has shot his expectation by a hundredfold by the budgeting he has done, but that Novartis is ready to support hundredfold more patients. They now have 35,000 patients 'round the world. So he is ready to absorb up to 70,000 to 80,000 patients without any problem. So that is looking for one more decade of, if the incidence remains the same, so, which we believe is not going to be changing. So in another decade we'll have another 35,000 patients.

KSR: That's interesting because even on Novartis's own website they claim that they were going to discontinue GIPAP in countries where generic versions are available.

RR: Yeah, yeah, but that never happened.

However, GIPAP is not Rao's first recourse, which is always to prescribe generic versions of imatinib mesylate unless the patient absolutely requires the free program. This means that almost every one of Rao's patients who is prescribed Novartis's drug gets it free through GIPAP:

RR: I don't offer it to patients. I will prescribe the medication to all patients, the generic medication to all patients. That is our standard practice. We do not offer the program to patients. We don't solicit patients. So only if the patient complains that he cannot any longer afford the drug or he cannot purchase even the first drug, or he has been evaluated by a physician anywhere in this or adjacent states and is recommended to us, then only we will put the patients on the program. We will not offer any patient—it's just like doing a clinical trial. We don't offer a patient a clinical trial unless the patient wants to enroll. So it is not our intention to say we will give the drug free to every patient. No, we don't. So we will always prescribe the generic drug. They are free to choose the brand they want. Or we will suggest what the priced brands are like. If they continue taking the drug, we have no problem. The moment they say I have run out of money, I don't have any further reimbursement, my lifetime reimbursement is over, or I have not been reimbursed by the state or my employer, but I would like your help in taking the drug, then we will enroll them onto the program. We don't offer the program as the patient walks in. That is taboo.

KSR: So there isn't a single person who is paying for the Novartis drug then? Either they pay for the generic versions, or . . . ?

RR: Only the third-party payment fellows are still taking. So patients who are on a reimbursement, or are supplied drug from other dispensaries where the product is approved, yes they take. That is 1 percent of my patients.

Contrary to Novartis's assertions, however, generics companies have also helped CML patients on a philanthropic basis (a point also referred to by Parikh in his affidavit). This help was not programmatically enshrined in the manner of GIPAP, and was often a response to individual requests from the physician:

KSR: But if they can't afford a drug, could you just ask a generic company to provide it?

RR: Yes, we do ask them. We ask Natco, if they have been on Veenat. I will just directly call up. So if the patient says I can probably afford half, if the drug was given at half the price, I'll make a request, can you give it at half the price? The patient says I can buy it at one-tenth the price, I'll make a request, can you supply at one-tenth the price? So I will fill out a form, give it to their field staff, who will collect it from me, and collect the drug from their depot. So the patient pays one-tenth the price, but collects the entire month's supply. If even that's not possible, I will ask Natco, can you give the drug free? I will ask Reddy's, can you give?

Natco has been offering a free program if the physician recommends it. So do all the other Indian manufacturing companies. Yes, together, they all have a sizeable number of patients which will be equivalent to the GIPAP program. So together, they probably have as many patients off the GIPAP program on other free assistance programs as you have. Did they offer [a] patient unconditional free drug? Yes, they did offer. They didn't ask the patient to buy two months of drug, I'll give you free, or you pay me half, I'll give you half free. No. So dependent on the physician's recommendation, they either accepted in toto or said no. They have never so far said no. None of the pharmaceutical companies in India have ever refused to give the imatinib free for any patient recommended by a physician. It has not been questioned as to what your intentions are of putting this patient on the free assistance program. They've never questioned anyone.

In 2004, the CPAA petition against EMR on Gleevec had pointed to the stark stakes of being able to access Gleevec or not, as a matter of life and death. In practice, over the subsequent six years, Rao's experience with providing access was less stark. Undoubtedly, this was facilitated by the continued presence of a generic market in imatinib mesylate. But it has also been enabled by Novartis's continuation of GIPAP in spite of earlier threats to the contrary. Indeed, for many of Rao's patients, philanthropic donation or at least considerable subsidy of the drug was necessary, even by generics providers. In terms of the practice of providing access then, Novartis's actions over a period of time have contrasted with the negative reputation they have garnered as the legal history of Gleevec played out in India.[22]

Nonetheless, Novartis's brinkmanship over the continuation of the program in 2003 justifies some of the negativity directed their way. Parikh's affidavit provides a sense of what was at stake in 2003–2004 in ways that corroborate CPAA's EMR petition:

At that time [2003] many of my patients were taking generic forms of imatinib mesylate. Luckily, not many of them had to stop the same, as some of the generic companies were allowed to continue to manufacture and sell the drug in India due to the order of the Bombay High Court [which refused to grant an injunction against three generics companies as demanded by Novartis under its EMR, and therefore allowed them to continue making the drug even as the Madras High Court forced seven other generics companies to stop doing so]. I say that if all the generic companies were made to stop manufacturing and selling the drug in India, a lot of my patients would have been forced to stop taking the drug, as Glivec is not affordable to the masses . . . based on the fact that about 11 of my patients have been denied the drug [through GIPAP]. Some of my patients would also have died as a result of such an eventuality.[23]

And further:

On 6.9.2004 I wrote a letter to Mr. Ranjit Sahani, the Vice Chairman and Managing Director of Novartis India Ltd. . . . , informing him that dozens of our patients had to stop treatment after the generics went out of market. I also informed him that a lot of poor workers . . . were refused assistance under the GIPAP program. They were poor persons earning a measly sum of income . . . and GIPAP . . . turned their back on them.[24]

The accounts of Rao and Parikh suggest mixed physician experiences with GIPAP, with some having smoother interactions with the program than others, at different periods of time. But it is important to remember that there is more at stake in health care than access to a drug. The stakes of access are often high when an essential medicine such as Gleevec, which is far better than the current standard of care for a particular disease, is in question. But pharmaceuticalization alone is hardly ever sufficient even to provide adequate treatment. Rao's real problems in treating CML patients in a post-Gleevec world, even when GIPAP was functioning smoothly, had to do with infrastructure on the one hand, and knowledge on the other. The former issues largely had to do with patient compliance problems resulting from logistical issues (hence Rao's insistence that Novartis implement mechanisms to deliver the drug to patients at their doorstep rather than requiring them to come to hospitals to collect it) but also from Gleevec's success as an anticancer therapeutic:

What we have realized is, logistics is still an issue. Patients do not want to come to the hospital even four times a year. Once in three months, we are giving the drug worth 3.6 lakhs on the GIPAP program, once in three months. But they still don't want to come to the center to collect. They just don't have enough money, or road or a rail connection which they can afford. They don't have money to travel in a city, stay one day for a blood test, collect the drug the next day and go home. So the default rate is surprisingly not low, it is quite high. So the default rate is as high as 15 to 20 percent even when the drug is given free. Poverty is the biggest problem in getting people here. In fact, [a] ticket from the railway station to the bus stand to here is costlier than the train ticket [to get to Hyderabad from surrounding rural areas]. Because you need to come by an auto, very expensive. Poverty, illiteracy, these are the issues.

So, this could be not just logistics and poverty; it could be a false sense of security which they get as soon as they take the drug. Because as soon as you start the drug, in about three months' time, all signs and symptoms of the disease disappear, and [the] patient feels that [he] is unnecessarily continuing the drug for nothing. So the same compliance problems, what you see in diabetes, hypertension, heart disease, or any chronic, other chronic illness, you will find in this disease also.

The problems concerning knowledge link questions of therapeutic access to those of epidemiology and experiment. While research and safety and efficacy tests on Gleevec were done in other countries, very little is known about the particular mechanisms of drug response and drug resistance in Indian populations. This involves monitoring patients to study the rate and nature of molecular and cellular remissions in response to the drug, for which tests are available but not covered under GIPAP. It also involves conducting molecular and clinical experiments to understand incidence and mechanisms of drug response and resistance. Gleevec is an example of a therapeutic molecule that has been derived from an understanding of cellular and molecular mechanism; but in a research resource-poor environment, even when the drug is made available and accessible, one is faced with the problem of therapy without adequate capacities to monitor patients and develop an understanding of local population and environment-based specificities that may be of importance in optimizing treatment outcomes. Rao therefore contrasted the positive "humanitarian" impact of GIPAP to its negligible "scientific impact":

Supplying the free drug, did it make an impact or did it not make an impact? Disappointed to say it did not make a real scientific impact. It may have done on a humanitarian basis. [Patients] do not have the money to do the monitoring investigations which are now highly recommended, at least to know whether they are in hematological remission, whether they are in cytogenetic remission, and of course whether they are in molecular remission. So all three are of an increasing expense to the patient. A hematological remission in a hospital like this would cost about six hundred bucks; a cytogenetic remission establishment would cost an additional eight hundred bucks, so sixteen hundred bucks [*sic*] together. But the molecular remission establishment is still very high. It will be between four and five thousand bucks for a patient. So [the] majority of them cannot afford it. So although we are giving the drug free to a large number of our patients, not more than 10 percent of our patients can actually afford to get themselves monitored for the effectiveness of the drug.

Any support that Rao has received for monitoring his patients has in fact not come from Novartis, but from other companies, including generics companies such as Natco:

> RR: I do get a lot of support for investigations from Natco. In fact, Novartis doesn't support any investigative work-up. But for mutation analysis, I get from Natco. Prior to Natco, I did lot of work with a company called Onconova, which just supported chronic myeloid leukemia work for couple of my PhD students who were registered with the Osmania University. So, we had a collaborator in the University of Hyderabad, while the center was supported from the U.S. from a group from Onconova, again a group fully of Indian scientists, which had some compounds which might in future have some use in drug resistance in chronic myeloid leukemia. So far we have not used any drugs, did not do any clinical trial in chronic myeloid leukemia. But they did support our work in mutation analysis. We discovered twenty-three new mutations, but we still don't know the significance of them. So we need to find out whether they are drug-resistant mutations, or mutations in the general population in this part of the world. So, is it a nonsense mutation, or a missense mutation, or does it make really sense, to imatinib? So, they are willing to support that part of the work also.
>
> So we would be able to clone the gene, put it into a cell, see whether it confers a drug resistance. That is one part, for imatinib. Second is identifying this in normal human beings, whether such mutation exists in *Bcr* in its native form or *abl* in its native form, on the 9 and 22 chromosomes. So whether they already exist, these mutations are population-based abnormalities, so which are inherited, so they are of no consequence to response to the drug. So that is still pending.

KSR: So this kind of research, Novartis doesn't support?

RR: No, it doesn't support any research. Novartis by itself does not have any clinical research group in India, or basic research group in India. So it doesn't do any clinical trials in India. It did not do any clinical trial for CML in India for this or subsequent compound, or for GIST, gastrointestinal stromal tumor—that is the tumor for which they have a large number of patients. So almost all of it is supported by Indian pharma.

Therefore under GIPAP, one sees a situation of access without the necessary experiments that would build a knowledge base of public health significance in the Indian context. Contrast to this chapter 2 concerning the HPV vaccine studies in India. These involved clinical experimentation in the cause of access, an attempt to incorporate vaccines that protect against HPV infection, and thereby cervical cancer, into India's national immunization program. However, this was done in the absence of adequate epidemiological data on cervical cancer in India. Hence, the vaccines themselves were seen as a purely pharmaceutical intervention into a disease problem whose contours were not adequately established epidemiologically; but this intervention required experimental subjection to the vaccine. It was, however, an experiment that was not designed to fill the gaps in the epidemiological knowledge base regarding cervical cancer, leading to a cycle of increasing pharmaceuticalization and experimentation without building the epidemiological evidence base that would justify either. This shows the complex, deeply situated relationships in practice between the politics of clinical research and access to medicines.

Some of these relationships manifested in the case of GIPAP as well, in spite of the fact that Novartis had not conducted clinical trials or invested in research on Gleevec in India. The company did however wish to build a database using GIPAP, which emerged as a source of controversy, as I describe next.

Controversies and Political Stakes

In his affidavit to the Madras High Court, Dr. Purvesh Parikh alleged that Novartis was using GIPAP as a means of postmarketing surveillance of the effects of the drug. Raghunada Rao had underscored to me the epidemiological importance of understanding drug effectiveness and outcomes, but was himself of the firm conviction that such studies were ethical only if conducted through public clinical research programs with proper institutional review, not if they were proprietary studies done without such oversight for corporate ends. He described his experience with Novartis's patient data collection to me as follows:

> Novartis wanted to start a database in India, which I, along with lots of other Indian physicians, opposed. Because one of the dictums on the informed consent form of participation cites when going on the GIPAP program is that no part of his data—not just personal identification, but his clinical data, his laboratory data—will *ever* be used by Novartis for *any* purpose. Either improving their marketing, or improving their biology, or science or . . . anything. So I vehemently opposed collection of data of patients on the GIPAP program because it is unethical and illegal. And because Novartis has signed an agreement with individual GIPAP physicians, and the patients sign an agreement saying that it will not use this data in *any* purpose related to *any* activity of Novartis. It specifically states that Novartis will not ask for any data.
>
> It still did establish a CML registry in India. I'm not part of it. There are physicians who are part of it, with whom I could not get in contact to convince them that what they are doing is totally illegal and you should not collect data because you have signed an agreement which says you will not part with this data to anybody. Except if you want to make a publication yourself and you have an ethics committee clearance, you can do it. But it is still collecting data. I am aware of that.
>
> This data is used for profiling Indian patients, for collecting their epidemiologic data, for collecting the incidence data, for collecting the response data at all three levels, i.e., hematologic remission, cytogenetic remission, molecular remission; relapse patterns, mutation analysis, everything they are collecting. Which is not justified to be done. Well, that is my viewpoint. I had a year argument with them—I did not agree. And nobody came back to me again to ask for the data.

Parikh described these data collection activities at length in his affidavit. Like Rao, he referred to these practices as "unethical and illegal." But he focused not just on the question of research or data collection practices, but also on institutional questions, specifically the nature of the relationship between the Max Foundation, which was administering GIPAP, and Novartis, which was providing the drug. Parikh insisted that if this was a corporate drug donation program, then Novartis's role should simply be donating the drug: beyond that, any kind of interaction with patients or their data needed to be the sole prerogative of the Max Foundation. Yet he found that institutional separation between the two organizations was lacking. It is worth quoting at length from Parikh's affidavit to describe the nature of his ethical and institutional concerns:

> In or around August 2002 I wrote a letter . . . to Novartis India Ltd., seeking clarifications on contradictory statements about Ms. Viji Venkatesh who was introduced as representing Max Station, India, as part of Max Foundation. However, in a letter dated 31.08.2002, it was stated that she was part of Novartis India Ltd. and her designation was GIPAP Consultant. I say that I was informed that Max Foundation and Novartis were separate and that they would be following strict ethical guidelines and confidentiality of the patients will be maintained. However, Viji Venkatesh appeared to be employed by Novartis and was working as a Consultant with Max Foundation, which would have compromised patient confidentiality [and] become unethical.[25]

My attempt here is not to cast personal aspersions on Venkatesh, who by all accounts has been a crusading advocate for and supporter of cancer patients in India, but rather to ask about the nature of institutional relationships between global patient advocacy groups and multinational pharmaceutical companies. (Recall that when I wrote to Venkatesh about GIPAP, I received a response from Novartis.) Organizations like the Max Foundation play important roles as brokers in global therapeutic economies, and acquire ethical legitimacy by virtue of being brokers for patients and their treatment and care. If in fact they are also acting as brokers for corporate interests, then questions of accountability, responsibility, and conflict of interest must be asked. Parikh proceeded to ask them as he elaborated upon his concerns:

> On 2.12.2003 I received an e-mail . . . from Mr. Tyagi of Novartis India. The e-mail stated that Max Foundation had informed him that GIPAP patient of Pin INRPRA000762 who was under my care passed away. The e-mail stated that they had to report any adverse event, and I was asked to fill an adverse event form and send it to one Mr. Sanjay Sane of the medical department of Novartis. Below the e-mail addressed to me was an e-mail sent by Max Foundation to Mr. Tyagi informing him about the death of the patient. First of all, I was shocked to get an e-mail from Novartis about the death of a patient, and was further shocked that Max Foundation was reporting to Novartis about the name, status and progress of the patients on the GIPAP program.[26]

This led to Parikh's suspicion that Novartis was engaged in the postmarketing surveillance of GIPAP patients, which itself can be considered a form of clinical experimentation (often referred to as a Phase 4 trial, though Parikh himself did not use that phrase):

> I have myself conducted about 50 clinical trials and I know the protocols and the ethical guidelines to be followed while conducting such trials. I say that a lot of permissions are required while conducting any kind of trial, including but not limited to the Drug Controller of India, from the institutional Ethics Committees, etc. I say that even where pharmaceutical companies sponsor the trial, they do not know the name of the patient or any other personal information that could identify a specific patient or his/her progress or outcome. The trials are conducted in an anonymous manner. I fear that Novartis and Max Foundation are conducting such trials without any kind of approval or permission and without any ethical guidelines. I say that if Novartis was only sponsoring the treatment for CML patients, there is no need for them to know the name and status of the patients. However, Novartis has access to all the records of the patients and their status and in fact want[s] to know the SAE [serious adverse events] from the physicians. I say, that this raises doubts as to the veracity of the free program of Max Foundation funded by Novartis.[27]

Parikh provided further examples:

> Even in March 2004 I received an e-mail from Charlene Balick of Max Foundation . . . thanking me for assisting Novartis India with reconciliation of Serious Adverse Events (SAE) that occurred with my patients in GIPAP. They provided me with a list of 10 names of my patients who had passed away and wanted me to fill a form for SAE. . . .
>
> Once again on 20 May 2004 I received an e-mail from Max Foundation . . . instructing me that serious and unexpected adverse events related to the use of Glivec must be reported to Novartis. The e-mail explained the term "serious" as an experience that results in death, permanent or substantial disability, in-patient hospitalization, prolongation of hospitalization or is a congenital anomaly, the result of overdose or life threatening. The term "unexpected" referred to a condition or development not listed in the current labeling for Glivec. It could also include an event related to an event in the list in the labeling, but differs from the event because of increased frequency or greater severity

or specificity. In fact, for the format provided to report such "serious" or "unexpected" condition clearly is entitled as "Novartis CTSO Non-Inverventional Clinical Trial SAE Query Follow up Form," it states Trial Drug Name as "glivec" and states the trial code as "GIPAP"—indicating that this is a clinical trial. . . .

On June 3, 2004 I received an email from the Max Foundation . . . informing me that they wanted to formalize their collaborations with physicians and medical institutions through which they reach patients. All GIPAP physicians were asked to sign on the agreement. The letter stated that Novartis Serious Adverse Event Report Form had to be filled and sent to Novartis local representative in the country—again confirming that the process to be followed would have been that generally used for clinical trials. Conducting such a trial without necessary regulatory and ethical approval makes it illegal and unethical. The explanation given to us by Novartis and Max Foundation had been that this GIPAP was not a clinical trial. In good faith and for the benefit of eligible patients, his [sic] was the assumption under which I was referring patients of CML for enrollment into GIPAP. Hence I refused to sign this unless Novartis and Max Foundation has clarified the true facts.[28]

The intricacies of following GIPAP's practice suggests a complicated story involving commitment and support in making free drug available (but not more so than generics companies); limitations in the nature of that support (extending to therapeutic access, but not subsequent clinical investigations or public clinical research); and controversy (having to do with blurred boundaries between corporate interests and philanthropic outreach, but also between drug donation and experimentation or surveillance). Indeed, India was not the only country in which GIPAP had run into controversy. A case was filed in Argentina in 2007 by a former worker in the Max Foundation, Zuma Pilar Labrana, alleging a premeditated attempt to use Argentina's social services to pay for sales of Gleevec. She stated that "GIPAP was implemented as an aggressive sales program that included payoffs, frauds and abuses of patients," with the Max Foundation only providing one month of free drug to eligible patients, after which they helped obtain legal help to get public social service programs to pay for a continuation of therapy.[29]

What do these intricacies of and controversies around GIPAP in practice have to do with the macrostructural issues and matters of policy that have been at stake in the legal interpretation of intellectual property issues in

India? Often, GIPAP has led to polarized positions that restrict themselves to diagnosing Novartis's character. As I have argued, Novartis has constantly used GIPAP as an ethical justification of its monopolistic practices. In contrast, activists for access to medicines have often pointed to the controversies as an indication that GIPAP is simply a cover for unethical practices driven by profit motives. While demands for moral accountability against any corporation are legitimate, I do not wish this account to simply be an exposé of Novartis's actions. Rather, I am interested in what if anything these normatively charged positions that ironically defend monopoly on the one hand and attack philanthropy as an act of bad faith on the other have to do with policy questions concerning the limits of patentability.

For this, it is important to think through the layers of politics that are at stake in GIPAP. This chapter has explored corporate philanthropy as a form of and space for politics, as it articulates both a particular form of social responsibility and a legitimation of monopoly. But the argument between Novartis and CPAA over the Gleevec EMR was not just over the extent or limits of legitimate monopoly; different things were at stake for each of the antagonists. Novartis was defending the terms of access to a single drug under specific circumstances, as it was ensured by a particular drug donation program; CPAA was arguing that as a principle of policy, free market competition makes essential medicines more accessible than market monopoly does. Politics here concerns a disagreement over the best mechanism for making a specific drug accessible, and the best mechanism for making drugs generally accessible. But as indicated through physicians' perspectives on GIPAP, there is also a layer of politics concerning health care beyond therapeutic access, which has to do with the broader relationship between the availability of a drug and that of medical and research infrastructure and practice, and the various norms and responsibilities enshrined within those relationships.

This is further layered onto other forms of politics. Novartis as a company operates within the financialized terrains of speculative capitalism described in chapter 1, which itself leads to the contradictory pressures to grow its markets while protecting its core Euro-American ones. This leads to strategic and ethical ways in which value comes to be imported into Indian markets as philanthropy, and then extracted from them as monopoly. This has not been without elements of public scandal and the mobilization of civil society advocacy (of the sort described in chapter 2 in relation to unethical clinical trials in India) as seen most visibly in the Drop the Case campaign orchestrated nationally and globally by MSF in 2006–2007. But advocates have repeatedly told me how difficult it has been to generate such social movements around as esoteric and technical a matter as intellectual property, which has lent itself more easily to judicial forms of remediation (see chapter 3).

This judicialization at one level resolves as a battle between multinational corporate capital and global civil society fighting for access to medicines. But it is also a competition between Euro-American R&D-driven pharmaceutical companies and Indian generics companies. The latter provides a major threat for the multinational pharmaceutical industry, not just in specific developing and emerging markets such as India but also in Euro-American markets in post–patent cliff scenarios (see chapter 1). Hence one of the stakes in this battle for the Euro-American industry is either the acquisition or liquidation of its generic competitors. This competition is not just national and sectoral but also pits different varieties of capitalism, the monopoly capitalism of the so-called innovator companies and the free market capitalism of the generics companies, against each other.

The registers of the ethical that are deployed by the adversaries are not the same. I have shown in this chapter how the Euro-American R&D-driven industry operates within an ethics based in philanthropy. In chapter 5, I show how in contrast, the Indian generics industry has operated within one based in a postcolonial noblesse oblige, itself adapted in recent years to articulate strategically with emergent global civil society movements for access to essential medicines. I do so through an account of the Indian pharmaceutical industry through the history of Cipla, India's oldest surviving pharmaceutical company. Cipla is exemplary of the Indian generics industry as representing a competitive industry that produced affordable medication for domestic markets due to the enablement of the 1970 Patent Act, but also as one that has come to be an important node in a global politics of access to essential medicines in the wake of the HIV-AIDS crisis in Africa in the 1990s. It is also exceptional in persisting with older strategies of generic production and resisting acquisition by the multinational industry in a post-WTO business environment where most other large Indian competitors have turned to R&D themselves or set themselves up as acquisition targets.

The rendering of each of these forms and strategies of the ethical, on the part of the Euro-American R&D-based industry and the Indian generic industry respectively, operates on unequal geopolitical terrains. After contrasting these two modalities of ethical incorporation, I show how they are underwritten by geopolitics of monopoly, enforced through multilateral free trade mechanisms and by the power and authority of the American state. This opens up further structural questions having to do with the situation of global pharmaceutical politics in relation to histories of imperialism and postcolonial nationalism, as I discuss in chapter 5.

POSTSCRIPT: PHARMASSIST

What are the implications of an institutionalization of corporate social responsibility (especially where multinational corporations are concerned) as a model of therapeutic access for national-state sovereignty and democracy? I address these questions by first discussing the limits of drug donation and corporate philanthropy as a modality of access to medicines, and then considering the moral economies at stake in these alternative political economic possibilities.

An MSF report in 2001 argued that drug donation programs were not the best mechanism for ensuring access to medicines (Guilloux and Moon 2001). The report traced an increase in multinational pharmaceutical drug donation programs since the late 1980s and pointed to their limitations.[30] These included the reliance that develops on such programs, which gives the appearance that problems of access have been solved when in fact they have not (think in this regard of the figures Novartis provided in its EMR counterpetition to the Supreme Court as somehow a solution in itself, compared to the in fact partial solution that GIPAP provided in addressing access to the drug and care of patients with CML); questions about the sustainability of such programs given that they are contingent on the will of the donor (think here of Novartis's threat to stop GIPAP in countries that allowed the marketing of generic imatinib mesylate); the fact that the scale of drug donation programs is often incommensurate with the scale of the disease problem in question; geographic and quantitative restrictions that are often placed on these programs (only supplying certain regions or hospitals, or a certain quantum of medication); the duration of donation; the distortion of public health priorities that such programs cause (both because they privilege pharmaceutical intervention in itself as the health care solution in the absence of broader infrastructural or research support, as has been seen in the case of GIPAP, but also because they result in the prioritized focus upon certain diseases to the exclusion of others); the need for public health structures and infrastructures for donation to work feasibly, resulting in burdens being placed upon them; and the implications of drug donation programs for generic competition, which the authors argue is the best long-term solution for access to essential medicines (thereby suggesting that donations do not only justify monopoly as ethical, but are actually a tool to further monopoly).

In addition, the report focused on the cost borne by donor countries for corporate drug donation programs, and estimated that the American public would pay more (through tax incentives and after-tax gains for donor companies) to support an American company's drug donation program in a developing country than it would to pay for alternative policy structures based on generic purchasing, concessionary pricing, or price reductions. Guilloux and Moon (2001) calculated that, in addition to the ethical value that companies would receive from their charitable act, and to the fact that by ensuring uniform pricing globally while giving away drug free in developing markets these companies could protect their pricing in Western markets, there were strong market incentives to give a drug away rather than engage in these alternative strategies that depended upon responding to what a free market in a developing country could bear.[31]

How do we think then of the moral economies of such philanthropy, if they feed into and sustain multinational corporate monopoly? Supporters of such practices would see no contradiction, but rather a win-win situation that sees benefit both to capital and to society. Indeed, there is no reason in this perspective for philanthropy to be an act of renunciation or of gifting without return.[32] Opponents meanwhile often employ cynical reasoning, suggesting that ethics in such programs is a purely profit-driven strategic calculation and therefore does not withstand normative scrutiny. Slavoj Žižek (2006) provides a third way of looking at corporate social responsibility that is based in structural rather than cynical reason. In an essay titled "Nobody Has to Be Vile," Žižek argues that the real evil of such practices is that they allow for an imaginary of moral action without structural political economic transformation.

Regardless of whether the company itself has acted in good or bad faith in implementing its philanthropic programs, this for me is the fundamental limit of a program such as GIPAP. Its use as a tool of ethical monopoly renders any argument about the merits of a patent system null and void, and, further, even dismisses the need to enforce the patent as a tool of public interest rather than of corporate monopoly, since it suggests that the latter can serve seamlessly as the means to attaining the former. Let alone not allowing the imagination of a world of therapeutic intervention outside or beyond capitalized pharmaceutical political economies, it does not even allow an imagination of worlds outside monopolized pharmaceutical political economies. The Indian courts' refusal of such arguments is in part an insistence on imagining such alternatives.

The stakes of the Gleevec High Court and Supreme Court verdicts went far beyond the question of the patentability of a single molecule and had to do with protecting the spirit of Section 3(d), the major health flexibility enacted in the 2005 Patent Act (see chapter 3). But I argue further that what is at stake in the battle between the desires of the multinational pharmaceutical industry *as driven by logics of surplus health, and the restrictions placed upon it by the Indian courts through bioconstitutional moments of intervention into those logics, are two very different imaginaries of property and social relations, respectively reflected in the corporate social responsibility that companies practice as opposed to the constitutional social responsibility to which the courts have held the Indian state. In terms of posing the problem of pharmocracy, it is worth thinking about the democratic potentials (but also limits) of allowing free market competition in therapeutics (and of invoking the spirit of the Indian Constitution in order to do so), as opposed to the most definitely undemocratic alternative of instituting monopolistic terrains in which corporations decide upon the extent and terms of access to medicines. I elaborate upon the alternative formations of the political that are afforded in these two capitalisms in chapter 5, thus suggesting that there is much more at stake here than simply a question of how much access or how much innovation is allowed under one kind of market regime as opposed to another.*

CHAPTER FIVE

Postcolonial Values

Nationalist Industries in Pharmaceutical Empire

First Conjuncture: Cipla Goes Global

This chapter turns to the history of the Indian generic industry, in order to show how the pre–World Trade Organization (WTO) terrain of pharmaceutical production and consumption in the country was constituted in a manner that enabled low drug prices through free market competition. I focus on the history of India's oldest surviving pharmaceutical company, Cipla, which has become a leading player in the opposition to WTO-mandated product patent regimes and hence an ally of global civil society groups fighting for access to medicines. Cipla's history is one that sees consistent action in its own market interests, and an attempt to define a market terrain in terms of those interests; but it also sees the articulation of certain explicit nationalist and (subsequently global) humanitarian sentiments, in ways that open up questions of postcolonial and welfare investments of these market actors. I situate Cipla's story in the context of the broader terrain of pharmaceutical geopolitics as seen from India.

Cipla's trajectory represents a larger organic story of an alternative to monopolistic forms of pharmaceutical capitalism as it has emerged in India through its generic drug industry.[1] This alternative is not an alternative to capitalism; indeed, it is nothing other than the free market. But it is marked by particular postcolonial nationalist histories and is embodied in the trajectories and biographies of certain capitalists. These free market alternatives are constrained by geopolitics that forcibly inscribe monopolistic forms in order to render them natural. Therefore, rather than seeing this as the exception to the norm of global pharmaceutical capital, I wish to use the case of Cipla to denaturalize and render particular the Euro-American pharmaceutical industry's monopolistic practices and show just how extreme they are even from the perspective of free market capitalism (if not from the perspective of speculative financialized capital that captures these industries; see chapter 1).

I focus on three moments of Cipla's trajectory: first, around late 2000 to early 2001, which was the time when the company emerged as a central actor in global civil society advocacy over antiretrovirals; second, the early 1990s, when it articulated a strong opposition to India's becoming a signatory to the TRIPS agreement; and third, the 1970s, when it earlier established its business subsequent to the new process patent regimes enacted under the 1970 Indian Patent Act. Each of these moments sees an intertwining of an articulation of public interest (initially as postcolonial nationalism, subsequently combined with global humanitarianism) with business interest. Cipla's actions are not incompatible with strategic calculations of market value but rather imbricated with them in complex and occasionally contradictory ways.

I then show how the kinds of actions undertaken by companies such as Cipla in alliance with certain arms of the state and with civil society actors advocating for access to essential medications leads to reconfigurations of global geopolitical terrains, not just destabilizing existing hierarchies but also leading to rearticulations of these hierarchies in new forms. I argue that this involves situating the postcolonial actions of Indian market actors in the context of global geopolitical configurations, which requires a conceptualization of imperialism that is adequate to our times. This is a structure of imperialism that is itself postcolonial, as it takes shape in a conjuncture where most nation-states are formally decolonized and self-determining. Yet it contains structures of Euro-American corporate hegemony underwritten by the (in today's time, especially American) state that show uncanny echoes of precolonial formations of mercantile imperialism that were driven by the expansionist interests of especially Dutch and English trading corporations.

"Cipla Shows HIV/AIDS Patients How to Live with Hope."[2] Such headlines were commonplace in writing about access to essential medicines in the early 2000s, and they were tied to others such as "One Man Gives Hope to Millions."[3] This referred to Yusuf Hamied, who took over the company in 1972 and ran it until 2013.[4] At a European Commission meeting on AIDS in Brussels on September 28, 2000, Cipla announced the development of Triomune, the first combination HIV therapy to be available in a single molecule. This was not a new drug, but a creative recombination of existing drugs; hence while not innovative in the way the term gets defined by the R&D-driven pharmaceutical industry, it was most certainly an innovation in the fight against AIDS.[5] Providing access to and compliance with triple therapy was particularly cumbersome and difficult in resource-poor environments, and a less rigorously enforced drug regimen (such as with two drugs rather than three) would lead more readily to drug resistance. The consequences of this were especially stark in Africa, which had emerged as a biomedical and political epicenter of AIDS by the end of the 1990s. Hence, Cipla's intervention with Triomune saw it emerging as a global player in the context of the AIDS crisis.[6]

In February 2001, the company offered to cut the price of the drug to make it affordable in African markets, a move that was hailed as combating the price gouging of the Euro-American innovator industry, and which thrust Cipla into the spotlight as an ally of patient advocacy and civil society groups fighting for access to essential medicines. These were groups that had themselves emerged as global advocates, at a time when global civil society was becoming a consequential actor in struggles against the inequalities engendered by global capital. The September 2000 meeting in Brussels led to Cipla forging alliances with organizations such as Médecins sans Frontières (MSF), which would endure throughout the judicialized battles around patent law interpretation and access to essential medicines that would play out in India over the next decade. In the process, the company took on a representative role, claiming to fight for the interests of Third World patients who would have otherwise died in spite of the fact that medications that could provide a cure to their disease existed. Hamied himself came to be figured globally either as a pirate or as Robin Hood, depending upon one's position in the debate that saw the Indian industry either as copycat or as savior. This continued an earlier role of representing Indian national interests that Cipla adopted more or less since its inception, as I subsequently describe.

This situation within a global political terrain of access to essential medicines led Hamied to articulate a strong ethical position. I provide a sense of this articulation in Hamied's own words.[7] Our conversations began with my asking Hamied about the impact of India's becoming party to the WTO on the national industry. His response was emphatic, but did not speak immediately to impacts on the industry per se. Rather, he said, "That's a silly question, professor. In fact, I have said, on TV I've said, the government has committed selective genocide. I've used the word *genocide*."

What is genocidal for Hamied is not the patent, but the monopoly—precisely the allowance that companies such as Novartis insisted was ethical because it provided the conditions of possibility for philanthropic drug donation (see chapter 4). At stake therefore is an absolute polarization around the ethics of monopoly. How can this polarization be explained? There is clearly something more to this than the contrary opinions of individuals or of particular companies, and it involves understanding the global structures within which different pharmaceutical industries operate. But one cannot reduce this explanation to a cynical one that is purely driven by rational interest either. After all, as discussed in chapter 4, Novartis's implementation of GIPAP was driven both by strategic calculation and likely by good faith. Hamied's antimonopolistic position meanwhile has been consistent for over half a century, and was articulated in the 1960s as he argued for a process patent regime in much the same terms as he was arguing against contemporary post-TRIPS product patent environments in the late 2000s. This position against monopoly was the bedrock of the Indian Drug Manufacturer's Association (IDMA), a lobbying group of the Indian pharmaceutical industry that Hamied founded in 1961, well before the passage of the 1970 Patent Act. As he said of his (and the group's) position then, "At that time we had meetings with the multinationals, saying that no, fellows, we have nothing against patents. Please, listen to me very carefully, what I'm saying. Even at that time, 1960s. I'm a scientist, I'd come back with a PhD degree. I'm a scientist. I have nothing against patents. I'm against monopoly. We are willing to give you a 4 percent royalty on sales, on our net sales. But no monopoly. And they told us, virtually, go to hell. Go to hell. And then we fought and fought and fought." This is a fight that melds concerns for public interest under monopoly with those of national industrial competitiveness, and that is still ongoing.

While ethical in this light, Cipla's 2001 humanitarian offer of Triomune was undoubtedly animated by business logics.[8] It offered the company a route to becoming a global brand even as it indicated the capacity that existed for low-cost generic manufacture of antiretrovirals to both the Indian government and global bodies such as the World Health Organization (WHO, which included Triomune in its prequalification program in 2003).[9] This continued the company's national business strategy, which was based on leveraging its brand value rather than on monopolistic protection of its products. But it also allowed Cipla to envisage and open new markets in Africa.[10] Yet business logics cannot explain everything, and strong moral imperatives were never far beneath the surface in Hamied's own explanation of the Triomune offer: "In Africa, in 2001, the prize of AIDS drugs in Africa was $12,000 per patient per year. Monopoly. There were only 4,000 patients that could afford to use those drugs. Then 2001, Cipla came out at $300. You should see the State of the Union speech of Bush in 2003. He said the world is given an opportunity because the price of AIDS drugs has come down from $12,000 to $300. These cost you a hundred dollars to make. Why the hell are you charging $12,000? Obscene."[11]

Cipla's antiretroviral offers in Africa were a factor in influencing subsequent debates over patent laws in India, since this demonstrated therapeutic possibilities and business alternatives to those that would prevail under TRIPS, even in combating contemporary epidemics that demanded new forms of therapeutic intervention. Hence, this was a political move rendered as ethical, and continued Cipla's long-standing crusade against a monopolistic patent regime in India. These politics had started prior to the enactment of the 1970 Act and continued throughout debates around TRIPS in the late 1980s and early 1990s; but an ethics articulated in terms of the morality of public access to essential medication through the free market was always present in these politics. I next move back to consider Hamied's opposition, and the broader political terrain that prevailed at the time when India decided to sign on to TRIPS.

Second Conjuncture: Cipla Opposes TRIPS

In late 1993, the Indian Parliament established a committee under the chairmanship of Inder Kumar Gujral in order to assess whether it would be in India's interests to become party to the TRIPS agreement on the terms that were provided. These terms were outlined in a draft agreement outlined by Arthur Dunkel, the director-general of the General Agreement on Tariffs and Trade (GATT) from 1980 to 1993. The Gujral Committee Report suggested that it was not, which means that the Indian delegation that signed on to TRIPS in 1994 did so against the advice of its own Parliament's committee.[12]

The context under which the Gujral Committee met itself reflects the ambivalent position of the Indian state with respect to TRIPS. As the Uruguay Round negotiations commenced in 1986, India was initially opposed to the American insistence that intellectual property rights be negotiated as part of the round. Yet subsequently, India acceded to this inclusion. Hence, the matter before the Gujral Committee concerned not the fact of inclusion itself, but the terms under which such inclusion would operate, which were outlined in the Dunkel Draft. The basic terms included the global application of a product patent regime for pharmaceuticals that would exist for twenty years. Under the 1970 Indian Patent Act, only process patents were allowed and they were only valid for seven years. But there were other contentious issues as well. One concerned the fact that there was no provision allowing a national government to issue compulsory licenses, which would force the holder of a product patent to license the patent to a local manufacturer if that was deemed in the national interest. The 1970 Act allowed for an automatic right to license. This meant that any company could get a license on a drug that had a process patent by paying royalties to the patent holder. Hence, the patent served not as an instrument of monopoly but as a source of revenue through royalties. The Dunkel Draft was therefore triply monopolistic compared to the 1970 Indian Patent Act. It replaced process patents with product patents; disallowed an automatic right to license; and, further, did not provide the Indian state an explicit allowance to enforce compulsory licensing in certain situations.[13] Furthermore, the Dunkel Draft had no provisions that would force a patent to be worked in the country of its issue. In other words, a company could get a product patent for a drug in India without having to manufacture that drug in India. Hence, this reduced the possibility of technology transfer through the development of local manufacturing capacities for patented medication.

All of these were points noted and raised by the Gujral Committee Report. The Commerce Ministry of India had by this time adopted a generally supportive position toward the Dunkel Draft, suggesting that compulsory licenses could still be issued since there were no express provisions against it, and that the impact of TRIPS on drug prices in India would be minimal because patented medication constituted a small proportion of drugs on the market. The committee disagreed with the ministry's position on both counts, making instead an explicit argument for upholding public interest over the primacy of patent holders. In the process, the report framed an opposition between monopoly and public interest that would endure in judicial articulations over the subsequent two decades.

The recommendations of the Gujral Committee Report unambiguously rejected many central facets of the Dunkel Draft. It stated, "(i) the Indian patent law has been rightly emphasising patenting the process and not the product. This should be maintained. (ii) the proposed extension to 20 years period virtually discourages any R&D and should not be conceded. (iii) India should insist on grant of automatic licensing in certain circumstances."[14] Yet India agreed entirely to the Dunkel Draft recommendations in the final round of negotiations in 1994 in Geneva, a complete reversal of the position advocated by the committee.

In the process of coming up with its recommendations, the committee heard a number of expert witnesses. The spectrum of positions on the table was reflected by three key witnesses. At one end of the spectrum was support for the Dunkel Draft resolutions, articulated more generally as a proglobalization position by Manmohan Singh, at the time India's finance minister and architect of its economic liberalization program, who would subsequently become prime minister in 2004. Singh's contention to the committee was, "We cannot afford to remain outside the global system."[15] This contrasted sharply to positions at the other end of the spectrum, such as that of M. D. Nanjundaswamy, president of the Karnataka Rajya Raitha Sangha, a powerful farmers' group that was at the forefront of antiglobalization protests in India in the mid- to late 1990s. Nanjundaswamy painted a Manichean opposition not just in terms of the well-established refrain of developing versus developed nations, or First World and Third, but between what he called "the White World and the Coloured World."[16] He termed the Dunkel Draft "the latest weapon of imperialism of the White World to collectively colonize the Third World through its various proposals."[17] A third position was provided by Yusuf Hamied. He also voiced strong opposition to the Dunkel Draft positions, but from the perspective of national interest, stating that "every country has a patent law to suit its own needs."[18] All three of these positions saw intellectual property and free trade not as goods in themselves, but as part of a consideration of strategic geopolitics and of an imagination of how the world was configured. But the imaginations and strategic interests were seen differently by each. While Singh saw the world as economically interconnected and India's interests as served through inclusion in those networks, Hamied was insistent upon India preserving its sovereign right to enact its own legislation in its own interests.

What constitutes its own interests from Hamied's perspective is complicated. On the one hand, national interest for him clearly mapped onto the interest of national industry, which he felt would be disadvantaged relative to the multinational pharmaceutical industry if India accepted the Dunkel Draft proposals. But on the other hand, it was also tied to public interest. This latter articulation was made through an explicit argument for the free market against monopoly of any sort, by anyone. In this regard, the end game for Hamied was less the broad issue of whether India would be under a product or a process patent regime than it was the terms under which a product patent regime would operate. His insistence to the committee was that India preserve the automatic license of right, thereby maintaining the patent system as one based in the incentive of royalties rather than of absolute monopoly. Indeed, Hamied articulated a fundamental position against monopoly, rather than of national industrial interest, as the basis of his opposition to the draft proposals, stating, "We do not want monopoly in India, either Indian or international monopolists."[19] Hamied's alternative was not to capital, not even to the patent; just to the monopoly. The model for him remains the 1969 Canadian Patent Act, which allowed patents not as an absolute monopoly right but as a licensing right. Under this act, developers of a drug would have a patent, but it would only entitle them to royalties from any competitor who made a generic version of the drug, and would not allow a competitor to prevent making the drug altogether. In contrast to the Schumpeterian rendering of the monopoly as ethical and essential that takes recourse to the fundamental value of innovation that it enables (see chapter 4), Hamied posits it as the fundamentally unethical antithesis to the free market—but also, in the process, to public interest: "A patent regime doesn't make sense unless you say—this is the product, this is the originator, the originator gets a royalty. *That's that.* I'm pushing for . . . read Canada 1969. There is nothing better than the Canadian Patent Act of 1969."[20]

For Hamied, the "genocidal" monopoly afforded by product patent regimes allows for the "obscene" pricing strategies of the Euro-American industry. But what allows for the monopoly in the first place is the state's role in restructuring the market in accordance with TRIPS, even as it was the state that afforded companies such as Cipla the possibility of becoming serious nationally (and later globally) competitive industrial actors through a restriction of monopoly under the 1970 Act. Hence the state itself does not act through a singular logic or even in one voice: even as its own Parliamentary Standing Committee was arguing against the terms of TRIPS, the executive was preparing to agree to the Dunkel Draft recommendations. The state's actions themselves become the site of politics, both in relation to the dichotomy between the interests of capital and public interest, and in mediating the interests of competing forms and sectors of capitalism. I explore this next through a rendering of Hamied's own understanding of state action. I further situate this in relation to the structure and geopolitics of global pharmaceutical capital within which the Indian state operates and by which it is constrained. I therefore move from the question of the relationship between ethical and business interests to ones concerning the geopolitics that inscribes such interests, by focusing on the period between the Uruguay Round negotiations and the passage of the 2005 Act.

For Hamied, India's agreement to the Dunkel Draft provisions in spite of the Gujral Committee's mandate to resist it was nothing other than the state selling out to multinational corporate interests. It was an agential failure, one that had happened before and would happen again. It is worth recounting Hamied's view of the Indian state's capture by multinational capital during the Uruguay Round negotiations. The foundational issue concerned whether intellectual property should be a part of free trade negotiations in the first place:

> What happened in '89? The commerce minister of India . . . India in 1989–90 had 0.4 percent of world trade. So whether we were party to GATT or not in GATT, I told the government, what difference does it make? It makes no difference. In 1989, commerce minister was Dinesh Singh. He was a Communist Party member. Card holder. But he was commerce minister, Indira Gandhi's favorite. To force intellectual property into GATT, WTO, took place in 1989. Whether intellectual property should be . . . Dinesh Singh said no, should not be. What has intellectual property got to do with trade? And he gave strict instructions to his team—secretary, joint secretary—that when you go to Geneva, you have to oppose this tooth and nail. So this team goes to Geneva. And what happens? Against Dinesh Singh's instructions, they sold the country out. And de facto, it was agreed that intellectual property should be part of GATT and that is how WTO was created. (Hamied interviews)

This set the stage for the Dunkel Draft and the Gujral Committee deliberations a few years hence:

> Okay? What did they do immediately? They called a chap called Dunkel. They appointed a guy called Dunkel to draft out Trade-Related Intellectual Property Rights, TRIPS. He drafted out TRIPS. And this was circulated worldwide for the debate. To India also. In 1993—or '92, '93—the Indian government appointed a committee of parliamentarians under the chairmanship of I. K. Gujral to discuss [the] Dunkel Draft. In their wisdom or stupidity, this committee asked me to come and give evidence before this committee. I gave evidence. They asked me questions. And they asked me a question on R&D, I remember answering. I said you have a choice. I said Indian government has a choice. Either you allow me to sell products at American prices and I can do research, or follow what we are doing today, which is giving drugs at the lowest possible prices to the masses in the country. You

can't do both. You can't do fundamental research like the Americans are doing with the prices that I'm getting today. So you have to decide. I can't decide—the Indian government decides. If you allow me to sell products at American prices, I will convert Parliament House into a research center. They all laughed.

The politics at stake for Hamied were about more than just agreeing to TRIPS. They also concerned the specificities of its implementation. For instance, Hamied wondered about the so-called ten-year transition period for less-developed countries, and the ways in which that opened up the possibilities for exclusive marketing rights as an intermediate state of monopoly that could prevail in the country prior to a formal adoption of a product patent regime:

> YH: Then comes '95. Critical. India then agrees to join WTO, '95. Then what happens? India says, we are not ready to join. Give us a grace period. So they were given a ten-year transition period. I still don't understand till today, professor, what is the meaning of the word "transition period." I still don't understand. So maybe you as a professor can understand what the word "transition period" means. Under what circumstances did India sign WTO and they were given a ten-year transition period? We were told at that time categorically by the Indian government—categorically—that product patents would kick in post-2005. Okay? So, they said *teek hai* [okay], we've got a ten-year transition period. Then what happened—this is important to understand—then what happened in the year December 2000, suddenly, the only country in the world, introduces EMR.[21] Exclusive marketing rights. Now how and why did that come up?
>
> KSR: So none of this was being talked about in 1995?
>
> YH: Nothing! [In] 1995 we did not know what exclusive marketing rights meant. You know what, then they introduced . . . and India accepted it! I'm coming to lots of things which are shocking.
>
> KSR: And these came out of WTO—it was WTO that was saying . . . ?
>
> YH: Naturally. Naturally. Exclusive marketing rights said that if you have patented anything post-'95 January, you will get exclusive marketing rights. I know for a fact that WTO rules cannot be retroactive. You can't backdate. So how in December 2000 you backdated this to 1995? Because from 1995 to 2000, you could only have process patents in India. So that is a very, very gray area. Nobody talks about

it. Why? Because it doesn't suit people to talk about it. I talk about it. I want to know. Even now I want to know. Why are you backdating to '95? In fact if you see WTO it says, those people who joined in '95 will be given one-year grace period to implement. So it should actually kick in from '96. If that is true, Roche's case is out, because their patent on erlotinib is March '95.[22] Are you understanding what I'm trying to say? So, how can you backdate transition period?

The game changer—which transformed the WTO from an institution that operated solely in the interests of the multinational pharmaceutical industry to one that allowed national governments the sovereign authority to enact flexibilities in their patent laws—was the Doha Declaration in November 2001. Hence, if the period from 1995 to 2000 saw the progressive consolidation of monopolistic interests through multilateral trade forums, it also saw such formations reach their breaking point—mainly because this was also the time when AIDS in Africa reached epidemic proportions, and such monopolies were making it impossible to provide antiretroviral medication to the continent at affordable prices. Yet according to Hamied, the negotiations in Doha were full of consequential geopolitical arm twisting:

YH: Then comes Doha. One clause you must understand in Doha. Can I read it to you? I know it by heart. "Every country has a right to decide for themselves what is a national crisis." Health crisis. See 5(c). 5(c).[23] This includes malaria, TB, AIDS, and other epidemics. This was passed by Doha. This was passed. Six months later, Doha Declaration came for ratification in Geneva. There were 144 countries present. And this point came up for discussion. And the Americans said we oppose the words "other epidemics." And there was a debate, and they put it to vote. The vote was 143 in favor, 1 vote against. Guess who won that vote? The one vote. The American vote. Veto.

Two thousand three, I think, August 2003. Americans asked for a meeting to discuss 5(c). And they said, instead of calling 144, let us call five countries. Who are the five countries? India, Brazil, South Africa, Kenya, America. They met in Geneva. What happened at this meeting? Because I was following this with a magnifying glass. None of those representatives were allowed to take the papers out of the meeting room. One of the representatives was a friend of ours and he told us afterwards what happened. Americans said, we concede to—here is 5(c). What does it say? Read it.

KSR: The right to determine what constitutes a national emergency and other circumstances of extreme urgency: it being understood that public health crises including those relating to HIV-AIDS, TB, malaria and other epidemics. . . .

YH: You can see "other epidemics." Now you concede to what we are asking. What are you asking? Point 1: the country must declare a crisis. Okay? This should be ratified by WTO. Number 2: the country should declare what drugs they require for that crisis. This should be ratified by WTO. Point 3: if any of these drugs are covered by international patents, the government must negotiate with the patent holder for suitable royalty. By which time, my dear friends, the epidemic will be over. How could the Indian delegate, or delegation, agree to this? You know that this has become law now? You know that European Parliament, these points have been accepted? For crisis? Are you aware of this? On what basis? On what basis? You don't know what is going to hit you by 2015 with the crisis of drugs in India. You have no idea. It's already started.[24]

What is important here is not an exposé of what "really" happened behind closed-door meetings. After all, Hamied's own information is secondhand and comes with its own interests, though it is hardly surprising to hear that the United States managed to successfully push solitary and unambiguous positions in favor of monopoly with direct input from the multinational pharmaceutical lobby.[25] Rather, I wish to highlight how the picture of global relations of power and production looks different from different situations. From the perspective of the Euro-American innovator industry, India has an inconsistent patent environment that does not respect innovation, a structure of public explanation that has received traction and become common sense in American political discourse. My own rendering of the trajectory of judicialization in India has shown how this is not the case: that India in fact fully respects a product patent regime, but also has allowed an interpretation of patent laws in ways that favor the implementation of public health flexibilities that exist in the law and that are allowed under TRIPS subsequent to Doha (see chapter 3). Hence, it is not a patent environment that is being denied to the Euro-American industry in India; it is simply an environment of absolute monopoly. From Hamied's perspective, however, even this denial is deeply contingent and constantly subject to geopolitical, corporate-mandated pressures, aided by an Indian state that has a history of selling itself out.

This sellout does not happen only at the level of policy. According to Hamied, it also happens at the level of the practice of granting patents. This adds complexity to the understanding of the Indian situation as one that sees limits to patentability. I have cataloged a number of cases of drugs that have patent protection throughout Euro-America and elsewhere that have been denied patents in India under its public health flexibilities. Yet these are in fact the very few drugs that have been made objects of concern and opposition by generic companies and civil society groups engaged in a constant triage of patent applications. According to Hamied, there are literally thousands of other drugs that slip through the cracks: "You know, the patent office in the last one year have issued in health alone, 5,000 patents? Who's reading them? Telephone call comes from Commerce Ministry, see that this patent is granted? *Arre bhai, kya hai yeh* [I say brother, what is this]? There is no examination." What I have discussed here is a relationship that Hamied has posited between the state and global geopolitics in terms of the state selling out. This is not quite malfeasance, nor quite failure, but rather an abdication of representative responsibility. This is not simply a function of a neoliberal turn, even though the events Hamied is discussing here have to do with a conjunctural moment that is widely regarded as one when the Indian state makes such a turn.[26]

Indeed, Hamied's critique goes back to one of the socialist, regulatory state: his is emphatically not a call for a socialist or socialized pharmaceutical regime. For instance, Hamied described the context within which he had to establish himself in his early years at Cipla as one of forced personal privation and "sacrifice":

> You know, when I came back in 1960, with a PhD from Cambridge University, you know, it took one year for the government to give me, to give Cipla permission to employ me, because I was related to one of the directors. It took one year. I worked one year here free. Then they sent a letter to Cipla: you can employ Dr. Hamied on monthly salary of 1,500 rupees a month for the next three years. That's how it started in '61. From '61, I worked in Cipla; till 1995, I had a personal negative income. Negative income, personal. I could entertain [a] thousand people, and sign on behalf of Cipla. But personally, nothing. So it was a big sacrifice. There was ration in India; to travel abroad you needed permission. You know, very difficult period. You couldn't buy a car. You know it took me three years to buy a car in Bombay.[27]

Yet even this regulatory state was one that could operate in the interests of multinational capital.[28] For instance, in the 1970s, even as the state had provided a boost to the Indian industry at the level of legislation through the passage of the 1970 Patent Act, it constrained the industry at the level of practice by levying excessive duties on raw materials and active pharmaceutical ingredients (APIs) that the Indian industry needed to import in order to manufacture drugs:

> We grew, in spite of the stepmotherly treatment of the Government of India. Import duties of APIs was 146 percent—yes sir, this was '70s—and import duty on the end product was 100 percent. The then secretary in [the Ministry of] Chemicals and Fertilizers . . . I went and said sir. . . . I was young those days and more aggressive than I am now. I've mellowed. I said sir, you are secretary. There's only one question I can't understand. How can you as an intelligent individual allow end product at 100 percent duty, and raw materials to make that end product at 146 percent duty? It just doesn't make sense to me. Unless you can change that, you shouldn't be where you are. They were all believing in supporting the multinationals left, right, and center. Exactly what is happening today. Exactly what is happening today.

Hamied's diagnosis of the sellout is unambiguous and largely plausible. But it elides certain complexities that are worth paying further attention to. First, even as the state consistently sells out, it is also the state that can be made accountable and responsible to public and national industrial interest, a fact that Hamied himself has recognized and leveraged over decades. This was notably evident in the passage of the 1970 Act, but there is a broader post-colonial trajectory here of the state's investment in its pharmaceutical industry in which the conjuncture of the 1970s is particularly important. Second, the state itself had contrary opinions of its actions around GATT. While the Gujral Committee felt that acceding to the Dunkel Draft recommendations was not in the national interest, the executive branch of government decided that it was. In other words, the government did not see this as a sellout, but as strategic leveraging of global economic and geopolitical terrains. As reflected in Manmohan Singh's assertion to the committee that India "could not afford" to remain outside GATT, this suggests an understanding of these terrains as both constraining and providing new kinds of opportunity.

Therefore, there was a shift in state emphasis from the 1970s to the 1990s that is worth tracing, with greater specificity than an epochal diagnosis of neoliberalism. Indeed, I will argue that it is important to locate the shift from a regulatory, socialist welfare state to a neoliberal globally oriented one within an understanding of enduring global structures of imperialism. Such shifts then become situated and strategic responses to perceived geopolitical structures and power relations. This involves turning to Nanjundaswamy's diagnosis of colonialism. Whether one accepts the stark First World–Third World opposition that he drew or not, there is something serious worth unpacking within it. In other words, I suggest that reading the three expert opinions to the Gujral Committee—of Singh, Nanjundaswamy, and Hamied—against each other requires something more than just a contingent understanding (these happened to be the opinions of three individuals with their points of view) or a cynical one (these are individuals operating to maximize their self-interest). It requires a situated understanding, thinking through how the world looks from particular (individual but also institutional) perspectives, and thus through how the terrain of globalization is constituted by striated realities that are interpreted differently, and arguing for different kinds of strategic response.

Third Conjuncture: From Cipla's High Noon to Its Vanishing Present

In April 1975, the Indian Ministry of Petroleum and Chemicals released the Report of the Committee on the Drugs and Pharmaceutical Industry. The committee was established under the stewardship of the parliamentarian Jaisukhlal Hathi, and hence was referred to as the Hathi Committee Report.[29] The Hathi Committee was appointed by the Indian Parliament in 1974 to look into promoting growth in the Indian drug industry and to rationalize price structures to facilitate access to medicines. This was not the first committee set up since Indian independence with such mandates: both the Tek Chand Committee (which gave its recommendations in 1950) and the Ayyangar Committee (which did so in 1959) had been given similar charges and came up with seminal recommendations (see table 3.1 ; Chaudhuri 2005). The difference was that these two prior committees were established at a time when the 1911 colonial Patent Law was in effect, allowing for product patents and pharmaceutical monopolies. Therefore the primary focus of both these committees was to mitigate the effects of such a structure. The Ayyangar Committee indeed recommended India's transition to a process patent regime and thus was an important antecedent to the 1970 Patent Act.

The Hathi Committee is particularly significant therefore not in terms of its impact on the Indian industry—the Ayyangar Committee Report arguably had more—but because of the conjuncture within which it must be situated.

It was established after India had passed the 1970 Patent Act, but only just after it became effective (which was in September 1972). Hence in many ways this represented a transitional period, when India was formally operating under a new legal and policy regime, but before such a regime had a chance to show its effects either on the Indian industry or on access to medicines. Further, the committee's report is of interest because it demands something more radical than a free market economy in pharmaceuticals—it actually recommended measures for ensuring a thriving public sector pharmaceutical industry, with therapeutic access socialized. This happened at a global moment when alternative social and geopolitical orderings were being imagined in the domain of health through multilateral forums such as the WHO.[30]

At this time, the importance of generic drugs in making medicines accessible was becoming evident. Hence, even though the question of generics per se was not part of the committee's initial terms of reference, it was a focal point of the report. But the report went well beyond rubber-stamping the centrality of the generic drug industry to India's public health prospects. Rather, it investigated the market conditions and constraints that would be required to ensure that a generic industry would adequately serve its social function. This included discussions about whether brand name drugs should be restricted or abolished altogether. As mentioned, branding was a major strategy employed by the larger generic companies such as Cipla to generate value in a competitive market environment; hence, while supporting the interests of a generic industry, the committee did not necessarily support the market structure as it was being consolidated in the 1970s, which allowed for competitive differentiations within the industry through branding (and which was consequential both in the rise of the subsequently globalizing Indian industry through companies such as Cipla, Ranbaxy, and Dr. Reddy's Laboratories, and in the relative devaluation of public sector alternatives as these large generics companies came to take on increasingly representative roles in providing solutions to the problem of therapeutic access). The committee also paid careful attention to corporate marketing practices, considering whether to stop distribution of drug samples to doctors by pharmaceutical medical representatives and direct-to-consumer advertising of drugs through All India Radio.[31]

In order to understand the committee's recommendations, it is worthwhile considering the state of play of the pharmaceutical industry in India at the time as outlined in the report, and situating it in relation to Cipla's own development within this trajectory. The report emphasized the important role of the industry in maintaining "the health of the nation," melding ideas of public health with postcolonial national robustness.[32] This "health" pointed simultaneously in two directions: toward the health of the population and toward the economy and industry. This was a national industry that had existed in varying forms since the late nineteenth century, when Acharya P. C. Ray established the first pharmaceutical laboratory in Calcutta. As in the West, major spurs to the development of the industry were provided by the world wars. The cessation of drug imports during World War I provided the first stimulus for local drug production; by the end of World War II, progress had been made in domestic manufacture of sera and vaccines.[33] But most of the activity of this industry still consisted of the processing of imported drugs for distribution in Indian markets.

Cipla was a child of the Indian freedom struggle, but was itself in significant ways born of the war effort. Its founder, K. A. Hamied, had obtained his PhD in chemistry in Germany in the 1920s, returning to India in the early 1930s to carry out his longtime wish of starting an indigenous pharmaceutical company.[34] Cipla was established in 1935, but the major milestone in the company's origin story as narrated by both Hamieds was Mahatma Gandhi's visit to the company in 1939. K. A. Hamied had already been influenced by Gandhi prior to his departure for higher studies in Germany. In the early 1920s, upon Gandhi's call for noncooperation, he had left university to go to Sabarmati Ashram.[35] Subsequently, on Gandhi's suggestion, he joined the newly constituted and nationalist Jamia Millia Islamia University in Aligarh as one of its founding faculty. In 1939, he was surprised by Gandhi's personal visit to his company:

> Then in 1939, this is very auspicious day for us. June 2, he rang up my father, and said, can I come and see you? And where he came downstairs is here.[36] Okay? And why did he come here, is the question. My father asked him, sir, why have you come to me? He said, because the British have contacted me, and have said that we will give you independence if you help us in the war effort. My father said, why've you come to me? He said, because drugs in Europe have stopped coming to India. Blockade. Fighting in Europe—where are you going to get German and Swiss drugs here? There's a tremendous drug shortage. So, Cipla started producing drugs for the war effort. Antimalarials . . . and that, specifically on the request of Mahatma Gandhi. And Sardar Patel, all of them. (Hamied interviews)

Hence, World War II saw Cipla's rise to prominence as a major national drug manufacturer. Nonetheless, at the time of India's independence, and subsequently through the 1950s, the entrenched players in the Indian market were still the multinational companies. This was facilitated by the continuance of the 1911 Patent Act that allowed them market monopoly, which meant that Cipla was primarily operating in the niches, making drugs such as steroids that were off patent. But it was also facilitated by physicians, who preferred prescribing better-known multinational brands than Indian ones.

There were other players in the marketplace too. Even as multinational companies were the powerful players, an Indian public sector industry was founded.[37] Roles were divided between these various actors, speaking to different modalities of pharmaceutical development at the time: reformulation versus bulk drug manufacture. Bulk drug manufacture speaks to the creation of an API; reformulation involves the recombination and packaging of active ingredients to create therapeutic products that are sold in the marketplace. Ironically, at the time, multinational companies were the strongest players in the bulk drug sector, because of high import duties on raw materials compared to finished products. This made it expensive for Indian companies to import the necessary materials to make APIs in India; in contrast, multinationals would make bulk drugs abroad and import them into India, including those for further reformulation.[38] Indeed, multinationals rarely manufactured bulk drugs in India; there was very little investment in building technology or manufacturing infrastructure within the country. Through the 1950s and 1960s, therefore, most high-value drugs from a market perspective were produced by the multinational industry, but invariably elsewhere. In India, multinationals operated primarily as trading rather than manufacturing concerns.[39] Indian companies did manufacture, but largely operated between the cracks. The committee pointed out that this was not an adequate division of labor from the perspective of the "needs of the country" and was explicit in criticizing the "anti-social role of the multinationals," which needed to be contained by "the laws of the land."[40]

Two possible trajectories existed as a solution to this problem. The one that was followed was facilitated in large measure by the 1970 Act and allied industrial policy that prioritized the interests of the domestic industry. But it was also enabled by the multinationals' response to the act, as they decided for the most part to leave India altogether rather than compete with Indian companies in a process patent–driven free market regime. This effectively gave companies like Cipla a "virgin market":

The biggest mistake the multinationals did in '72, when the patent laws changed . . . they had a meeting, I remember. In Geneva. Six, seven of them. And they decided, goodbye India. And they walked out. All of them walked out. They absolutely didn't care a damn about India's health—all walked out. Some of them stayed like Glaxo and all, who had older products. But most of them walked out. And you will see . . . top fifty companies in India, 1971. Who are the top companies? Top fifty companies? Out of the top fifty, multinationals were thirty-three. Seventeen Indians. Cipla did not feature, top fifty. Top fifty companies, 1996? Indian companies, twenty-eight. In 2004, multinationals, fourteen. Indian companies, thirty-six. See the change there. Now those idiots, if they'd hung on in India, if you accept what the Indians have done and you live by the laws of the land, then today they would have been top. They left the field open for people like us. All the Indian companies— Ranbaxy, Reddy, ourselves—it was like a virgin market. (Hamied interviews)

The 1970 Act therefore enabled the restructuring of the market in ways that allowed the Indian industry to become the high-value drug producer. But it was the private, generic industry that did so, often (in the case of the larger companies especially) through leveraging brand value. The committee, however, unambiguously posited the solution to the problems facing drug manufacture and therapeutic access in India as coming from a public pharmaceutical sector. It deemed health care a "national charge" and recommended that public sector capacity be built to obtain a leadership role in both bulk drug manufacture and reformulation, insisting that this was the only way to "make essential medicines available to large masses of our people at reasonable prices."[41] In order to build this capacity, the committee proposed the establishment of a National Drug Authority, a central authority that would establish and coordinate policies for drug manufacturing programs. These would only be nonbranded drugs: the committee argued against allowing branded medication altogether, even if manufactured by private industry. There was an ethics to this, an "ethics of production" that "should have essentially the character of meeting national . . . as distinct from trade and commercial needs."[42] The committee therefore posited an opposition between market needs and social needs (the role of the public sector being to fulfill the latter). In contrast, the contemporary terrain of pharmaceutical access politics provides a choice of which kind of market need best serves social needs: there are no options available beyond market alternatives.

In making a call for a socialized medicine with a central role for the public sector, the committee was doing more than arguing for an industrial policy.

Not unlike the Indian judiciary more recently (albeit in a different context and through different solutions; see chapter 3), the committee was emphasizing the social responsibility of the state. It insisted that the "leading role for the production of drugs and pharmaceuticals should rest with the state" (66), asked for a policy philosophy of "socializing drug production and distribution" (85), and stated that the government should decide "acceptable profit margins" for companies that could be enforced through price controls (182). The justification for this came from a reading of the Indian Constitution, and specifically its directive principles (see chapter 3).

How did these principles disappear so radically from Indian state action within two decades of this report, as the government signed on to GATT? After all, some of the ethos of the Hathi Committee Report endured in the Gujral Committee Report of 1993, but it went unheeded. This switch in perspectives and priorities involves understanding both global corporate power, articulated through American state free trade policy (as implemented through bilateral as well as multilateral forums), and the strategic rationality of the Indian executive in 1994 that saw value in being a global player. I explore the Indian state rationale in the mid-1990s next, before turning to the question of corporate power and global geopolitics.

Fourth Conjuncture: India Signs on to TRIPS

I next explain the Indian state's rationales in the 1990s and its strategy behind agreeing to the terms of the Dunkel Draft. This speaks to then Finance Minister Manmohan Singh's sentiments as expressed to the Gujral Committee, which insisted that India could not afford to be left out of multilateral trade forums and emergent terrains of global capital. In order to elaborate this, I draw upon A. V. Ganesan's (1994) account of the government's thinking at the time, *The GATT Uruguay Round Agreement*. Ganesan was the chief negotiator for India at the Uruguay Round in 1989, and was commerce secretary (the highest bureaucratic position in the Ministry of Commerce, which oversaw the GATT negotiations) from 1991 to 1993. Therefore, he was directly involved in conversations around TRIPS and the Dunkel Draft, policymaking situations in which the role of the bureaucrat as a representative of national-state positions was central. Ganesan did have prior experience with the United Nations on issues of global trade, having been a regional adviser to the UN Centre on Transnational Corporations from 1980 to 1985. However, it is worth remembering that the Indian bureaucracy, modeled on the British Civil Service, is explicitly constituted by generalist rather than technocratic expertise. Hence, while Ganesan was arguably the most important bureaucrat to oversee the transition from India's state socialism to neoliberalism, developing considerable expertise in economic and trade policy and its multilateral dimensions, he was not an economic expert of the sort that would normally perform a similar role in an American context.[43] While from Yusuf Hamied's perspective the Indian delegation simply sold the country out, there is a more complex story here about bureaucratic expertise, perceptions, and investments at a significant conjuncture.[44]

The transition to a more globally oriented Indian economy, while often associated with the liberalization programs initiated by the Narasimha Rao government in 1991, had commenced in earnest under Rajiv Gandhi. Ganesan starts his book with an epigraph that encapsulates this vision:

> Should India retreat into a shell like we have in the past in a way, protect ourselves and let the world go by, or are we going to come out and fight for our rightful place in the globe? Are we going to have the guts to come out into the open? That is the real question that is in front of us. And if we are to take this step, and in my mind I am very clear there is no alternative, then the challenge very definitely is in exports, in a competitive industry, an industry which can compare with any other industry on the globe. (1994, 1)

This represents a break from an earlier Nehruvian idea of India, based strongly in socialist principles (Khilnani 1999). Investments in national industrial competitiveness remained, but this was now no longer articulated (as it was in the Hathi Committee Report) in terms of finding niches where the industry could thrive. Rather, it was about directly competing with other national industries, an aspiration that would come to fruition over the next two decades most strongly in India's information technology industry. The bigger question, however, concerns the *we*: Rajiv Gandhi's *we* as he speaks of India is not the same as the Hathi Committee's. The committee's imagination of the state was as an entity that served a representative function toward its people, especially those who fell out of a therapeutic market. Gandhi's *we* concerns a state that speaks for the interests of capital—but not all capital, as Hamied's interests were certainly excluded in this formulation. Who or what would get represented in terms of the national interest itself came to be at stake in this transitional moment.

The specific moment at which Ganesan wrote *The Uruguay Round GATT Agreement* is noteworthy. The Uruguay Round negotiations concluded on December 15, 1993 (just days after the demolition of the Babri Masjid in

Ayodhya by Hindu nationalists). It had intervened in domains beyond its traditional purview, specifically intellectual property rights (through the TRIPS agreement), but also investments (through the agreement on Trade-Related Investment Measures) and services, through the General Agreement on Trade in Services. Together, these constituted an agenda for the establishment of the WTO. Ganesan wrote his book just before the final signing of these agreements in Marrakesh in April 1994. He was therefore fully cognizant of the enormous opposition GATT had already raised by that time in India, and the book in some measure was a response to it.

Ganesan's perspective on the negotiations was informed by both primary issues that were at stake in it. While the politics of GATT were largely around pharmaceutical patents and its implications for drug prices, there was an important dimension of agricultural policy at stake as well (hence Nanjundaswamy's deposition before the Gujral Committee). This specifically related to restricting agricultural subsidies that governments would give to their farmers. Ganesan argued that the Uruguay Round attempted to tackle international trade distortions brought about by the subsidizations of industrialized countries. He suggested that this would provide greater access to global markets for developing countries, especially providing opportunities in exports of rice, wheat, and cotton for Indian farmers. This was an argument to move from a supply-side agricultural export policy to an (international market-driven) demand-side one, which would necessarily require greater corporate participation and investment.

The negative impacts that corporatization of agriculture would have on food security was the basis of Nanjundaswamy's opposition to GATT; but Ganesan insisted that GATT would lead to investments in agriculture and adoption of modern technologies, further leading to increased money flowing to the agricultural sector and to villages, and greater rural purchasing power.[45] In this rendering, the village becomes the site of investment even as rural India becomes a potential consumer market. This signifies an articulation of rural interest with market interest that would recur in subsequent years in other domains such as public health (for instance, in the National Rural Health Mission introduced by the Indian government in 2005; see chapter 2).[46] What is at stake here is not simply a question of economics or access, but of who provides rural India with its food and therapeutic essentials, and on what terms. Ganesan himself conceded the trade-offs that a more corporatized agricultural policy direction presented in terms of increased domestic food prices and pressures on a public distribution system that depended significantly upon the provision of subsidies. But he felt that these trade-offs were worth making for the development that would ensue.

Ganesan's points about agriculture were no doubt important to Indian strategy toward GATT, but this did not concern TRIPS or intellectual property per se. This is the arena in which, according to Hamied, the Indian bureaucracy explicitly acted against then commerce minister Dinesh Singh's directive in 1989, and Ganesan was the head of the delegation that did so. In his justification for India's acquiescence to TRIPS, Ganesan explicitly acknowledged the global power differentials and geopolitics that were at play, while also suggesting that the positions taken especially by American negotiators in the Uruguay Round were a direct reflection of multinational corporate interests. Indeed, Ganesan's stated reasons for the American insistence on bringing intellectual property rights into the ambit of trade negotiations were quite similar, if more diplomatic, than Hamied's diagnosis that the United States was entirely driven by the multinational pharmaceutical lobby. He traced the broader historical shift in Western industry from industrial manufacture to knowledge-based goods; described the "clamor of their industry" (not just pharmaceutical, but also the film and software industries) regarding "piracy"; and the (especially American) sense that the global forum that existed for the regulation and enforcement of intellectual property, the World Intellectual Property Organization, was "toothless" (Ganesan 1994, 14). At the end of the day, however, what won the day was power: the industrialized countries "with their greater economic clout and identity of interest . . . could prevail upon developing countries" to bring intellectual property rights under GATT's purview (14). Ganesan pointed out that the explicit threat of American trade sanctions was a major contributing factor in developing countries acquiescing to the inclusion of intellectual property rights under GATT.

Therefore it was not the case that Hamied or Nanjundaswamy recognized a hierarchical geopolitics that the Indian government was blind to. On the contrary: even those who saw the Uruguay Round as on balance in the national interest did not think that the world was flat or that they had free choice in the matter. The political positions that were articulated were instead a reflection of different strategic sensibilities in response to the striations that existed. Ganesan's position (reflected by Manmohan Singh before the Gujral Committee) was that it was better to join them than to try to beat them. Even as Hamied articulated a representative position on behalf of the Indian generics industry at the time, most large generics companies adopted a similar mentality of strategic resignation by the 2000s, hoping to become attractive acquisition targets for the multinational industry. Indeed, Hamied expressed his own sense of loneliness in this regard:

> YH: Do you know, professor, there is not one generic company in the world today, not one, that is supporting me in what I am doing? All my friends with whom I started, IDMA [Indian Drug Manufacturers' Association, the pharmaceutical lobby group of the national industry] in 1961, don't even talk to me now.
>
> KSR: Why is that?
>
> YH: They're all sold to the multinationals. You take it from me that in the next ten years, 90 percent of the so-called Indian companies as such, as we are today, will not exist. Dr. Reddy's, Ranbaxy, Cipla will not exist as such by 2020. (Hamied interviews)

Indeed, Hamied insisted that Cipla's resistance to being acquired was entirely a function of his individual nationalist principles, and "did not make business sense."

Free Trade and Pharmaceutical Imperialism

Ganesan's account of India's reasons for joining TRIPS portrays a constrained geopolitical playing field that is anything but level, and that is structured in significant measure by the interests of the Euro-American multinational pharmaceutical industry. But it also portrays this as a field that could be strategically leveraged to advantage, in which being part of a multilateral forum would be more nationally beneficial than being left out. But another situated perspective was operational at the time, articulated most starkly by Nanjundaswamy's diagnosis of colonialism and imperialism before the Gujral Committee. It is worth exploring the operation of this worldly understanding in relation to the debate around pharmaceuticals and TRIPS.[47] This involves understanding some of the historical geopolitical context of the Uruguay Round of GATT negotiations, which eventually led to the signing of the TRIPS agreement and the establishment of the WTO.

It is important to note the substantial difference between the Uruguay Round and any previous attempt at multilateral trade negotiations, which concerns the unprecedented and hardly intuitive incorporation of intellectual property rights into a free trade agreement (FTA). But what were the broader geopolitical stakes of such an inclusion and the contexts within which this came to occur? The related conceptual question concerns the "freedom" of free trade. Whether or not the Uruguay Round led to institutions that would genuinely allow trade to be free in all contexts—clearly it did not—it did lead to a freedom of transnational corporate capital to realize value and to engage, especially through the capture of the American state, in particular forms of global governance that were not earlier available to it.

Chakravarti Raghavan (1990) has argued that the Uruguay Round was not just a trade negotiation but a means for the structural reorganization of the world economy in the interests of American geopolitical and Euro-American (and Japanese) multinational corporate interests.[48] But GATT itself was an instrument of post–World War II global economic restructuring. It came into being in 1948 and was assumed to be a temporary agreement until the International Trade Organization (ITO) envisaged under it came into being. The ITO, which never materialized, was to be a quintessentially Keynesian instrument of global governance. Its charter, called the Final Act of the United Nations Conference on Trade and Employment (or the Havana Charter) was proposed by Keynes and signed by fifty-three countries on March 24, 1948. The focus of the charter was to promote global economic cooperation and curtail anticompetitive business practices. The charter never came into force because of the United States' refusal to submit it for ratification by its Senate. This refusal was a function of American unwillingness to cede its capacity for sovereign economic action to a multilateral trade governance regime. Consequently, the Havana Charter itself was dead in the water before it could be implemented.

The GATT agreements were therefore never institutionalized in an organizational form such as the ITO (until they were, subsequent to the Uruguay Round, in the WTO). Instead, they operated through multiple rounds of negotiations. Seven rounds were held in the four decades between the establishment of GATT and the Uruguay Round, and most of these facilitated the trading interests of multinational corporations. Initially, GATT was very much a northern arrangement, unlike the ITO, which was envisaged as a more thoroughly global forum, at a moment of decolonization when the possibilities for globalization included alternatives based on South-South cooperation.[49] Indeed, initially, there were very few Third World countries in GATT.[50]

What one saw in the Uruguay Round was an inversion of global power relations in the sense that it was now northern (especially American) interests that were pushing a truly global economic order that would incorporate the Third World into it.[51] How and why did this reversal happen? Raghavan attributes this to northern, and again especially American, economic crisis. He traces this to a number of moments and factors through the 1970s and early 1980s, of which perhaps the most important were the OPEC actions of 1973–1974 following the breakdown of the Bretton Woods regime.[52] This represented a possibility for a restructuring of global economic relations, if not from the South, then at least from the Middle East, and marked a flashpoint that would lead to northern counterreaction. Alongside this, it is worth mentioning the Club of Rome's 1972 report, *The Limits of Growth*, which predicted the impossibility of indefinite economic growth because of finite natural resources, especially oil (Meadows et al. 1972). In *Life as Surplus*, Melinda Cooper (2008) has identified the neoliberal response to this report as critical in marking the contours of an emergent economic ideology and governance regime, one that would begin to attain its full fruition with the coming to power of Ronald Reagan in 1980. The epistemic crisis that the Club of Rome diagnosed meshes with the geopolitical crisis that Raghavan recognizes as crucial in mobilizing significant global economic restructuring from the North.[53]

The 1980s would not just bring Reagan to power, but would also see the continuation of chronic American economic crisis, especially with Japan establishing itself as a competing economic power.[54] This made for a contradictory geopolitical structure, which saw the United States, Europe, and Japan as economic competitors on the one hand, but with common interests as industrialized economies in Third World resources, labor, and markets on the other. This of course mirrors the structure of corporate interests, marked by simultaneous competition between companies and their consolidated actions (for instance, the lobbying of governments) in the interests of capital accumulation and appreciation. What this led to was a northern lobby in the GATT negotiations, influenced itself by corporate lobbies within northern nations, of which the pharmaceutical lobby was particularly powerful going into the Uruguay Round. The disproportion of North-South power was mirrored by the formal fiction that GATT was a contractual arrangement constituted by equal contracting parties—though it was precisely the ability to strategically activate that fiction which would subsequently lead to the occasional instances of southern countries using the multilateral forum of the WTO to their advantage. The most significant example of this in relation to pharmaceutical politics was the ability to pass the Doha Declaration of 2001.

The Uruguay Round was therefore intimately linked to American geopolitical interests, which were themselves closely articulated to northern or industrialized economic interests in relation to a formally mostly decolonized Third World, at a time when the Cold War and competing world economic ideologies were still very much a reality. The subsequent two decades have seen the consolidation of capitalism as, in Slavoj Žižek's (2004) terms, "the concrete universal of our historical epoch." In other words, unlike in 1986, we now live in a world that is safe for capitalism. The question of which capitalism the world has become safe for, however, remains an acutely political question, one that constitutes the contemporary geopolitical terrain of access to essential medicines.

The structure of this geopolitical configuration looks very different depending on one's perspective. From the perspective of the Euro-American R&D-driven industry that demands and requires absolute monopoly, the flexibilities afforded by the Doha Declaration and the activation of those flexibilities in (especially Indian) legislation since the declaration represents a fundamental threat to market interests, articulated as a threat to innovation itself (see chapters 1, 3, and 4). In this perspective, what one sees is an Indian state running riot, creating exceptions to normative patent regimes left, right, and center. Gleevec is the tip of the iceberg, and Section 3(d) a dangerous precedent, one that might be followed by other countries.[55] From Hamied's perspective, however, there has been just a series of losses over the past thirty years. In the mid-1980s, even the question of whether intellectual property rights should come under the purview of an FTA was debatable. By 2013, the upholding of a public health flexibility that prevents pharmaceutical evergreening while fully respecting a product patent regime was being hailed either as a major victory or as a concession, depending upon one's position in the debate.

Even the enactment and upholding of such limited flexibilities has led to northern backlash through the institution of measures and regimes that have been termed TRIPS-plus. The *plus* here suggests intensification and excess—an attempt to enforce the most monopolistic aspects of TRIPS, with fewer exceptions and flexibilities, but also to institute monopoly by means that go beyond anything envisaged under TRIPS. The primary mechanisms of TRIPS-plus have been bilateral FTAs, mainly involving the United States but also the European Union, which layer upon TRIPS but also go beyond it.[56] The ambitious exception to this is the Trans-Pacific Partnership (TPP), which seeks to be a new multilateral TRIPS-plus framework. The TPP Agreement (TPPA) is an FTA between the United States and ten Pacific Rim nations: Australia, New Zealand, Singapore, Malaysia, Brunei, Vietnam, Peru, Chile, Canada, and Mexico. Other countries could subsequently join this arrangement, even after the agreement is signed, but without the right to change whatever has been agreed to through these negotiations. These countries together represent

34 percent of U.S. trade (Maxmen 2012). Negotiations toward this agreement began in 2008 and concluded in October 2015. The United States has stated that it wishes the TPPA to "set the standard" for future trade agreements (Office of the USTR 2009). The negotiations themselves were largely conducted in secret, and whatever was known to civil society about their content as the agreement was being negotiated was obtained through leaked documents. Significant among these for pharmaceutical politics are two versions of an intellectual property rights chapter, drafted in February and September 2011 respectively.[57]

The TPPA draft chapters propose some of the most monopolistic intellectual property measures ever instituted in any kind of bilateral or multilateral free trade framework. They demand instruments that strictly link patents to regulatory structures (through mechanisms such as data exclusivity, patent linkage, and border enforcement of the transit of generic drugs globally), endowing other kinds of enforcement authorities (such as drug regulators or customs officials) with the authority to enforce intellectual property in the interests of corporate monopoly. Hence, these provisions also explicitly link domains of intellectual property rights and access to medicines with those of clinical trials.[58] There are specific provisions concerning evergreening and pregrant oppositions that target the kinds of public health flexibilities that India incorporated into its 2005 Patent Act, as TPP member nations are prevented from enacting similar flexibilities.

Within the framework of global civil society discourse concerning access to medicines, the TPP signifies everything that is wrong with monopolistic intellectual property regimes.[59] The draft provisions contain mechanisms that increase the effective monopoly on patented pharmaceuticals even beyond the duration of formal patents, raise the bar for generic entry into the market, enforce more stringent border policing of global trade in generics in a manner that curtails rather than enables free trade, and severely restrict the flexibilities individual governments possess to enact modifications or exceptions to the demands of this regime. I am in solidarity with all of these points of opposition, but wish to focus on the implications of the simultaneous appropriation of health by capital with the appropriation of national-state and global governance by corporate interests. In other words, I am interested in the nature of the political at a moment when national-state sovereignty itself comes to be at stake, where questions of democratic accountability come to the fore, and where institutional questions concerning the corporation as an agent of governance at national and global scales must be asked and confronted.

There are two immediate questions to be asked of the TPP in this regard. The first concerns the secrecy surrounding the negotiations and the way in which they were kept out of the purview of democratic accountability. And the second concerns the implications of an agreement that disallows nation-states from defining and acting in any sovereign definition of public interest that is at odds with monopolistic corporate interests as defended by the agreement. This leads to broader questions concerning the nature of the state, the corporation, and their interrelationships in frameworks of national-state and global governance itself, which are ultimately questions of democracy.

The American draft proposals for the TPP were deemed confidential.[60] And yet corporate interests had access and likely input into these proposals through their membership in trade advisory committees. The advisory committee system was established by the U.S. Congress to 1974 to provide input into American trade policy and negotiating objectives. There are currently twenty-eight advisory committees, consisting, according to the U.S. Trade Representative (USTR), of approximately 700 "citizen advisors."[61] As pointed out by a fact sheet outlining civil society concerns about the TPP, these citizens are primarily persons from the private sector.[62] Nonetheless, the USTR has insisted that the TPP negotiations have been transparent and even put out a fact sheet to this effect in 2012 in response to civil society criticism of its procedures, which states, "To ensure public input on TPP from the start, USTR solicited written comments from interested individuals, organizations, and businesses before entering into the talks."[63] "Public input" here is circumscribed by the stated need for confidentiality, on the grounds that "major trade and investment negotiations address a broad range of often complex and commercially sensitive sectors and issues and often take many months or even years to conclude. In order to reach agreements that each participating government can fully embrace, negotiators need to communicate with each other with a high degree of candor, creativity, and mutual trust."[64] Nonetheless, it was claimed that "USTR will publish the full text of the TPP—as we do with all FTAS we negotiate—well before it is signed to invite further comments from Congress, trade advisors, and the public."[65] This is potentially at odds with the negotiation's own classification guidelines, which state that the draft provisions will only be made public four years after the agreement is signed.[66]

What does it mean for a document to be simultaneously transparent yet confidential? How is this related to a public input that is restricted to interested parties? What does it mean for a document to be potentially available for public input when the process by which that document comes to be is explicitly kept confidential? All of these questions concern the ways in which the secret comes to be legitimately enfolded into the operation of the democratic state.[67] The drive of the American investor-state to make corporate monopoly an end in itself is evident in the TPP draft negotiations—but its drive is also to do so in secret, even while claiming transparency.

What does it mean to imagine that public knowledge of the content of TPP negotiations will threaten the "candor, creativity, and mutual trust" between negotiating parties? One sees here an inversion of the basis of Weberian legitimate authority (Weber [1922] 1978), which in the rendering of public sphere theorists such as Jürgen Habermas (1984, 1985) operates through communicative action. In Habermas's account, it is precisely communication, the publicity of knowledge, which renders state authority legitimate through the engendering of trust. Yet the USTR assumes that public knowledge of the content of negotiations will render mistrust and suspicion—not among the public, but rather among the interested parties involved in the negotiations. In other words, who the state claims accountability toward is itself inverted; this is not about garnering legitimate public authority, but about providing negotiating parties with security from public scrutiny and accountability. The interests really being protected here are corporate ones, not even necessarily those of other negotiating states. Indeed, the TPP American draft provisions have faced considerable opposition from a number of other states that are party to the negotiations, including New Zealand (which raised concerns over TRIPS-plus provisions in the draft) and Malaysia (which emerged as the most vocal opponent of the American position in the negotiations).[68]

The democratic comes to be at stake in negotiations such as the TPP, then, at the level of knowledge—or, more precisely, nonknowledge. One sees here the explicit sanctioning, indeed mandating, of ignorance, ostensibly in order to protect the trust of negotiating parties, but also clearly in order to protect the ability of (certain) governments to push corporate interests without public interference. The sanctioning of nonknowledge as part of an institutional epistemic apparatus has been analyzed in terms of what Robert Proctor and Lorna Schiebinger (2008) have called "agnotology." Proctor (2012) elaborates upon how agnotology functions in relation to the corporate interests of the tobacco industry in *Golden Holocaust*. Proctor's is a stunningly broad and meticulously detailed account, but the forms of nonknowledge that he traces primarily focus on explicit acts of agential occlusion of knowledge by corporate interests. His is ultimately an understanding of nonknowledge based in cynical reason.[69] I suggest that we need to go beyond a diagnosis of cynical reason alone, beyond an understanding that assumes purely calculating rational corporate actors effectively buying the state, in order to understand the politics of nonknowledge that are at stake here. This is not to say that strategic calculation is absent, just that it cannot be the point at which explanations run out. Purely rationalist explanations based in cynical reason cannot account for the seamless naturalization of in fact absurd inversions that one sees in relation to the TPP negotiations—such as confidential transparency, or the incentivizing of public disclosure through the mandating of nondisclosure. Such naturalization can only be understood through the paranoid reason of a state that sees publicity and disclosure, indeed knowledge itself, as threatening to corporate interests. It becomes important to theorize such a state, the corporate interests that possess it, and the global relations of production and power that such states engender, as a counterpoint to the Indian state that has contended with the judicialized and publicized trajectories of the political.

This chapter has explored corporate alliance making on the part of Indian generics companies with civil society groups for access to medicines in the context of geopolitics that are both postcolonial and imperialist; indeed, a conjuncture in which imperialist relations of power and production remain a part of the formally postcolonial global condition. Cipla's place within such a conjuncture is both exemplary and exceptional. It is exemplary because the company has itself played a significant role in the development of the Indian pharmaceutical industry as a nationally and globally competitive industry, both through the development of industrial capacity and through decades of organizing domestic industrial interests and lobbying the Indian government to support those interests. The value of the actions taken by the Indian industry in the imaginary of global civil society advocacy around access to medicines is represented in significant measure by Cipla's position and actions, even as civil society actors recognize that this alliance is, among other things, a strategic one that has allowed Cipla to carve out a certain market position. It comes to be an increasingly exceptional position as the strength of India's own industry becomes diluted under emergent post-TRIPS global market reconfigurations that have seen Yusuf Hamied, in his last few years as head of the company, often beating a lone path as other major Indian companies have also sought to position themselves as attractive targets for acquisition.

Hamied's own stubborn insistence in sticking to an antimonopolistic stance therefore involves understanding a value system that goes beyond strategic market interests (even as it incorporates an assessment of those interests) and incorporates his own biography. As with the story of judicialization (chapter 3), a generational capitalist ethos is at play here, one that is likely in the process of vanishing but that might leave its own traces and legacies.[70] It is important to situate the alliance making of Indian companies in terms of their pragmatics but also in terms of their individual and institutional post-colonial inheritances.

Whether one is trying to understand the monopolistic strategies of the multinational industry that operate through emergent transnational governance mechanisms underwritten by American economic and political hegemony, or the free market strategies of Indian firms that are simultaneously resisting this hegemony as they carve out their own global market niches and position themselves as potential targets of acquisition by their adversaries, it is important to conceptualize the kind of state that mediates these corporate interests. The socialized imaginaries of the 1970s as articulated in the Hathi Committee Report never came to pass, in part because of the success of Indian companies such as Cipla to orient the state toward free market interests. This constrained possibilities for the consolidation of a genuinely strong public sector alternative to free market pharmaceuticals, but still involved some measure of representative accountability for generics companies themselves, at least to the extent that they needed to compete and make their drugs affordable to the markets they operated within. A seizure of the state by the vested interests of monopolistic multinational corporate capital, however, precludes any possibility of such representative accountability; if even jurisdiction for infringements of monopoly passes into their hands as envisaged by the TPP, it further precludes democratic possibilities. While the trajectories of pharmaceutical politics in India described in this book gesture toward deeply conflicted but nonetheless promissory horizons of the political, those envisaged by the TPP dream of an appropriated state that would, from the perspective of democratic accountability, be a deceased state.

POSTSCRIPT: PHARMA'S MARKETS

The fiction that capitalism implies democracy is a major source of ideological sustenance for capitalist interests. The implicit assumptions that underlie this fiction are those of freedom: that capitalism implies free markets and consumer choice. The reduction of democratic freedom to the freedom of consumer choice is problematic enough; this book has further attempted to show how in the domain of pharmaceuticals every aspect of this fiction is ludicrous. Free consumer choice is hardly relevant to situations where large segments of potential consumers are excluded from the market altogether because essential medication is priced higher than markets can bear (chapters 1, 3), even as certain populations come to be therapeutically saturated as their drug consumption comes to be the source of market growth (Dumit 2012a, 2012b). Free markets can hardly be assumed when one of the fundamental contestations in the terrain of global pharmaceuticals pits free market capitalism against monopoly capitalism, with the former the geopolitically more vulnerable form. And therefore, capitalism itself is a fictional concept, because what is at stake is never a singular capitalism but always competing entities and forms of capitalism operating under similar logics, battling for the establishment and instantiation of different kinds of market terrains. Rather than making simplistic determinations of the democratic nature of capitalism or otherwise, it is worth unpacking the kinds of pharmocratic structures that are in competition. One (represented by the multinational Euro-American R&D-driven pharmaceutical corporation) is a structure of corporate imperialism, which comes to possess the state such that it becomes an investor-state. The second is a structure of representative obligation on the part of the capitalist elite (represented by figures such as Yusuf Hamied), which has been a feature of postcolonial Indian capitalism and governance.

The former structure requires attention to corporate power, for which it is useful to think with Thorstein Veblen's ([1919] 2005) argument in The Vested Interests and the Common Man.[71] *There are three questions that I wish to consider through a reading of Veblen. First, what is the nature of corporate power, and how does it come to be a vested interest whose self-perpetuation trumps the preservation of public interest? Second, what does this have to do with the sanctity of liberal principles of ownership and property? And third, how might we think about the patent as a monopolistic instrument of corporate rather than public interest in this regard?*

These are not questions that can be answered discretely or sequentially, because the point of Veblen's analysis in The Vested Interests *is their mutual imbrication. Indeed, his very definition of the corporation is "a formal coalition of ownership" (Veblen [1919] 2005, 24). This is related to a modality of business enterprise that is distinct from industrial production, and that increasingly makes the latter subsidiary to it. This means that progressively, the production of value comes to be uncoupled from industrial production to become a function of investment and financial enterprise.[72] In the process of ownership coalescing institutionally in the corporate form, however, Veblen argues for the "denaturing" of ownership itself, "so that it no longer carries its earlier duties and responsibilities" (44). Veblen is suggesting here that the liberal legal consolidation of ownership assumes it to be the industrialist's legitimate protection of his "industrial arts."*

One sees this in the rationality of the patent, for instance, which assumes a direct relationship between inventor and invention. The mediation of the corporate form in this structure of ownership, Veblen argues, subverts the very rationality of ownership itself; but the law does not acknowledge this subversion, and acts as if the protection of corporate ownership is the same as the protection of the ownership of invention by inventor, or product by the industry that manufactures it. Veblen refers to this as the transition to "absentee ownership of anonymous corporate capital" (44). In other words, corporate ownership maintains the figure of the inventor-industrialist as central to its rationality, but no longer requires his actual body as the source of value. Invention itself comes to be about the production of capitalized value rather than the production of the product itself—but always justified with recourse to the idea of a transparent relationship between corporate ownership and the production of the product. In such a situation of corporatized ownership, the owners of property operate purely as vested interests. Their very raison d'être is the perpetuation of their ownership. Law that sanctifies ownership in such a context is one that "translates into legal decisions bearing on the inviolability of vested interests and intangible assets" (60). If he had been talking about free trade and intellectual property rights, Veblen could have in this statement been describing the TPP.

At issue here is a structure that is purely about the representation of vested interests, hence thoroughly undemocratic even as it operates in the name of democracy. But how does one understand the latter pharmocratic structure, the one seen in postcolonial India as manifested by capitalist stewards of public interest such as Yusuf Hamied?

To answer this question, it is worth thinking about Hamied's strategic and situated opposition to TRIPS. This is an opposition that articulates and defends Cipla's business interests, which thrived under free market competition facilitated by the 1970 Patent Act. But it is not just the interests of an individual company in a competitive market terrain that are upheld; so too are those of a national industrial sector, which Hamied claims to represent. At the same time, it reflects Hamied's nationalist (and more recently global) humanitarianism. I wish to mark the manner in which Hamied discursively articulates antimonopolistic free market sentiment with public interest and national interest; but how, further, he renders national interest in terms of an elite postcolonial responsibility for a national destiny, of which individuals like him are custodians. As he told the Gujral Committee, "After all, we are responsible for India's destiny and we should not, under any circumstances, budge on the stand of monopoly."[73]

There is an echo here of a Nehruvian sensibility of a national "tryst with destiny," one that can be met only if the postcolonial elite bears its responsibility. In his famous speech to the Constituent Assembly at the moment of independence from the British, India's first prime minister, Jawaharlal Nehru, emphasized the responsibility of the elite toward the nation:

> Long years ago we made a tryst with destiny, and now the time comes when we shall redeem our pledge, not wholly or in full measure, but very substantially. At the stroke of the midnight hour, when the world sleeps, India will awake to life and freedom. A moment comes, which comes but rarely in history, when we step out from the old to the new, when an age ends, and when the soul of a nation, long suppressed, finds utterance. . . . Freedom and power bring responsibility. The responsibility rests upon this Assembly, a sovereign body representing the sovereign people of India.[74]

Nehru himself was speaking of the responsibility of the Constituent Assembly, a representative state body. But there is a history of Indian capitalism that sees this representative responsibility articulated and embodied in the self-fashioning of certain Indian industrialists (such as the Tatas and Birlas, and certainly the Hamieds).

"Freedom and power bring responsibility." This is the critical sentiment that I wish to emphasize here. I do not want to make a romantic argument for Indian pharmaceutical capitalists as inherently noble in comparison to evil multinationals: after all, Indian companies are strategic actors who leverage their market interests, just as multinational corporations have undertaken their own forms of philanthropy at least occasionally or to some extent in good faith. But the burden of responsibility that Hamied bears exceeds strategic calculation; it is his biographical inheritance, a function of the time and place and family he grew up in. Just as judicial cultures are important to note in order to understand the interpretive strategies of Indian higher courts as they decide upon issues of health and therapeutic access (see chapter 3), so too are cultures of capitalisms important to attend to even as one recognizes that logics of capital underlie them all.[75]

It is precisely this sentiment of responsibility that is so lacking in the kinds of world making the monopolist pharmaceutical industry is attempting to instantiate. It is not the case that European or American capitalism is incapable of such an ethos: the mid-twentieth-century image of Merck, for instance, is intimately tied to the figure of its then head George Merck, who articulated a sense of public responsibility for the pharmaceutical industry which was not that different from that espoused by Hamied.[76] But such an ethos can only survive in a managerial corporation. As the especially American corporation has come to be progressively captured by financial capital, its operation as a purely vested interest has intensified in a manner that was diagnosed and anticipated by Veblen. In stark contrast to Hamied's sensibility, the only thing that a corporation would be responsible to in the kinds of market structures the TPP envisages is its own financial interests. If the former keeps open the possibility of a (self-interested yet vanguard representative) democratic capitalism, the latter makes a mockery of any democratic pretense.

Constitutions of Health, Responsibility, and Democracy

Three Moments of Rescripting

First moment: in September 2012, the Delhi High Court passed a judgment denying a patent to the Swiss pharmaceutical company Hoffmann-La Roche and the New York–based OSI Pharmaceuticals for their anticancer drug erlotinib. Erlotinib is a human epidermal growth factor receptor that has provided a major breakthrough in the targeted treatment of metastatic non–small cell lung cancer. The verdict, issued by Justice Manmohan Singh, followed the precedent that was established by the Madras High Court in denying a patent on Gleevec, in that it was an instance of an Indian court utilizing the public health flexibilities that existed in its 2005 TRIPS-compliant patent legislation to impose limits on the extent and scope of intellectual property rights in the cause of access to essential medicines. However, unlike Gleevec, erlotinib had already been granted a patent, which the court proceeded to revoke.

A patent application for erlotinib was jointly filed in 1996 by OSI and Pfizer.[1] The drug was approved for market by the U.S. Food and Drug Administration (FDA) in 2004 and by the European Union in 2005. It was marketed under its trade name, Tarceva, by Roche, which had entered into a licensing agreement with OSI in 2001 that allowed it to market and sell a number of drugs covered by the agreement, including erlotinib. Roche introduced

Tarceva into the Indian market in 2006, and the patent office in Delhi issued a patent on the drug in July 2007. Nonetheless, Cipla began manufacturing generic erlotinib (trade name Erlocip) in December 2007 in violation of the patent, knowing full well that it would be sued for its transgression. Sure enough, Roche and OSI took Cipla to the Delhi High Court to dispute the infringement on January 15, 2008.[2] Cipla responded with the claim that growth factor inhibitors had already been used in the treatment of cancers; hence erlotinib was building on known prior art and was simply derivative of known compounds. It pointed to a European patent issued to Zeneca Ltd. in August 1995 for quinazoline derivatives (EP 0566226), to which family erlotinib belongs. One of the examples of pharmaceutically acceptable salts covered by EP '226, Cipla claimed, bore deep structural similarities to erlotinib, providing a basis from which a person skilled in the prior art could have anticipated the latter. What one sees here is a new mechanism employed by Cipla to dispute a patent: unlike the case of Gleevec, which involved the filing of pregrant oppositions to the Patent Office that led to the denial of the patent, the Tarceva case saw a granted patent being disputed simply through its violation—which allowed for a subsequent opposition to the granting of the patent to be mounted through the courts, as a defense of the violation. In the process, Cipla filed its own counterclaims (C.C. No. 52/2008) to substantiate its arguments against the granting of the patent, going so far as to ask that the patent be revoked.

In a verdict that built upon the Gleevec precedent but extended its scope, the High Court upheld Cipla's right to manufacture the generic medication on the grounds that a right to health trumps property rights. If the Gleevec verdict was a technical verdict that read the spirit of the constitution through a historicization of legislative intent regarding the scope of patenting drugs, the Tarceva verdict was an explicitly normative statement about the relative values of these two kinds of rights. What one sees here is the judiciary restructuring the terrain of global pharmaceuticals away from one of absolute monopoly. This could be seen as a case of Indian resistance to multinational pharmaceutical hegemony.

Second moment: in May 2012, a Parliamentary Standing Committee on Health and Family Welfare produced a scathing report on the functioning of India's Central Drugs Standards Control Organization (CDSCO), which is the primary regulatory authority for drug evaluation and approval. It suggested that the very priorities of CDSCO were skewed. Whereas comparable regulatory authorities in other countries such as the U.S. FDA had an explicit mandate to protect the public interest, the Ministry of Health and Family Welfare informed the Parliamentary Standing Committee that CDSCO's mission was to "meet the aspirations . . . demands and requirements of the pharmaceutical industry."[3]

The report did not itself touch upon either the question of unethical clinical trials or of access to essential medicines. In fact, on the face of it, it concerned itself with the opposite—the approval of drugs for market in India without the adequate conduct of late-stage clinical trials on Indian populations, leading to an excessive marketing of drugs that might potentially not be safe and efficacious in the Indian context. This indicates the ease with which pharmaceuticalization can occur alongside the proliferation of cases of unethical clinical trials and of situations where accessing essential medications under new patent regimes becomes potentially more difficult.

In reviewing the recent history of drug approvals by the CDSCO, the Parliamentary Standing Committee found files pointing to the regulatory history of three controversial drugs—perfloxacin, lomafloxacin, and sparfloxacin—missing. These drugs had been either not approved or withdrawn from the market in a number of Western countries, but were still being marketed in India. It was further determined that between 2008 and 2010, thirty-three drugs had been approved for marketing without any clinical trials being conducted on Indian patients; even trials that were conducted often did not include representative sample sizes across a wide demographic range. Expert inputs into drug approvals were also found to be inadequate or dubious, suggesting an "apparent nexus between drug manufacturers and many experts."[4]

While the report made depressing reading in terms of the state of drug regulation in India, it was significant in emphasizing different normative priorities than those being pushed by the CRO industry in the mid-2000s (see chapter 2). For instance, the CROs' idea of regulatory capacity building primarily involved devising guidelines for good clinical practice that were harmonized with international norms and that were in the interests of facilitating the influx of global clinical trials. In contrast, protecting public interest and public health was the primary aim of the report. The CDSCO Report contributed to the emerging civil society dialogue on how clinical trials in the country should be regulated.

Third moment: in December 2013, the U.S. FDA approved sofasbuvir (brand name Sovaldi), developed by the American company Gilead Biosciences, to treat hepatitis C. As part of a combination therapy with other drugs, Sovaldi has been found to cure hepatitis in 90 percent of patients treated, with significantly reduced side effects compared to the previous standard of care, interferon. However the price of the drug, $84,000 for a twelve-week course of treatment in the United States, generated controversy.[5] This has not been just among advocates fighting for access to medicines; for instance, the chief management officer of Express Scripts, the world's largest pharmacy benefits management organization, stated that such pricing is "simply unsustainable" (Express Scripts 2014). Sovaldi represents in a particularly stark manner the ethics and politics of prescribing an extremely expensive drug that has a much greater potential for safe and efficacious therapeutic intervention. Hepatitis C affects millions of people worldwide, with an estimated 3 million cases in the United States alone. This makes it difficult for public health and private third-party systems to contemplate procuring the drug. For instance, while the United Kingdom's National Institute for Health Care and Excellence approved the purchase of Sovaldi by the National Health Service, doubts have been expressed about whether the state can bear the cost burden of treating its hepatitis C population with the drug (Helfand 2014b; Staton 2014).

In response, Gilead entered into discussions with Indian generic manufacturers in January 2014 to market the drug at significantly lower prices in developing countries. A licensing deal struck in September 2014 allowed generics companies to market the drug at a lower price in ninety-one developing countries, with Gilead itself selling its drug in these countries for just $900 for a twelve-week course (Helfand 2014a). The potential market in these countries amounts to over 100 million hepatitis C patients. This suggested the possibility that a multinational pharmaceutical company would consider differentially pricing cutting-edge drugs globally as an alternative market strategy to the aggressive defense of monopoly rights and single global price points that was a feature of Novartis's strategy around Gleevec.[6] Gilead's move sought to tap into large markets with low capacity to pay, in spite of the economic and political risks associated with such a strategy (see chapter 1). [7] This book has outlined the ways in which the appropriation of health by capital has led on the one hand to the self-fashioning of India by the CRO industry as a global experimental site, leading to a spate of scandals surrounding allegations of unethical clinical trials; and on the other hand to the aggressive insistence on monopoly regimes for drugs by the multinational pharmaceutical industry, potentially putting access to essential medicines at stake. Yet here are three examples of trajectories of judicial politics, state oversight, and market strategy that suggest the possibilities for rescripting the power hierarchies that operate in global pharmaceutical politics.

Or do they?

My purpose in this book is neither to diagnose a desperate or hopeless state of pharmaceutical politics captured by logics of capital, nor to end with predictions for the possibility of better futures consequent to resistance from the South. The ways in which logics materialize and trajectories of the political develop are always contingent and situated. What I wish to do instead is to think about the terrain of politics as it is constituted through the articulations of its multiple emergent and constitutive forms with value and knowledge in all their multiple senses. I argue in these concluding reflections that this raises crucial questions for a praxis toward pharmocracy, which involves thinking about the impacts of political economic structures of global biomedicine on both health and democracy, and further involves considering democracy in terms of forms of responsibility and the structures of accountability that they engender. This is not an attempt to be superficially prescriptive or to suggest that socialized health is better than capitalized health in any simple sense.[8] It is rather to note that a spectrum of biomedical, social, and political imaginaries emerge through particular spaces for and forms of pharmaceutical politics, with consequences not just for health but also for democracy.

Compare for instance the range of political possibilities that were imagined in the Hathi Committee Report of 1975 (see chapter 5) with those that are imaginable today. The Hathi Report was arguing, as a realistic principle of policy, for the establishment of a strong public sector pharmaceutical industry even as it made a case for situating pharmaceuticals within the context of broader policy interventions into providing basic health care for citizens. Now, the best bet for access to essential medicines is seen as the survival of a private generic drug industry, including especially in southern countries such as India. Even imagining a viable mechanism for drug access through building institutional capacity in the public sector seems inconceivable. And the long-term prospects of Indian generics companies seem tenuous at best in a changing market landscape that makes them attractive targets for acquisition by the multinational pharmaceutical industry. The question therefore is not whether public sector pharmaceutical companies are better or worse than private sector ones—that would be an overly simplistic and hypothetical question, meaningless unless situated in relation to particular conjunctures, histories, trajectories, and locations. Rather, the question we face concerns the consequences of living in a world where a public sector alternative to the acutely felt problems of health care access is not even on the table. This is not just a problem of distributive justice and of the limited incentives that capital has to concern itself beyond its markets (except in search of raw materials or labor, such as that of experimental subjectivity). It also speaks to the kinds of innovation that come to be incentivized and valorized. In the capitalized health that we increasingly experience through current moves of global harmonization, innovation comes to be narrowly framed in terms of the production of new drugs, many of which are themselves not particularly novel (often modifications of existing drugs, or drugs that belong to well-researched families of molecules, and invariably drugs that can be marketed to populations that can pay for diseases that can be chronically managed with therapeutic intervention for extended periods of time). Reverse engineering generic drugs, which requires considerable ingenuity in developing novel manufacturing processes, is not just devalued in such an imaginary: it is likened to copying and piracy.[9] And the genuinely transformative innovations, such as Gleevec, themselves tend to be a function of decades of largely public-funded fundamental research on cellular and molecular mechanisms that were undertaken without specific drug-development goals in mind, subsequently interacting and collaborating with industrial drug development programs in often serendipitous ways (see chapter 3).[10]

Meanwhile, Indian judicial interventions into curtailing the extent and scope of multinational corporate monopolies might seem like a major act of resistance, and certainly their importance should not be underestimated. But it is worth tempering this with the realization that the Gleevec verdict in itself was a fight to maintain the strength of a single clause in a section of policy that provides for the enactment of public health flexibilities that curtail the monopolistic institution of product patent regimes. The possibility of imagining a situation in which a country with a major pharmaceutical industry could prevent patents on drug molecules altogether now seems inconceivable. Indeed, Section 3(d) does not even prevent pharmaceutical evergreening, its stated purpose, in any absolute sense—only in situations in which the modified molecule does not show increased efficacy.[11]

Even this limited protection has come under attack. The Indian executive has always been ambivalent about Section 3(d), which was only enacted because of the exigencies of coalition politics that prevailed in 2005 and the pressure exerted by the communist parties on the ruling Congress government of the time (see chapter 3). As just one illustrative example, the chief economic advisor in the Narendra Modi–led BJP government, Arvind Subramanian, has been publicly on record stating that the United States should take India to the WTO's Dispute Settlement Board because of its utilization of public health flexibilities in its patent legislation ("Modi's Chief Economic Adviser" 2014).

First India did away with process patents. Then it introduced a crucial public health flexibility to limit evergreening (without in any way questioning the authority or sanctity of product patents, only their utilization as pure instruments of corporate monopoly)—a flexibility that has significant but limited import, and one that has only been upheld in letter and spirit after years of legal battle. And now even such flexibilities are under attack: not just those such as Section 3(d) that are relatively unique to India, but even others such as the invocation of compulsory licensing, which is an instrument used to limit monopolies on drugs in instances of nationally determined public health needs across the world for decades. India's first compulsory license, on Bayer's anticancer drug Nexavar, was disputed by the company and had to be upheld by the Intellectual Property Appellate Board. Attempts to issue a compulsory license on the next-generation treatment for chronic myeloid leukemia, dasatinib, came under attack from the U.S. Trade Representative.[12] Manufactured under the brand name Sprycel by Bristol-Myers Squibb, dasatinib is an important drug for the treatment of patients who have developed resistance to Gleevec/imatinib. But since it is a new drug that was manufactured after 1995, it has qualified for a product patent and generic versions of the drug do not exist.[13]

Gaining the wiggle room to institute a patent regime that is not tied into absolutely monopolist imperatives has involved enormous struggle against hegemonic corporate interests; the possibility of imagining a regime of pharmaceutical manufacture and distribution that is outside or beyond patents altogether (unless such a system furthers monopolistic corporate interest through other means) seems impossible. The Indian judicial verdicts curtailing the scope of intellectual property rights have provided vital room for political maneuver for those fighting for access to essential medicines; but they do not transform the political economic structures under which drug development and access operate. Again the question here is not simply one of whether monopoly or the free market is better in terms of drug access, as that question can have different answers depending on the situation (see chapter 4); in any case, the narrowing of the problem of health to one of drug access is itself limiting. Instead, the question I would like to emphasize concerns the consequences for both health and democracy of living in a world in which the structure of monopolistic drug development becomes the norm in relation to which alternatives have to be carved out through expensive, contentious, and contingent political battles, to the extent that the initial rationale of patents as a purely instrumental monopoly existing in the public interest itself comes to be subverted and forgotten.

In a similar vein, while advocacy against unethical clinical trials has raised vital awareness about a significant problem, it has found itself caught in its own Catch-22 situation in which failures to implement the current regulation lead to demands for more punitive regulation. The intent behind the regulatory changes enacted in 2013 by the Health Ministry in response to civil society and judicial concerns was good, but its consequences potentially mixed. After all, the institutional capacity for implementation remains as limited as before. Meanwhile, the reactive tightening of regulations made India a potentially unattractive destination for clinical research, affecting even studies that might be important for epidemiology, public health, or basic research. Further, if the political economies of intellectual property are constituted by monopolistic interests whose power endures in spite of occasional setbacks and recalibrations, then those of clinical trials are constituted by brokerage economies all the way down. The situation of clinical trials in India might have changed to some extent consequent to the scandalous events discussed in chapter 2, but the structures of brokerage remain.

This book has explored a number of forms of and spaces for politics: financialization, advocacy around public scandal, judicialization, philanthropic monopoly, strategic free market alliances, and imperialist and postcolonial geopolitics, all operating in India in relation to a contemporary conjuncture of global policy harmonization that I have suggested is actually a battle for hegemony. Each of these political forms and spaces shows different relationships between situational change and structural transformation. The most evidently politicized pharmaceutical trajectories in India over the past decade, which have seen limits on monopoly regimes through legislative public health flexibilities that have been activated and upheld by the courts and advocacy that has brought unethical clinical trials to light, have been important, even historic, in shaping contemporary global biomedical terrains. But they have largely been situational responses that have not managed to reverse more foundational structural transformations that have been underway over the past half-century toward more capitalized, corporatized, financialized forms of health. The actions of Indian generics companies have in their own way been structurally transformative, enabled by national legislation such as the 1970 Patent Act and a broader global conjuncture of the 1970s that envisioned other kinds of internationalist public health alliances than those driven by American geopolitical hegemony. At the same time, the 1970 Act itself served private interests, just Indian national as opposed to Euro-

American multinational ones; and in spite of the recommendations of the Hathi Committee, deep investment in building and sustaining public sector infrastructure for drug development in India never came to pass.

The real structural transformations of our times in biomedicine have been driven by the financialization of multinational pharmaceutical capital. Ongoing TRIPS-plus negotiations about the extent to which monopoly capital will run its writ through emergent regimes of global governance are equally consequential in terms of long-term structural configurations under which health comes to be defined and institutionalized (see chapter 5). But again, the stakes here go beyond health care as one considers the kinds of democratic curtailments that will be effected if, as the Trans-Pacific Partnership Agreement envisages, the jurisdiction for enforcing monopoly regimes passes from the hands of nation-states where it is currently held to those of corporate monopoly holders themselves.

I am arguing that the most structurally transformative forms of global pharmaceutical politics over the past half-century have been those that have facilitated the capitalization of health in various forms, especially those that have facilitated a financialized, monopolistic corporatization of pharmaceutical production. This is not just about an appropriation of drug production or distribution by capital; it has entailed a concomitant attempt to appropriate the regimes of governance that shape the modes and relations of production, distribution, and consumption of biomedicine. The role of hegemonic nation-states, and especially the role of American geopolitical power, is of particular importance to conceptualize here; but so too is the role of other forms of transnational governance that have the power to set industrial, commercial, and health policy agendas, whether through international forums (free trade agreements such as the WTO or TPP, or various other TRIPS-plus agreements that have been negotiated bilaterally) or through technocratic bodies of expertise (organizations such as the Gates Foundation or PATH). Forms of judicialization or public advocacy from the South that have resisted such corporate and geopolitical hegemony have been of vital importance and have won significant victories, but have not managed to transform or reverse the structural appropriation of health by capital.

But has politics failed if structures are not transformed? Or, in other words, what might the stakes of the political be even in the absence of structural transformation? I argue that answering this question involves thinking through the question of representation and theorizing the representative state at a moment when the value and validity of the state itself have come under increasing attack both from progressive quarters and from neoliberal interests. In order to do so, I consider the articulations of value, politics, and knowledge in global pharmaceuticals in relation to questions of democracy and responsibility.

Democracy and Responsibility

It is not the case that capitalized, corporatized, financialized, monopolist capitalism cannot be benevolent. Capitalized health in fact consistently operates through idioms of value that are ethical as much as they are about the generation of surplus. Sometimes, this ethics is programmatically enshrined as philanthropy (corporate drug donation programs, for instance). At other times, they take the form of public health interventions (such as PATH's demonstration studies to roll out HPV vaccines in a national immunization program). More generally, the trajectories of global harmonization that facilitate capital flows in biomedicine were underwritten from the outside by normative value systems having to do with biomedical ethics or innovation. One cannot afford to be cynical about the normative impulses that animate these value systems; rather, it is important to look at their structural limits, not just in terms of providing health care to those who need it but also in terms of enabling democracy. In order to elaborate this, I wish to think further about the question of responsibility.

I argue that the responsibility articulated by corporatized structures such as corporate social responsibility or public-private partnerships is limited in at least four ways. First, such forms of responsibility, through a focus on ethics, often evacuate the political. Second, they render market systems and logics in place by putting forth logics of win-win.[14] Third, such acts of responsibility can be withdrawn at will (consider Novartis's threats to withdraw the Gleevec International Patient Assistance Program in countries that offered generic alternatives to the drug; see chapter 4). And fourth, there is often a notable lack of public accountability in such regimes of capitalized and limited responsibility. In this sense, the limited responsibility of corporatized philanthropy sits comfortably with an idea of Responsibility Ltd. It is a form of responsibility that is completely appropriable and appropriated by the interests and instruments of global capital.

I contrast this to Jacques Derrida's (1992) idea of responsibility without limit. This is central to Derrida's call for a notion of justice that includes but goes beyond the force of law. It animates the 2013 revisions to the Indian Drugs and Cosmetics Act, which stipulates that trial sponsors be held responsible for continuing medical care for those who suffer trial-related adverse events (see chapter 2). This extends the responsibility for the trial both outward (beyond the brokers who conduct the trials to the actual agencies who sponsor them) and forward (beyond immediate emergency medical care for trial-related injury to long-term responsibility for the well-being of trial participants). And it speaks to the kinds of constitutional social responsibility that the Indian courts have tried to invoke repeatedly in relation to questions of access to medicines, which is one that is unlimited relative to its more corporate and corporatized varieties.

The idea of a responsibility without limit might seem impractical to legalize or institutionalize. Indeed, the proposal that trial sponsors be held responsible for adverse events over a long term drew both ire and ridicule from many researchers, and might well have been a factor in the recent ambivalence of many agencies, public and private, to conduct clinical studies in India. As a pragmatic principle of policy, responsibility without limits has its limits. But Derrida articulates this not in such narrow pragmatist terms, but as a horizon of the political: is it possible to imagine a politics that demands and entails responsibilities without limits? It is worth remembering that the regime of limited responsibility that global capital embraces and demands manages, without any qualms, to think of profitability without limits as both desirable and natural. And it is worth remembering, again, that a world constituted by limited (corporate) profitability and unlimited (state) responsibility was precisely that which was envisaged in the Hathi Committee Report just four decades ago. This is a structure that seems impossible to even imagine today.

I argue that this has something significant to do with the possibilities and limits of imagining the democratic. For all of its limitations and failures, a structure of limited profitability and unlimited responsibility can only be conceivable in relation to a state, and indeed to a democratic state, accountable to all its citizens. For all its productive potential, a structure of limited responsibility is precisely the limit of a nonstate actor; even a noncorporate actor that is not in search of unlimited profitability such as MSF, for instance, could not possibly conceive surviving a situation where it is held responsible for the long-term medical care of an indeterminate number of people in different parts of the world who might have been affected by clinical studies that they are involved in sponsoring. The responsibility that is institutionally articulated to the norms and forms of a state constitution is necessarily more expansive and unlimited than one that is not. And yet, the state has failed and continues to fail, and the failures of the welfare state have undoubtedly been responsible at least in part for its utter discrediting by neoliberal corporatized logics, which in today's India have come to occupy a valorized and hegemonic position. How then might we conceptualize the democratic? My own interest lies in thinking about the possibilities for a democratic politics in the context of the operation of radically different stakes and across glaring power differentials, which keeps open the possibility of structural transformation through engagements—including strategically agonistic ones with powerfully situated entities—in which the end game is not necessarily consensus, but is rather the promise of justice.[15] This could materialize in specific, highly differentiated and situated articulations and investments of politics; but it commits to an idea and ideal of politics that manages to hold together the disparate scales and stakes of agonistic tactical and strategic engagement with an imagination of the possibility of structural transformation. This necessarily involves thinking politics in relation to the state.

Seizing the State

Given what I have just said, I suggest that the horizon of progressive politics today must at some level involve seizing the state.[16] Indeed, I believe that the success of corporatized, financialized capital, especially in the American context, has been achieved through such seizure that has rendered the state more and more accountable to such interests even as it has asphyxiated those functions of the state that could or should be held publicly accountable. In this section, I briefly think through the possibilities, limits, and contradictions involved in seizing the state in the two trajectories of politics I have described that have attempted to resist and rescript hegemonic formations of global pharmaceutical capital, those of judicialization and the public scandal.

The higher courts in India have not just become a bulwark for ensuring access to essential medicines or for pushing a broader public interest agenda; their actions have opened up the possibility of pushing the state toward enacting its constitutional responsibilities toward its citizens. Indeed, their very conceptualization as citizens who are entitled to essential therapy at affordable cost rather than simply as consumers who might under certain circumstances be beneficiaries of ethical benevolence is significant. This reflects a broader judicial turn in Indian politics through the mechanism of public interest litigation.[17] In spite of notable exceptions, the Indian judiciary has tended since the late 1970s to pursue the goals of social justice in an activist manner, which is certainly reflected in its stance on access to medicines. This is animated not just by a spirit of public interest but often by an affirmative reading of the Indian Constitution as a document that enjoins both positive and negative obligations upon the state toward its citizens (see chapter 3).

Mobilization based on public scandal such as that seen around unethical clinical trials, like judicialization, also represents an important site for the expression of democratic political sensibilities. This has led to concerted civil society engagement in deliberative processes concerning the conduct of clinical research in India, even resulting in policy changes (as indicated earlier).[18] The ambitions of such a politics go beyond the narrow regulation of a sphere of unethical activity: there is an attempt in the process to forge a people-centered clinical research agenda in place of one that is driven by corporate interests. There may well be limits and contradictions to the specific policy changes enacted in 2013 in response to such mobilization; but the impulse of such politics is to imagine a political horizon in which health care is not accountable only to logics of capital.

Imagining a political horizon is a process that always has to contend with its inherent contradictions. I have pointed to one already: how the regulation of unethical clinical trials has moved toward instituting more punitive measures for violators, without the concomitant building of institutional capacity to implement the regulations that do exist. This means that the problem of regulation remains in practice, even as clinical researchers with a range of investments (including those that might encompass people-centered research) have become wary of India as a site for their work. This is reflective of a larger problem in relation to seizing the state. It is one thing to demand that the state ensure accountability for the actions of both state and nonstate actors involved in clinical research of all kinds, which is a demand that has been consistently articulated in the course of the politics of public scandal surrounding clinical trials over the past few years. But it is an altogether more complex task to imagine the building of public institutions that are structurally accountable to civil society in a manner that nonstate institutions are not. At a time when the state's role as a steward of public interest has come under attack from both the Right and the Left, a sustained conversation about building public capacity is often untenable and always interrupted.

Indeed, there was an interesting if predictable split among members at the 2011 consultation regarding the role of the state in relation to the civil society mobilization that was emerging. Generally, members with more formal Communist Party affiliations were more open to thinking about a politics that engaged the state and its institutions; those that had affiliations to grassroots nongovernmental organizations that had earlier mobilized around issues such as genetically modified organisms articulated a more antagonistic stance toward the state. A number of feminists in the consultation were also wary of the state, but it was a wariness borne out of the particular historical experience of the state's coercive family planning programs of the 1970s—a concern with a biopolitical state in which care of the population was articulated as a means of control over reproductive bodies.[19] The question of whether to demand state accountability from the outside or whether to engage in institutional endeavors from the inside was a vexed one that was itself subject to the historical trajectories of politics that individuals and groups brought to the table along with their concerns about unethical clinical trials. Seizing the state is all very well, but what that might tangibly mean is itself a deeply political issue.

Further, a critical question of representation is at stake in the imagining of a people-centered health through elite, globally articulated, largely metropolitan and cosmopolitan civil society movements. Who gets to decide what constitutes people-centered research? What relations with expert biomedical communities would need to be forged to facilitate such a conversation, and on what and whose terms? Often, concerns were voiced that only clinical research in the public interest or in the national interest should be allowed. Who would decide? While a relationship between public and national interest was aggressively posited and pursued by the Indian pharmaceutical industry in relation to the 1970 Patent Act (see chapter 5), what might such a relationship look like in relation to clinical research and clinical trials? Particularly vexed were questions about whether and on what terms clinical research should be allowed on vulnerable populations. How one might consider the articulation of the need to protect the vulnerable from clinical research (even as a component of people-centered research would necessarily involve ensuring that research was conducted on diseases and conditions afflicting the most vulnerable) provides particularly difficult and poignant considerations for a representative politics.[20]

All of this constitutes a fraught, tenuous, and contradictory space for the articulation of a democratic politics driven by civil society and in concert with the judiciary. But the state can also be seized by corporate capital to become an investor-state, which is what is imagined as a corporate horizon of the politics in TRIPS-plus arrangements such as the Trans-Pacific Partnership Agreement (see chapter 5). A contradictory democratic politics to seize the state seems infinitely preferable to one that cedes ground to its appropriation by corporate capital.

As a book about pharmaceutical politics, this was meant to be about health and its reconfigurations as it gets appropriated by logics of capital. Yet it has ended up in equal measure being about the political as it gets constituted in contemporary India, its explanations resting, if provisionally, upon questions of the democratic. Indeed, my linkage of the political to the democratic is a conscious conceptual move away from a lineage of social theory about the contemporary life sciences that, following Michel Foucault, articulates the political to "life itself."[21] *Even as pharmaceutical politics in India are repeatedly overdetermined by questions of health and illness, life and death, life itself suggests a sacralization of such politics that does not do empirical justice to the stakes of the political as they emerge in the domains that I am concerned with.*[22] *Yet of course health matters, not just as a structural abstraction but in deeply embodied, subjective, and experience-proximal ways.*

My father passed away from stomach cancer as this book was under review. He was virtually asymptomatic; only a stomachache that did not respond to treatment for gastritis led to the sequence of tests that diagnosed the cancer. He was immediately hospitalized for a total gastrectomy, in a private hospital in Chennai. He was operated upon by the city's most renowned gastric surgeon. He was recovering well from his surgery and due to be discharged in a couple of days, though the biopsy of his stomach suggested a cancer far more advanced than we had expected, with poor prognosis. One evening, his oxygen levels suddenly started dropping precipitously. In spite of desperate attempts to revive him, he had a sequence of cardiac arrests. Within an hour, he had passed away. I had spent nearly a decade researching and writing about the politics surrounding an anticancer drug, but nothing prepared me for the visceral proximity of the disease, even though this encounter with it was all too fleeting. I miss him.

There was no evident malpractice on the part of the hospital. A cardiac arrest can happen to anyone, and this one was possibly caused by a pulmonary embolism. My father had all three major risk factors—old age, postoperative, cancer—for developing such an embolism. Nonetheless, my family and I have felt a lack of closure, an inarticulate anger, toward the hospital. As a former government employee, my father's surgery had been approved for reimbursement by the Central Government Health Scheme. Yet the hospital decided that the amount approved was insufficient and refused to conduct any preoperative tests or even attend to him until we changed his status to a private, full-paying patient. They did not deign to inform us of this, however; so he spent his first day in the hospital wondering why no one was coming to see him, already worrying that this was a bad omen. Since he had been a smoker for five decades, the doctors knew (and constantly reminded him) that their biggest concern was his poor pulmonary function. Yet not once did a pulmonologist deign to see him, either before or after his surgery. When we insisted upon the routine pulmonary tests that needed to be conducted before he could be considered fit for surgery, the pulmonologist responded, "If they want to see me so badly, let them come to my department and I'll see them." And so after a morning full of strenuous cardiac function tests, he tottered over to the pulmonologist, utterly exhausted; we had to obsequiously plead with the pulmonologist to conduct the tests. When he was transferred to his ward from the intensive care unit after his surgery, the surgeon asked the nurses to ensure that oxygen supply be constantly available to him; it took an entire day for it to be arranged. The day before he passed, the consulting doctor on morning rounds asked the nurse to have an X-ray taken; when he returned for evening rounds that day, the X-ray still had not been done in spite of our constantly badgering the nurse. At one point she helplessly proclaimed, "We are trying, but the radiologist is not coming." Once my father passed away, the hospital ensured that the money owed for his surgery and hospitalization was paid before his body was released. Not once did any of the doctors follow up—let alone to condole, but even to explain what had caused his death. It was only when members of our family reviewed the sequence of events that we concluded that it might have been because of an embolism.

All the while, relentlessly, closed-circuit TV screens around the hospital blared with public relations announcements, as the hospital owner's son bleated on about how the only thing that mattered at this hospital was the care of the patient. And indeed, this hospital was a major destination for medical tourists from around the world. A French couple in the room across from our father's stood with us in the corridor, in sympathy and horror, during those last moments when futile attempts were made to revive him. In those few days, my family and I experienced a personal tragedy, but also felt the limits and apathies of elite profit-driven private medical care in contemporary India.

The structural analysis that I have developed in this book seeks to highlight the differentiations of global biomedicine. From that perspective, the case of clinical research on marginalized populations, or denial of access to medicines to those who cannot afford it, represents one kind of limit. But I bring up the case of my father in the conclusion to this book as another kind of limit—the limits that the experiential dimensions of health pose to structural political considerations. When the first suspicions of cancer were voiced, I found myself wishing that if my father had to have cancer, that it might be gastrointestinal stromal tumor, which could be treated by Gleevec. It was not. After the surgery, we asked for his resected sample to be tested for her-2, the marker that manifests in certain breast cancers but also in a subset of gastric adenocarcinomas, in the hope that a her-2-positive diagnosis would open up the possibility of treatment with Herceptin. Before the results could come in, he had passed. Nonetheless, the developments of targeted anticancer therapy beckoned to us as a genuine possibility, inscribing us if all too fleetingly into a political economy of hope (Good et al. 1990; Novas and Rose 2005). Needless to say, structural considerations are always present in such an inscription, which would not have been possible had we not had the capacity to pay—for his surgery, for the tests, and indeed for treatment in a private hospital in the first place. Indeed, knowing full well the likely apathies of private medical care in India, it still seemed like a preferable and more comfortable option than being treated in a more democratized public hospital.

One can think easily about the relationship between health and capital (in the argument of this book, in terms of the appropriation of the former by the latter). One can also think easily about the relationship between capital and democracy (in the argument of this book, the severe limits placed upon the latter by the former, especially in its corporatized, financialized form). But it is harder to think across the gap between health as deeply experiential and embodied, operating at the level of intimate relations of care, and the democratic as structural, differentiated, and operating across scales that extend up to the global. Experience proximity humanizes the stakes of a politics of health and illness, even as it blurs structural and situational distinctions. How does one think about health across this huge scale from experience proximity to distance, in ways that are sensitive both to the deeply individualized stories of suffering and loss that are felt across contexts, and to the longue durée and spatially differentiated structures that result in international and intranational divisions of health? A story that simply creates a hierarchy of suffering based on structural inequity is as insufficient as one that fails to take structural inequity into account in its attention to the individual narrative.

One solution to this conceptual and methodological challenge is to begin with the experience-proximal narrative and situate it across structural contexts. This is a strategy that has fruitfully been employed by medical anthropologists. But the relationship between the individual (or even collective biosocial) experience of suffering and its rendering in structural terms is not just a theoretical question; it can also be an intensely political one. Hence the gap I am referring to is something more complex than one between the personal and the political.

For instance, the battle to control the price of Gleevec in Korea saw an alliance between leukemia patient advocacy groups and HIV-AIDS groups in the country.[23] However, once Novartis offered a compromise that involved them subsidizing the cost of the drug for patients while maintaining the actual price of the drug, differences of opinion arose among these allies. Leukemia groups were happy with the compromise because it would ensure easier access and availability of the drug for suffering patients. Groups for HIV-AIDS were not, because what was at stake for them was a principle of drug pricing policy, a structural concern that would go beyond the availability of a single drug for a single suffering group of patients.

Capital literally operates within such cracks that emerge between experiential and structural politics of health and illness, prying them apart. Sometimes capitalist interests are adept at sprinkling a good dose of ethics into the mix while positioning their solutions as win-win, as Novartis managed to do in Korea, and as it tried and failed to do in India as it attempted to institute an ethical monopoly through GIPAP (see chapter 4). When it can, capital simply uses its power to coerce (as in the case of the TPP, where the interests of corporate capital are underwritten by the geopolitical power of the American state). At other times, it walks away (as in the case of PATH's refusal to engage Indian actors in the HPV vaccine controversy).

The empirical scales at which the capitalized politics of health operate are often simultaneously too close and too far to easily allow for a simultaneous conceptualization of the experiential and the structural, except occasionally in situational and contingent fashion. Across these scales, lives continue to be lived, loved ones continue to be lost, and health and democracy in all their contradictory complexity remain very much at stake. The problem space of pharmocracy is as immediate and proximal as it is global and dispersed.

INTRODUCTION

1. Conversation with the author, Qazi Camp, Bhopal, November 23, 2011 (translated from Hindi).

2. Satinath Sarangi, conversation with the author, October 31, 2012. See also Hanna (2006).

3. Yusuf Hamied, interview with the author, August 28, 2008.

4. Interview with the author, November 2, 2012.

5. Current industry estimates put the cost of developing a new drug molecule in excess of $2 billion, with a failure rate of nearly 80 percent. While such figures have been disputed in some corners, they are widely accepted and form a basis for the justification of patent monopolies and high drug prices in the United States. I discuss this in greater detail in chapter 1, and unpack the ideology of innovation that underlies assumptions such as these through the course of this book.

6. Gramsci developed the notion of hegemony through a series of observations, many of which were recorded when he was imprisoned by the Italian Fascist government in the late 1920s and 1930s, and subsequently compiled into his famous *Prison Notebooks* (Hoare and Nowell-Smith 1971). Therefore this is not a term that he describes with a single definition, but is rather a problematic that he developed through fragmentary writings on a range of contemporary political issues over a number of years.

7. Even though I am uncomfortable with the term *harmonization*, I use it here as an actor's category that describes the processes I am interesting in unpacking.

8. I am referring here to pharmaceutical clinical trials, that is, the conduct of clinical trials to approve new drugs for market. There are many other forms of clinical research that may not be about drug approval: for example, epidemiological, outcomes-based public health research. While it is important to distinguish between the two, it is not always easy to make clean-cut distinctions (see chapter 2).

9. Important ethnographic work describing the rise of the CRO industry in the United States and globally includes Adriana Petryna's (2009) *When Experiments Travel* and Jill Fisher's (2008) *Medical Research for Hire*. Petryna is especially concerned with the globalization of clinical trials, a process that started in earnest in the mid-1990s, and the consequent "ethical variability" that has emerged in the conduct

of trials in different parts of the world. Fisher is more concerned with the privatization of trials as a function of broader neoliberal transformations in health care in the United States.

10. See Wen-Hua Kuo (2005, 2012) for an ethnographic account of ICH deliberations in the first decade of the 2000s in the context of establishing drug regulatory frameworks in Japan, Taiwan, and Singapore.

11. For an elaboration of the lobbying power of the multinational pharmaceutical industry in the Uruguay Round of TRIPS negotiations, see Sell (2003).

12. See Lawrence Cohen's (1999) elaboration of what he calls ethical and scandalous publicity as forms of publicity that operate alongside each other in the context of the debate around the organ trade, and João Biehl and Adriana Petryna's (2011) elaboration of the judicialization of pharmaceutical politics in Brazil. I elaborate upon these notions in chapters 2 and 3 respectively.

13. There is now a body of ethnographic work on science and technology that takes the hypercomplexity of the worlds it studies as a starting point and attempts to wade through and unpack that complexity rather than analytically reduce it. For some exemplary works in this regard (by no means a comprehensive list), see Lochlann Jain's (2013) *Malignant* (on cancer), Joseph Masco's (2014) *The Theater of Operations* (on the American security state), Michelle Murphy's (2017) *The Economization of Life* (a transnational history of U.S.-funded demography); Jake Kosek's forthcoming *Homo-Apians* (a critical history of the modern honey-bee), and Kim Fortun's book in progress, *Late Industrialism: Making Environmental Sense* (on environmental knowledge making over the past two decades). The strategies and entry point into studying complex worlds in these works are all different, but they all operate in various ways across sites, scales, and domains in their analysis. Kim Fortun's (2001) *Advocacy after Bhopal*, to me, remains an early template and model of such ambitious work.

14. The drug in question has been marketed by Novartis as Gleevec in the United States, and as Glivec in the rest of the world. For the sake of consistency, I use Gleevec throughout the book, even though as the drug become a site of legal and political contestation in India, it was referred to as Glivec.

15. See Wailoo et al. (2010) for a collection of essays addressing the biomedical and political significance of the HPV vaccine.

16. See Mukherjee (2010) and Keating and Cambrosio (2012) for accounts of Gleevec's importance in the history of cancer research and therapy.

17. There is a rich body of work that theorizes reproductive politics in the context of biotechnology and biomedicine (see for instance Clarke 1998; Cooper and Waldby 2014; Franklin 2013; Ginsburg and Rapp 1995; Murphy 2012, 2017; Thompson 2006, 2013; Rapp 2000).

18. While the trajectory of access to medicines politics in India is marked by judicialization and that of clinical trials politics by public scandal, this distinction is not absolute. In 2007, there was significant civil society mobilization in India and elsewhere against Novartis taking the Indian Patent Office to the Madras High Court, which manifested as a Drop the Case campaign orchestrated by MSF and explicitly framed Novartis's actions as scandalously denying essential medications to poor

people who needed them by insisting upon monopoly rights for Gleevec. And conversely, clinical trials politics have subsequently come to be judicialized, subsequent to the filing of public interest litigation in the Indian Supreme Court in 2013 that demanded further investigation into the HPV vaccine studies.

19. Biehl and Petryna develop their notion in relation to empirical material from Brazil. The processes that I trace in India show similar trajectories but also empirical and contextual specificities. A broader comparison of pharmaceutical politics in different parts of the Global South would be an essential exercise, and is being undertaken by Jean-Paul Gaudilliere, Laurent Pordie, and Maurice Cassier and colleagues (see for instance Cassier 2012). Biehl and Petryna's concept itself draws upon Jean and John Comaroff's account of the judicialization of politics in South Africa, another critical node in Global Southern politics around health (Comaroff and Comaroff 2006). While they consider politics in a broad sense, the Comaroffs specifically point to the domain of pharmaceutical and especially antiretroviral politics in their account of judicialization.

20. In her account of the Ameena case, Rajeswari Sunder Rajan uses the case as a problem space of "having to think *beyond* exemplarity yet well *before* an untheorizable particularity" (R. Sunder Rajan 2003, 41–71, esp. 42). Sunder Rajan describes the rescue of a girl, Ameena, who had been married to an elderly Saudi national by her parents in Hyderabad. When situated alongside another seminal case from a few years earlier that Sunder Rajan (with Zakia Pathak) has also written about, the Shahbano case (Pathak and R. Sunder Rajan 1989), the value of the case as elucidating the terrain of the political becomes particularly resonant. Taken together, the Shahbano and Ameena cases, while significant critical events in and of themselves, also frame a broader political conjuncture of importance. I will elaborate upon the importance of the notion of conjuncture for my analysis subsequently.

21. He says as much in *The Grundrisse*: "To develop the concept of capital it is necessary to begin not with labour but with value, and precisely, with exchange value in an already developed movement of circulation" (Marx [1857] 1993, 259). This does not mean that labor is unimportant; just that one can only understand how it comes to be at stake, alienated, and exploited if one begins one's analysis from the question of value.

22. My readings of value theory in Marx have been influenced greatly Louis Althusser and Etienne Balibar's ([1970] 2009) *Reading Capital*, Balibar's (1995) *Philosophy of Marx*, Antonio Negri's ([1973] 1992) *Marx beyond Marx*, Gayatri Spivak's (1985) "Scattered Speculations on the Question of Value," and Moishe Postone's (1993) *Time, Labor and Social Domination*. Each of these authors has different specific inflections and investments in their reading of Marx; but all of them develop the critical potential of his labor theory of value through a close attention to his analytic method.

23. Marx writes this at precisely the moment when he introduces the concept of surplus value in volume 1 of *Capital*.

24. Other work that discusses the political economy of health in the context of capitalist modes and relations of production includes Vicente Navarro's (1976) *Medicine under Capitalism*, Lesley Doyal's (1979) *The Political Economy of Health*, and Milton

Silverman and Philip Lee's (1974) *Pills, Profits and Politics.* See also Michael Taussig's (1980) "Reification and the Consciousness of the Patient" for a more conceptual development of these issues that anticipates elements of the argument Dumit makes three decades later.

25. In this regard, see also Dumit's "BioMarx" experiment, a search-and-replace in volume 1 of *Capital*, at http://dumit.net/biomarx-experiment/ (last accessed September 2, 2015).

26. While my own conceptualization of value is deeply influenced by Dumit's reading of Marx, it should be emphasized that his is just one mode of conceptualizing value in relation to health and pharmaceuticals. There are a number of other modes of analysis that are complementary to Dumit's, all interested in modes and relations of production but using different entry points and foregrounding different conceptual questions. A (by no means comprehensive) list of some of these other approaches includes Laurent Pordie and Jean-Paul Gaudilliere's (2014) focus on use values in pharmaceutical development through a study of reformulation practices in Ayurveda; Kristin Peterson's (2014a, 2014b) focus on the constitution of different kinds of markets in Nigeria, from monopoly markets in patent medications controlled by Euro-American pharmaceutical companies to free markets in generic drugs controlled by Indian companies to informal markets in fake and counterfeit drugs, all often operating in the same physical spaces of exchange; Maurice Cassier's (forthcoming) ongoing study of the reconstitution of modes of production and industrial organization of pharmaceutical manufacture; Cori Hayden's (2007, 2010) analysis of "the politics of the copy," focusing on the values and politics entailed in the constitution of novelty, similarity, and genericity in pharmaceuticals in different national and global contexts; Vinh-Kim Nguyen's (2010) analysis of the ways in which diseased bodies come to be valued in biomedical situations that demand emergency care, such as the HIV-AIDS epidemic in Africa in the 1990s; work that thinks about pharmaceutical value in terms of embodiment and bodily relations (in very different ways, Julie Livingston's [2012] and Lochlann Jain's [2013] analysis of cancer as bodily and political economic relation, or Emilia Sanabria's work on sex hormones in Brazil [Sanabria 2016; Edmonds and Sanabria 2014]); work that elaborates value in relation to institutions of national and global health ([Mahajan 2008, forthcoming; Brotherton 2012; McGoey 2015]; Veena Das's focus on everyday practices of pharmaceutical consumption and the experience of health and illness [Das and Das 2006; Das 2015]; Judith Farquhar and Lili Lai's [2014] focus on relating value to questions of epistemology in their work on ethnic Chinese medicine); and the various kinds of what Donna Haraway (2007) calls "encounter value" that mediate transspecies and multispecies interactions in the life sciences (also see Gail Davies's [2012a, 2012b, 2013a, 2013b] work on geographies of mouse research; Natalie Porter [2013, 2015] on securitized economies of research into and exchanges of virus in the context of the management of bird flu; and Jake Kosek [forthcoming] on the history of the industrialized honeybee, for examples of multispecies work that explicitly reconceptualizes value).

27. But also very much in relation to new reproductive technologies, which is why Melinda Cooper and Catherine Waldby (2014) think about experimental subjectivity

and new forms of reproductive labor together in their conceptualization of clinical labor. See Mezzadra and Neilson (2013) for the notion of multiplication of labor, which I discuss at greater length in chapter 2.

28. For an extraordinary manual that provides an example of one way in which this can be done, see Edward Grefe and Martin Linsky (1995), *New Corporate Activism*.

29. The former move is to be found in the trajectory of Bruno Latour's work, starting with *We Have Never Been Modern* (Latour 1993) and perhaps most explicitly in *Politics of Nature* (Latour 2004). The latter is at the heart of Marshall Sahlins's conceptualizations of value (for a recent exposition of which, see his essay "On the Culture of Material Value and the Cosmography of Riches" [Sahlins 2013]; see also his well-known reflections, "Cosmologies of Capitalism" [Sahlins 1988]). For elaborations of both investments, see the summer 2014 issue of *Hau: Journal of Ethnographic Theory*.

30. Of course, this leads to vexed questions for progressive politics around health in India, given on the one hand the deeply failed history of the postcolonial Indian state in providing adequate health care for large segments of its population, and on the other hand the fact that the state does remain an institution that can potentially be made structurally accountable to its citizenry in a way that institutions purely serving the interests of capital cannot. The structure of this dilemma, which inhabits every activist political engagement with the state in India around the question of health, is identical to that traced by Rajeswari Sunder Rajan (2003) in relation to feminist politics in India over the past three decades in *The Scandal of the State*. The parallels of politics around health to feminist politics in India are considerable, certainly in terms of the question of how such politics should engage and orient itself toward the state. But there are more than just parallels at stake. Some of the most important civil society initiatives against unethical clinical trials in India have been driven by feminist groups concerned with questions of women and health. While they might articulate with other groups that organize around these issues in less explicitly gendered terms (those concerned with biomedical ethics, or people's health and science movements), there are long histories of feminist engagements with the state around issues of women's health and reproductive rights that provide essential context to these struggles. Of relevance here are feminist engagements with the state's coercive family planning programs of the 1970s, extending all the way forward to contemporary engagements with new reproductive technologies, for instance, around the global political economies of surrogacy that, like clinical trials, have come to be outsourced to India with greater frequency in recent years (Sama 2010). It is not just in the domain of activist engagement that feminist histories matter: understanding Indian legal and judicial cultures in India in relation to the politics of health also requires an appreciation of the context of postcolonial engagements between women and the state. For instance, Lawyers Collective, the group that has been at the forefront of legal battles against Novartis around the Gleevec case, has a wing devoted to women's issues, and the collective's founding secretary, Indira Jaising, has a long record of involvement in feminist legal politics. The judge who delivered the Madras High Court verdict against Novartis in the Gleevec case, Prabha Sridevan, also has a record of seminal rulings on issues of women's rights.

31. Raymond Williams's (1978) formulation of residual, dominant, and emergent cultural formations is resonant here.

32. A dominant contemporary mode of theorizing the politics of health and illness is in terms of Michel Foucault's ([1976] 1990, 2008) notion of biopolitics, which has been developed by a range of theorists concerned with questions of life itself. Biopolitics speaks to the question of governmental rationalities engaged in the care of the population, to the singular power of the modern nation-state to "make live and let die" (Foucault [1976] 1990, 137–140). This book is obviously concerned with dimensions of the biopolitical, and the specter of Foucault constantly haunts the conceptualization of politics that it undertakes. However, I am ambivalent about the term in that too often it functions, too quickly, as the point at which explanations run out. There are at least three ways in which a biopolitical framework, while necessary, proves insufficient to the analysis this book undertakes. First, Foucault himself develops this term in the context of advanced liberal modernity, and some of the most faithful developments of the concept in relation to contemporary life sciences (such as Rose 2006) fail to attend to the question of whether and how it might be applicable to non-Euro-American contexts. The very different trajectories of modern governmental rationality in the context of colonial law and governance in particular are often completely elided. This is not to say that biopolitics is inapplicable to contexts outside Euro-American advanced liberalism (see, for instance, Biehl 2005, 2009; Mezzadra, Reed, and Samaddar 2013); just that one has to be careful not to extrapolate Foucault to other contexts in ways that evacuate historical and situational specificity. Second, there are limits of a biopolitical analysis to understanding logics of capital. In *The Birth of Biopolitics*, Foucault articulates biopolitical governance to forms of neoliberal economic rationality, but economic rationality is not the same as logics of capital. One of Marx's moves in volume 1 of *Capital* was precisely to explicate the relationship between the two as he undertook a critique of bourgeois political economy alongside his development of the labor theory of value. Hence, biopolitics is centrally relevant to an understanding of what myself and others have called biocapital (K. Sunder Rajan 2006; Helmreich 2008). But an analysis of biocapital cannot be reduced to one of biopolitics. Third, perhaps of most relevance to the ways in which I consider politics in this book, Foucault's theorization of governance thinks of the modern state entirely in terms of sovereign power. In contrast, my own interest in institutions of governance (including and other than the state) is in terms of their representative power.

33. Of course theorizations of the democratic go well beyond the Jurgen Habermas–Partha Chatterjee duality that I state here; but they are important touchstones for me because there is an empirical resonance of their conceptualizations of democracy in the material that I study. Global harmonization has echoes of a Habermasian ethic, which makes me additionally uncomfortable with his model of deliberative democracy: not only is it poorly suited to understanding the realities of democracy in what Chatterjee (2004) would call "most of the world," it also potentially blinds us to those situations of consensual harmonization that are in fact about the consolidation of hegemony. For an important critique of theories of deliberative democracy, see Bonnie Honig's (2009) *Emergency Politics*. Meanwhile, I do not think that one can discuss

theories of South Asian democracy today without taking into account Chatterjee's conception of it in terms of the popular.

34. To be sure, Chatterjee (2008, 2011) does complicate and specify this as he distinguishes corporate from noncorporate capitalism in discussing democracy in relation to economic transformation. In the process, he acknowledges an important democratic space within civil society and representative political arenas; it is just that those spaces are not the ones from which he develops his democratic theory. In relation to biomedicine, a similar limit is encountered in Veena Das's conceptualization of the experience of health and illness in India in terms of what she calls "the everyday" (Das 2006, 2011, 2015; Das and Das 2006).

35. Of course, many theorists of the political in India pay attention to the representative sphere in empirically rigorous ways. Sudipta Kaviraj (see especially 1997, 2010) over the arc of his work has perhaps been the most influential to my overall thinking on this. This influence extends all the way back to high school, when I studied a civics textbook that he had authored, which shaped many of my formative interests in and ideas of politics in India (Kaviraj 1989).

36. These are relationships that I have collectively investigated with a number of colleagues through a series of conferences organized at the University of Chicago and elsewhere under the rubric "Knowledge/Value" (see http://knowledge-value.org/, accessed October 10, 2015).

37. See Jasanoff (1997, 2015) for her notion of "serviceable truths" as scientific knowledge that operates in legal and policy domains. For an account of the very different ways in which knowing is structured in laboratory science as opposed to clinical medicine, see Ludwik Fleck's ([1927] 1986) essay "Some Specific Features of the Medical Way of Thinking." For an important theorization of knowledge in terms of its mobility, see Sabina Leonelli's (2016) analysis of big data in contemporary life sciences in terms of what she calls "data journeys." Also see Howlett and Morgan (2010) and K. Sunder Rajan and Leonelli (2013) for further theorizations of knowledge in terms of its mobility.

38. See note 32 for an elaboration of my thinking with and against Foucault's notion of biopolitics.

39. Foucault ([1970] 1994) himself has a more differentiated classification of knowledge in The Order of Things, wherein he describes knowledge in terms of attribution, articulation, designation, and derivation. But it is in his formulation of Power/ Knowledge and his articulation of the relationship between truth and power that Foucault develops his most explicit conceptualization of knowledge to politics.

40. One important genealogy for theorizing knowledge as translation within science and technology studies (STS) is actor-network theory, developed by Michel Callon (1986) and Bruno Latour (1987, 1988). However, the conceptualization of politics in Callon's and Latour's rendering is altogether too flat, reduced to a recruitment of interests by rational actors. Emily Martin (1998) provides an important anthropological and feminist counter to their model of knowledge production, taking into account the fundamentally differentiated power structures and cultural contexts within which knowledge is produced. More recently, Kim Fortun (2014) and Michael Fischer (2014)

have critiqued the "ontological turn" that Latour's actor-network model has taken. I organized a conference around the question of the translations of knowledge, value, and politics with colleagues at the University of Chicago in 2012, called "Trans-science." A relevant bibliography that relates to such questions, going beyond actor-network theory to think through conceptualizations of translation in STS, linguistic anthropology, and postcolonial studies, can be found on the conference webpage (Department of Anthropology 2012).

41. The term "knowledge-for-itself" follows Marx's ([1852] 1977) distinction in *The Eighteenth Brumaire of Louis Bonaparte* between a class-in-itself and for-itself. By "class-in-itself," Marx refers to the structural subject-position of a given social group within particular modes of production; by "class-for-itself," he refers to the ways in which that subject-position is acted out through materializations of relations of production, which need not correspond in any simple way to structural positions at all but is rather thoroughly political. Similarly, I am interested less in arriving at a definition of knowledge adequate to contemporary biomedicine than I am in seeing how knowledge gets acted out.

42. I develop the idea of situation in conclusion to this introductory chapter. Again, because of the fragmentary nature of his writings, it is difficult to pinpoint an exact citation within Gramsci for a concern that in fact pervades his writing. However, there are writings where Gramsci specifically develops his ideas of knowledge in relation to the problem of what constitutes the intellectual (see especially "Intellectuals," Gramsci 2000, 300–311). These writings are central to understanding how he thinks about the function of knowledge, intellectuals, and expertise in the constitution of hegemony.

43. This follows Gregory Bateson's ([1936] 1958) demonstration of the analytic potential of ethnographic situation in his account of the Naven. Situated attentiveness is reflected in the structure of this book and in the organization of its chapters, as already described. If Bateson uses situation as a device of comparison and juxtaposition to generate a thick account, then there is additionally the possibility of using it as the ground from which politics can be theorized. Situated analysis of this sort is central to Karl Marx's ([1852] 1977, [1871] 2009) historical writings, such as *The Eighteenth Brumaire of Louis Bonaparte* and *The Civil War in France*, and to Gramsci's ([1926] 2000) accounts of contemporary Italian politics in the 1920s, such as on "the Southern Question." Ethnographies that theorize politics out of situated analysis include Michael Fischer and Mehdi Abedi's conceptualizations of relationships between Islam and politics in Iran (Fischer 1980; Fischer and Abedi 1990). Donna Haraway's (1991) call for situated knowledge in relation to practices of feminist objectivity has been foundational to subsequent thinking in STS.

44. This figure is based on conversations with members of MSF's Access to Medicines and Treatment Campaign in New Delhi and Geneva over the past few years. For MSF, the survival of India's generic industry is vital.

45. The question of how to generate an adequate "anthropology of the contemporary" is a lively source of debate. See Paul Rabinow's (2003) *Anthropos Today* for a provocative methodological guide and Michael Fischer's (2003, 2009) *Emergent Forms of Life and the Anthropological Voice* for an alternative methodological and

conceptual modality. Rabinow's method is grounded in the notion of assemblage, referring to the contingent articulation of heterogenous elements. The anthropologist's task then becomes one of mapping this radical contingency. The notion of assemblage has received much traction in contemporary anthropological social theory, especially as developed in Bruno Latour's (2005) influential program for actor-network theory, *Reassembling the Social*. Fischer's method in contrast is more historically grounded, drawing upon Raymond Williams's (1978) formulation concerning residual, dominant, and emergent horizons and articulating it to Ludwig Wittgenstein's (1972) notion of a "form of life," invoking socialities of action. For Fischer, understanding these socialities involves being attentive to the ghosts of formations past that endure and to the traces of emergent possibilities yet to come, even as it involves tracing the dominant modes of production and forms of social relation prevalent in a particular place and time. This does not mean that any given event is not contingent; it just means that the conceptual project of understanding the contemporary must go beyond the mere mapping and declaration of contingency to include a deeper historical sensibility. It is this latter sense of the conjuncture that I adopt in my own reading of contemporary global pharmaceutical politics as situated in India.

46. In this section, I am drawing upon Gramsci's (2000, 200–209) notes on "Analysis of Situations: Relations of Force."

47. All of these could be seen as attributes of neoliberalism. As representative (but no means comprehensive) examples of analyses of neoliberalism, see Melinda Cooper's (2008) account of the capitalization and neoliberalization of the life sciences; David Harvey's (2003, 2007) diagnoses of neoliberalism and its relationship to accumulation by dispossession; Neil Brenner, Jamie Peck, and Nik Theodor's (2010) analyses of the spatialities of neoliberalism; work by scholars following and developing Michel Foucault's notion of governmentality and applying it to questions of contemporary neoliberal governance (Rose 2006); the work of anthropologists involved in the elucidation of the "global assemblages" of neoliberalism (Ong and Collier 2005); and Michel Foucault's (2008) theorization of *homo economicus* as the subject of neoliberalism, elaborated upon by Wendy Brown (2015). While in broad agreement with this range of scholarship, my own interest is less in the diagnosis of neoliberalism than in the question of the specificities and intricacies of this capitalist moment in India and of how global capital is constructed, perceived, and experienced from the situation of these specificities.

48. While beyond the scope of this book, the question of how poverty gets measured is absolutely central in this regard, and has indeed been an important facet of policy debates in Indian economics (Subramanian 2001), alongside more neoliberal concerns and articulations such as the obsession with economic growth.

49. The Right to Information Act and the National Rural Employment Guarantee Act were passed in India in 2005. The Right to Education Act was enacted in 2009. The National Food Security Act, popularly known as the Right to Food bill, was proposed in 2011. While an account of the NRHM is beyond the scope of this book, the HPV vaccine studies described in chapter 2 are an example of a public-private partnership that operates under its aegis.

50. Kim Fortun describes discursive gaps as emerging "when there are conditions to deal with for which there is no available idiom, no way of thinking that can grasp what is at hand" (2012, 452). In the case that I am describing, the discursive gaps were not so much because "there was no way of thinking" of an ethics that included therapeutic access, but because of the particular institutional investments that were structuring this moment, investments focused on maximizing the amount of clinical experimentation coming to India but not coupling that to therapeutic access or building broader health care infrastructures.

51. See the report put out by the Sama resource group on women and health that highlights some of these scandals (Sarojini, Anjali, and Ashalata 2011).

CHAPTER ONE. **Speculative Values**

1. In this regard, it is worth thinking about three registers of time that Jacques Derrida (1994) has alluded to: *histoire, le temps,* and *le monde,* referring respectively to specific histories, the time in which we live, and the time of "the world." See also Paul Rabinow's (2003) similar development of notions of epoch, present, and event. While Rabinow's aim is to develop the utility of these notions for an anthropology of the contemporary (ultimately privileging attentiveness to the radical contingency of the assemblage), Derrida's interest is in precisely avoiding such definitive resolution. Rather, following the method of deconstruction, he wishes to show how time is "out of joint." He was thinking of this precisely in a moment of crisis, in this case of Marxism after the dissolution of the Soviet Union. This was a moment when the old had died and the new had not yet been born, when Francis Fukuyama ([1991] 2006) was proclaiming "the end of history," and when the world historical importance of particular events was recognized even as the question of their long-term structural causes and implications was rife.

2. See the analysis of the 2008 financial crisis by Moishe Postone (2012). For an exploration of the humanitarian crisis in relation to contemporary pharmaceutical economies, see especially Peter Redfield's (2013) ethnography of MSF in relation to situations of "life in crisis." Redfield is interested in the work of an organization that has emerged at a historical moment when humanitarianism has become a dominant register through which the global gets thought and acted upon—a moment (starting in the 1970s) that also happens to be one that has witnessed the disintegration of the Keynesian welfare state and its replacement by neoliberal avatars in most of the developed world. See Kosselleck and Richter (2006) for an important overview of the philosophy of crisis, and Roitman (2013) for an important ethnographic conceptualization.

3. Of course, categories such as "developing" and "developed" countries are provisional, given the wide disparities in access to health care within most national contexts. Still, the distinction is not entirely invalid if one considers global power relations and geopolitical configurations that witness, more often than not, First World hegemony over Third World interests (even if many people within the former are denied the benefits of such hegemony). See chapter 5 for an elaboration of such geopolitics.

4. This was in part a function of pressure from emergent patient advocacy groups, especially around HIV-AIDS (see Epstein 1996). Patient activism in relation to the urgency of experimental therapy would subsequently develop in a number of other arenas, especially around cancer treatment.

5. These figures have been periodically updated, and a recent Tufts estimate puts the cost of drug development at nearly $2.6 billion per molecule (see Tufts University 2014).

6. Examples of off-label use go back to the 1970s. An example is minoxidil, approved initially to lower high blood pressure, but famous now as the over-the-counter hair-growth treatment Rogaine. But it was in the 1990s that off-label use started to boom as a business model that could consistently expand the markets of and revenues from a drug.

7. This of course was the time when massive structural and regulatory changes were happening in India, and the question of the structural relationship between financial indicators for Euro-American R&D-driven companies on Wall Street and policy transformations underway in India is precisely the problem-space of this analysis. I am not suggesting that these relationships are of cause and effect; what is at stake here is capturing a sense of the political economic terrain. Earnings per share and return on equity are two different growth metrics used to measure the performance of companies on the stock market. The EPS involves calculating gross revenues of a company, subtracting expenditures, and dividing the balance by the number of public shares it has issued. It is calculated on a quarterly basis. Return on equity is calculated annually, and involves dividing earnings by average shareholder equity rather than the number of shares. Figures regarding EPS expectations and actualities are from Norton (2001). The Arca Index, which shows return on equity, is a price-weighted index of companies in different sectors listed on the U.S. stock exchange; the pharmaceutical index includes major pharmaceutical companies (see www.nyse.com).

8. This term was introduced by Jurgen Drews and Stefan Ryser (1996), and acquired considerable traction in pharmaceutical industry literature in subsequent years.

9. Barbara Ryan, cited in E. Silverman (2010).

10. Of course, streamlining is rarely smooth, and there are often culture clashes in the process of merging two company cultures. Downsizing is never straightforward.

11. This opens up the question of what the frontiers of medicine might be from the perspective of pharmaceutical development. This is complicated. One could crudely periodize the history of pharmaceutical development as follows. From the mid-twentieth century, when the pharmaceutical industry became a major industry, till the 1980s, the major modality of pharmaceutical development was based in natural products chemistry, which depended upon the serendipitous discovery of natural products (either chemical or microbiological) that might have therapeutic effect. This became progressively less reliable as most of the low-hanging fruit were picked. The period from the 1980s saw the development of an R&D-based blockbuster model, which has shaded into a model that has come to increasingly depend upon off-label use and therapeutic saturation. This is the trajectory I have focused upon in this chapter, one that is marked by a constant increase in me-too drugs for similar indications and

an innovation lag. The horizon of medicine, in this model, sees the creation of new diseases in situations where those diseases have a market that can be envisaged, even as it sees a continuing inattention to unmet medical needs in cases where a market is difficult to imagine—such as, for instance, most developing country diseases. The notable exception over the past two decades in this regard has been in oncology therapeutics, which has seen the emergence of novel drugs for indications such as certain forms of breast cancer, or chronic myeloid leukemia, consequent to R&D efforts out of the pharmaceutical industry, which have significantly improved the standard of care previously existing for those diseases in terms of therapeutic efficacy, reduced toxicity, and chances of survival. Novartis's drug Gleevec, which forms the cornerstone of my account of intellectual property politics in this book, falls in this category. For an account of developments in oncology therapeutics and how those have created changes in the structure of clinical trials, see Keating and Cambrosio (2012).

12. These logics of bioavailability, where Indian subjects are not consumers but rather laboring bodies in circuits of biocapital, are also seen in the ways in which India emerged as a global destination for surrogacy, and the parallels between clinical trials economies and the economies of global reproductive politics are essential to think about here. See Cohen (1999) for an elaboration of the notion of bioavailability in relation to the organ trade in India. Catherine Waldby and Melinda Cooper develop the idea that experimental subjectivity in clinical trials and surrogacy are both forms of clinical labor (Waldby and Cooper 2008; Cooper and Waldby 2014).

13. This is a more complex terrain, however, than just one-way acquisitions of Indian companies by Western (or Japanese) ones. For instance, Ranbaxy itself had earlier acquired companies in the United States and Europe, in part to acquire the R&D capacity it felt was necessary to be competitive in post-WTO environments. However, the point about structural logics impacting the industry remains: as India's largest and most powerful pharmaceutical company, Ranbaxy also faced global pressures to consolidate and grow even as it emerged as an attractive target for acquisition.

14. The calculability of financial risk is itself a complex issue and one that has been the subject of interest among anthropologists and sociologists of finance. It is therefore worth qualifying this statement in two ways. First, it is important to emphasize the fiction of calculability and to stay attentive to the kinds of speculative activities that are calculable, the kinds that can be brought into the realm of probability and the kinds that are fundamentally beyond calculability. It is as unhelpful to read this fiction cynically as it is to assume that all financial risk is calculable and therefore potentially manageable and mitigatable. Zia Haider Rahman's *In the Light of What We Know* provides an evocative novelistic portrayal of this terrain of in/calculability, developing among other things a reflection of the activities of contemporary financial capitalism through a meditation on the mathematician Kurt Gödel's incompleteness theorem, which states that any effective theorem for expressing elementary mathematics cannot be both consistent and complete (Rahman 2014). Second, it is important to recognize that financialization is not singular but has many different practices and threads with different calculative rationalities and speculative intensities. I return to this point toward the end of the chapter. The point I wish to emphasize here concerns the power

of the imaginary of financial risk relative to uncertainties of other kinds of (especially biomedical) unknowability that pharmaceutical companies face in the process of drug development. See Appadurai (2011, 2013) for an analysis of risk as opposed to uncertainty within financial capitalism.

15. This argument, and my description of global drug pricing in the remainder of this section, is a distillation of Ed Schoonveld's (2011) analysis of global drug pricing, *The Price of Global Health*. Written as a textbook for the pharmaceutical industry, this is an elaborate description of the challenges companies face in formulating global drug pricing strategies through an in-depth look at the market terrains that they face in different parts of the world. Though global drug pricing is an intensely political issue and a fundamental strategic one for pharmaceutical companies, Schoonveld's is the only comprehensive treatment of the topic that I am aware of.

16. A pioneer in the adoption of differential pricing strategies among the R&D-driven pharmaceutical industry is GlaxoSmithKline, whose approach still remains the exception rather than norm. For an analysis of GSK's global pricing strategy, and how that makes business and financial sense, see Froud and Sukhdev (2006, 149–224).

17. The agency tasked with making these determinations is the National Institute for Health and Care Excellence (initially set up as the National Institute for Clinical Excellence in 1999) of the National Health Service.

18. Those justifications themselves involve arguably exaggerated figures for drug development costs. James Love (2003), for instance, has contested Novartis's claims about the expense of developing Gleevec by pointing to public investments in initial discovery research, to the tax breaks the company got by virtue of Gleevec getting orphan drug status as a treatment for a rare disease, and to the fast-track approval the drug received from the U.S. Food and Drug Administration, which reduced the time to market. Nonetheless, the principle stands—while monopolistic pricing opens pharmaceutical companies to charges of price gouging, especially in the developing world, differential pricing potentially makes them vulnerable to the economics and politics of pricing in advanced Western markets.

19. However, see Outterson (2005), who suggests that the fear of arbitrage is still largely a theoretical one. For an anthropological development of the relationship between arbitrage and speculation which attends to sensibilities such as belief and doubt that animate the work of arbitrage through an ethnography of Japanese arbitrageurs, see Miyazaki (2007, 2013).

20. In this regard, the writings of Thorstein Veblen are an essential counterpart to Marxian theories of value. See especially *The Theory of Business Enterprise* and *The Vested Interests and the Common Man* (Veblen [1904] 1978, [1919] 2005). I elaborate upon Veblen's importance in understanding the nature and specificity of American power in global pharmaceutical political terrains in chapter 5.

21. A comprehensive analysis of contemporary financial capitalism is beyond the scope of this book. Work in the sociology and anthropology of finance is useful in this regard. For a (by no means comprehensive) list of such work, see for instance Callon (1998), Callon, Millo, and Muniesa (2007), Knorr Cetina and Preda (2005, 2007, 2013), and MacKenzie (2006) for foundational sociological analyses of financial markets

and instruments; Hart (2000), Maurer (2002, 2012), Miyazaki (2007, 2013), and Riles (2004) for an anthropological analysis of financial forms; LiPuma and Lee (2004) and Riles (2011) for important epistemic analyses of financialization; Appadurai (2011, 2013), Ho (2009), and Zaloom (2006) for theorizations of finance through a focus on financial cultures; Lewis (2010) and Tett (2009) for popular critical accounts of contemporary finance capital especially as related to the 2008 financial crisis; and Meister (2011) for a Marxian analysis of financialization.

22. This is not to suggest that the patent cliff is over, though there are signs that the worst is over. See an Accenture Life Sciences (2012) report on signs of recovery in the biopharmaceutical sector "beyond the patent cliff." Regardless, what is clear is that post-2012, we are in the intensified acquisitions environment of generic companies as a hedge against decline in revenues from patented drugs.

23. This is why insurance companies typically do not insure against catastrophic events that are likely to affect large number of policyholders simultaneously, unless they have some form of reinsurance protection. Reinsurance is the process by which insurers transfer some portion of their risk portfolio onto other parties to avoid having to pay a large obligation from an insurance claim.

24. A securitized instrument typically involves different tiers or tranches, each of which have different risk profiles and which are marketed to different kinds of investors. Fernandez, Stein, and Lo (2012) propose three levels of tranches, the senior tranche having the lowest risk and lowest yield (likely to be offered to investors in money market funds or small pension funds), and the most junior tranche having the highest risk and highest potential yield (offered to hedge funds and very high-net-worth private investors, consisting of more equity investments than bonds).

25. Of course, the risk-pooling assumptions that underlay mortgage-backed securities did not account for the incentives that would accrue from such instruments to engage in the issuance of subprime mortgages by lenders, leading to the existence of a large number of mortgages in these funds from people who did not have the capacity to repay their debt. Hence, the crash in the U.S. housing market in 2008. See Gillian Tett's (2009) *Fool's Gold* for the mistakenness of these assumptions. Tett shows how these models falsely allowed for an idea that by dividing into different tranches of risk, risks could be so distributed that they would be minimized to any one holder of a particular form of risk.

26. Lazonick (2010) explains how the repurchase is the inverse mode of distributing corporate revenue to shareholders from the more traditional dividend. Dividends provide return on investment by holding stock, while repurchases provide such by selling stock. In other words, repurchases by definition cause volatility, and corporate management, not just external financial actors, have been increasingly induced to engage in such practices.

27. In this regard, Lazonick (2010) points to a letter written by four congressional Democrats to oil industry executives in 2008, which took aim at the industry's repurchasing practices and asked them to focus their energies on production and research into alternative energy sources instead. See U.S. Congress, "Democrats Tell Big Oil: Spend More on Production and Renewable Energy, Less on Stock Buybacks before

Making Demands for New Drilling Leases" (Washington, DC, July 31, 2008), cited in Lazonick (2010, 697). Their call went entirely unheeded.

28. It even emerged as an issue in the 2016 American presidential race as both Hillary Clinton and Bernie Sanders brought up the issue of controlling drug prices during their campaigns.

29. This goes hand in hand with the recognition that a blockbuster model of drug development—a one-size-fits-all model where value generation is a function of maximizing the number of people on a treatment and the time that each person takes that treatment—is less and less tenable, with a gradual shift toward a model that is based on personalized medicine, based on tailoring therapies to individual genetic and molecular profiles. The shift from R&D to M&A in large pharmaceutical companies often layers on shifts from blockbuster drug development to personalized medicine, since this kind of tailored pharmaceutical development often occurs in biotechnology companies that get acquired by major pharmaceutical companies if they develop promising drug candidates. Personalized medicine has hardly taken over the blockbuster model, and it is likely to be more or less promising depending upon the disease being researched, as well as the target populations for which the drug is being developed. But it might be considered an emergent horizon of therapeutic R&D—one where value considerations hardly go away (quite the contrary), but where the particular relationships between biomedical research modalities and speculative financial modalities will likely be reconfigured through new types of business models.

30. Good's notion has been developed by Carlos Novas and Nikolas Rose (2005). For the operation of obligation, commitment, and indebtedness in biomedical economies in relation to organ trade in India, see Cohen (1999). For an analysis of the place of love in biomedical economies, see Chloe Silverman's (2011) account of parent advocacy groups for children affected with autism. Both Cohen and Silverman provide moving accounts of emergent kinds of labor in biomedical economies. In Cohen's case, obligation, commitment, and indebtedness can never be simple liberal constructs, because they are founded upon differential forms and relations of bioavailability. In Silverman's case, the love of parents toward their autism-afflicted child often goes hand in hand with having to make painful decisions about subjecting their child to experimental therapeutic interventions. The affective entanglements of capital are never innocent.

31. This is a simplified account of the debate that Marx ([1857] 1993, 117–128) engaged with at the start of the "Chapter on Money" in *The Grundrisse*. Marx's specific critique is of the response of the socialist Alfred Darimon to the Banque de France making credit more difficult to obtain consequent to the progressive dilution of its reserves in 1855. Darimon cited the problem as being the importance attributed to the role of precious metals in circulation and exchange. Marx showed that there was in fact no relationship between metal assets and the bank's portfolio. Darimon lamented that the bank withdrew its services from the public precisely when they were most needed. This was the point at which Marx explained that they did so because they were banks ("And the bank should be made an exception to . . . general economic laws?," 120). This meant they were subject to laws of supply and demand, but also that

they engaged in financially speculative ventures, which he pointed out were as much responsible for their problems as anything else. These speculations were inherent to their institutional character and role, and would have led to crisis regardless of whether the medium of monetary exchange consisted of precious metals or not. The reason why banks made credit more difficult for people when they most needed it, Marx argued, was because of the structural logics inherent to credit itself, and these are tied into institutional rationalities of speculation. This argument would be as relevant in its basic logic in regard to the 2008 financial crisis as it was in 1855.

CHAPTER TWO. **Bioethical Values**

1. And so, articles with headlines such as the following have become common fare: "Indian Drug Trials Fuel Consent Controversy" (Lakshmi 2012); "In India, Oversight Lacking in Outsourced Drug Trials" (Sandler 2012); "Centre Must Take Corrective Steps on Illegal Clinical Trials: Supreme Court" (Venkatesan 2012); "10 Die per Week in Drug Trials in India" (*Indian Express*, July 9, 2012); "Drug Trials Claimed 30 Lives in January This Year" (Singh 2012). Perhaps the most detailed media coverage in this period was provided by the U.K.'s *Independent*, for which journalist Nina Lakhani conducted a two-part exposé. The first part ("Without Consent: How Drug Companies Exploit Indian 'guinea pigs,'" November 14, 2011) looked at the spate of unethical clinical trials that were coming to light, while the second ("From Tragedy to Travesty: Drugs Tested on Survivors of Bhopal," November 15, 2011) focused on reports of clinical trials conducted on victims of the Bhopal gas tragedy (the subject, also, of Gulhati's [2010] MIMS editorial). These were prefaced by an editorial published in the *Independent* on November 14, 2011, headlined "Drugs Firms Must Not Prey on Poverty."

2. As cited by the India Brand Equity Federation (www.ibef.org, accessed March 1, 2007). These figures include contract work that is generated domestically as well as by foreign sponsors—not just clinical trial activity, but also the manufacturing of active pharmaceutical ingredients.

3. Based on personal conversations of the author with leaders of the Indian CRO industry, 2006–2007.

4. In addition to the CROs, some key actors included regulatory agents of the state. The immediately responsible body in India was the Drug Controller General of India, roughly equivalent to the U.S. Food and Drug Administration. The ICMR has also been involved in setting regulatory guidelines. Other key actors were educational and training institutes for clinical research. Building the human resource capability to conduct and monitor trials in India was a key challenge, and a number of entrepreneurial ventures engaged in training the labor force required to undertake this work. A third group was the physicians who actually conduct the trials, though in the Indian context they have had a relatively marginal presence compared to the CROs in setting the infrastructural and regulatory agenda for research.

5. The largest such multinational in India has been the North Carolina–based Quintiles, which opened its first Asia office in Japan in 1993 and had become a

major presence in the Indian clinical research landscape at the time of Schedule Y harmonization.

6. For instance, in my research I met a twenty-one-year-old from Chandigarh who decided to learn about the clinical research field because he felt there was money to be made in it. He talked to people in the industry about the kinds of services they would find useful and learned that there was a potential niche in providing data management services for those conducting clinical trials. He hired thirty people with experience in advanced statistical analysis and set up a company. Another person I met was concurrently running a private detective firm. This speaks to the human resource–driven aspect of conducting much clinical research, especially as a large-scale outsourced service.

7. Many thanks to Rakhi Jain, an independent consultant who played a big role in setting up clinical research at Ranbaxy before moving to establish Wellquest, for conversations that have helped me understand Ranbaxy's role in spurring clinical research in India. This account is based on an interview with Jain (March 3, 2006) and subsequent conversations in 2006 and 2007.

8. I had conversations at FHI in 2006 that suggested how a combination of their existing expertise in biomedical outreach in "developing world" communities combined with their own changing structures of funding had contributed to their working for pharmaceutical companies. Often public-private partnerships with developing country governments have proven attractive and led to their adopting this CRO-like form. I thank Karen Haneke for facilitating my conversations at FHI. My attempts to have conversations with people at PATH who were involved with the HPV vaccine study drew a blank.

9. All of these quotes come from different leaders of the Indian CRO industry, obtained in interviews I conducted with them in 2006 and 2007. I keep individual quotes anonymous, since a number of my interviewees at the time preferred not to be named.

10. Interview with the author, February 24, 2006.

11. I put *vulnerable* in quotes because it is an actor's category that emerges in the context of the representative politics around unethical clinical trials and not a term that I adopt or embrace myself.

12. It is important to remember that this emergent advocacy was not on the part of experimental subjects themselves, but rather on the part of concerned civil society groups, members of Parliament, and journalists. What one is seeing, starting in mid-2011, is a confluence of feminists, biomedical ethicists, and groups involved in battles around access to essential medicines, coming together in India to campaign against unethical clinical trials, at the same time as it became a matter of concern in the Indian Parliament. The reasons why the latter two groups would be concerned about this issue should be obvious; the reasons why feminist groups are involved in these struggles have to do with broader contexts and histories of population and family planning politics in India from the 1970s and 1980s, which are marked (and marred) by unethical, government-run contraceptive trials on women, and also of forced male sterilizations during the time of the Emergency (1975–1977). Hence, it is important to

think about the politicization of clinical trials not just in its own terms, but in relation to politics around access to essential medicines and around gender and reproductive politics. This is why Catherine Waldby and Melinda Cooper's move of considering clinical trials and reproductive technologies together under the rubric of clinical labor is so important (Cooper and Waldby 2014). For an excellent collection that documents and analyzes issues of pertinence to reproductive politics in India in the context of new biomedical technologies, see Sama (2010).

13. The central place that the Gates Foundation has acquired in establishing public health infrastructures throughout the developing world deserves attention in its own right but is beyond the scope of this book. See Linsey McGoey's (2015) *No Such Thing as a Free Gift*, which discusses the huge consequences of Gates Foundation power for structuring the political economy and governance of global biomedicine. Manjari Mahajan is currently researching the history and role of the Gates Foundation in India.

14. For a self-rendering of PATH's own history, see http://www.path.org/about/birth -of-path.php, accessed October 16, 2011.

15. The privatization of public health is certainly not a movement restricted to the Indian context. For work that shows the operation of this process in the context of therapeutic access in Nigeria, see Peterson (2014b); for the operation of the Cuban socialist public health regime operating as-if capitalist, see Brotherton (2008, 2012).

16. For news reports on the shutting down of the study, see Dhar (2010), Mallikar-jun (2010), Sharma (2010), Thacker (2010).

17. Of course, a history of experimentation upon marginal populations is not unique to India. Until it was virtually outlawed (barring exceptional circumstances) in 1980, a major pool for the recruitment of experimental subjects in the United States was the prisoner population. There is also a disproportionate history of experimentation on African American subjects, the most notorious instance of which were the Tuskegee syphilis experiments that were conducted for nearly four decades, from 1932 to 1972. For an account of the history of twentieth-century clinical experimentation in the United States, see Marks (2000). For accounts of the Tuskegee scandal, see Jones and Tuskegee Institute (1981), Reverby (2000). See Duster (2006) for a historical overview of race in biomedical research, and Epstein (2007), Montoya (2011), and Kahn (2014) for its persistent importance in contemporary biomedical research in the United States.

18. The national immunization program was initially launched as the Expanded Programme on Immunization in 1978, with a primary focus on immunizing children in urban areas of India. In 1985, the program was expanded and renamed the Univer-sal Immunization Programme (UIP). The UIP is one of the largest immunization pro-grams in the world in terms of the number of vaccines used, and is now an important component of the National Rural Health Mission, which is the signature public health initiative launched by the Congress government in 2005.

19. A similar project was also launched in three districts of the state of Gujarat on August 13, 2009, but in this case with an HPV vaccine developed by GlaxoSmithKline, Cervarix. See "Gujarat Launches Cervical Cancer Vaccine" (2009).

20. While this war is taking place in large parts of central and eastern India, the situation in Chattisgarh has been particularly grave. This is because in 2005, the Chattisgarh state government abetted the establishment of an anti-Maoist, extrajudicial militia, the Salwa Judum, whose own violent atrocities added to those committed by Maoists and state forces. Salwa Judum was deemed an illegal organization by the Supreme Court of India in 2011.

21. "Update: PATH's HPV Vaccine Project in India," PATH, http://www.path.org/news/an100422-hpv-india.php, accessed October 17, 2011.

22. The two Indian-based ethics committees were the National AIDS Research Institute (NARI) IRB in Pune, and committees set up by the Andhra Pradesh and Gujarat governments. NARI was involved in conducting the first phase of the study assessing vaccine introduction in India. The committees set up by the state governments were not really IRBs, but were rather called "state advisory groups." What a state advisory group might be is unclear, but it was something that was assumed to have the authority to approve the study.

23. "Update: PATH's HPV Vaccine Project in India," PATH, http://www.path.org/news/an100422-hpv-india.php, accessed October 17, 2011.

24. The details of the HPV immunization card are outlined in Sama's report, which was authored by N. B. Sarojini, S. Anjali, and S. Ashalata (2010).

25. For the importance of screening as a preventive mechanism against cervical cancer, see the Centers for Disease Control and Prevention (2014).

26. Note that the Sama report is based specifically on a visit to Bhadrachalam. The rest of my account in this section is based on Sarojini, Anjali, and Ashalata (2010).

27. Of course, it is ironic that the consent form was clearly framed to suggest that parents were giving consent for their daughters to be administered the vaccine, when in fact in Bhadrachalam teachers and hostel wardens often ended up giving consent. As a former member of one of the University of Chicago's IRBs myself, I am confident that an informed consent form with such ambiguous wording would not have been approved at my institution. This raises questions of the institutional review process as well—it should have been the prerogative of the IRBs, one of which was based in the United States, to ensure much clearer wording so as to leave no doubt that the study was an experiment.

28. Having said this, I do not want to conflate the "gift" of public health immunization with the "gifting" that one sees in programs of corporate social responsibility. After all, the subjects of immunization do not really have autonomous choice-making capabilities, especially since they are invariably minors.

29. In this regard, see Chloe Silverman's (2011) *Understanding Autism*, a historical and ethnographic account of parent advocacy around autism research in the United States. Silverman vividly and piquantly opens up questions of the relationship between particular forms of biomedical expertise (and nonexpertise) and the love and responsibility of parenting in contexts when children are the subjects of experimental therapeutic intervention.

30. In the American regulatory context, these were enshrined in the Belmont Report, published in 1978, which summarizes ethical principles and guidelines for

the conduct of clinical research (National Commission for the Protection of Human Subjects of Biomedical and Behavioral Research 1978). The third pillar is justice.

31. Sarita died in January 2010, and the interview was conducted by the Sama group during their visit to Bhadrachalam in March 2011. Officially, Sarita's death was attributed to consumption of pesticide (and hence listed as suicide). According to her parents, she did not consume pesticide. They also stated that they were not told about the vaccination by Sarita's hostel wardens before its administration. The interaction between the Sama team and Sarita's parents was facilitated by local members of AIDWA, which is the women's wing of the Communist Party of India (Marxist). The interview was translated into English by the Sama team, and I quote the interview from their report, since that is now part of the public domain, but also with their permission. The Sama report includes the names of Sarita's parents, who provided permission for their names to be used. But since that permission was given to Sama, and since I do not need to use their names to make my point here, I keep them anonymous. I name Sarita because her name is also mentioned in the government report.

32. Final report of the committee appointed by the Government of India (vide notification no. V. 25011/160/2010-HR, April 15, 2010) to enquire into "Alleged irregularities in the conduct of studies using Human Papilloma Virus (HPV) vaccine" by PATH in India (February 15, 2011). Henceforth "Government report."

33. See the memorandum of Jan Swasthya Abhiyan (People's Health Movement—India) to Ghulam Nabi Azad, Union Minister for Health and Family Welfare, February 21, 2011, which raises concerns regarding the report.

34. The third, Rani Kumar (dean, All India Institute of Medical Sciences, New Delhi), focused on questions of ethical malpractice. I will not read this closely, except to say that ethical malpractice and lack of adherence to GCP was clearly established in her assessment.

35. Unlike the Sama report (Sarojini, Anjali, and Ashalata 2010), which focused on the deaths in Bhadrachalam, the ambit of the government report was to look at the study in both Andhra Pradesh and Gujarat.

36. Government report.

37. Government report.

38. An FIR is a written document prepared by the police in India when they first receive information about the commission of a cognizable offense.

39. In the Sama report, this girl is referred to as Sode Sayamma.

40. She is not mentioned in the Sama report.

41. Government report.

42. Government report.

43. Government report.

44. Government report.

45. For conversations concerning how arrows function as representational devices in biomedical infrastructure, I am indebted to the artist Helen Scalway. Scalway is interested in these questions in a context quite different from establishing the cause of death in a clinical trial; her current work involves thinking about these issues in relation to building mouse research infrastructure. She is, to this end, involved in drawing

the work of geographer Gail Davies, who is herself involved in a project that studies mouse research in the United States, the United Kingdom, and Singapore (see Mice Space, www.micespace.org, accessed September 12, 2015).

46. Government report, emphasis added.

47. Government report.

48. Government report.

49. Government report.

50. For a history of evidence-based medicine emerging as the gold standard of biomedicine, see Timmermans and Berg (2003).

51. Government report, 16.

52. Government report, 17, emphasis added.

53. Gupta produced this report on September 11, 2010. I admire the thoroughness and care of Gupta's reading of the evidence, which I think offers a contrast to the far more speculative and, in my opinion, irresponsible conclusions that Dutta drew. Hence, in the interests of full disclosure, I should mention that Gupta was one of my teachers when I was an undergraduate at AIIMS. He has never taught me in any formal advisory capacity, and probably does not even remember me from my time as a student there. He was also held in very high regard as a teacher, and indeed is held in high regard as a pharmacologist. So while there is no bias in my reading of Gupta's commentary, I want to make clear that I do know him in a context before and outside this episode.

54. Government report, 38.

55. Government report.

56. Government report, 42. Compare this to Dutta's conclusion: "was bitten in the leg by a venomous snake and died."

57. Government report, 44, emphasis added.

58. A well-known example of this is in the United States is Pfizer's antibiotic Trovan, which had to be pulled from the market after the postmarketing discovery of severe liver damage in a very small percentage of patients who were on the drug. The incidence of this side effect was too small to pick up in the clinical trials. But Trovan became a blockbuster drug and, in the much larger population of consumers of the drug, it became a significant problem.

59. For a broader analysis of the history and politics of HPV vaccines in the United States and globally (though not in India) see Wailoo et al. (2011).

60. Bachmann made a statement in September 2011 concerning an account given to her by the mother of a girl who had been vaccinated against HPV. Bachmann said, "She told me that her little daughter took that vaccine, that injection. And she suffered from mental retardation thereafter. The mother was crying when she came up to me last night. I didn't know who she was before the debate. This is the very real concern and people have to draw their own conclusions" (Rob Stein, "Bachmann Questions Safety of HPV Vaccine for Girls, *Washington Post*, September 13, 2011, https://www .washingtonpost.com/national/health-science/after-debate-bachmann-questions -safety-of-hpv-vaccine-for-girls/2011/09/13/gIQAynNfPK_story.html, accessed July 9, 2016). The American Association of Pediatrics responded thus:

The American Academy of Pediatrics would like to correct false statements made in the Republican presidential campaign that HPV vaccine is dangerous and can cause mental retardation. There is absolutely no scientific validity to this statement. Since the vaccine has been introduced, more than 35 million doses have been administered, and it has an excellent safety record.

The American Academy of Pediatrics, the Centers for Disease Control and Prevention, and the American Academy of Family Physicians all recommend that girls receive HPV vaccine around age 11 or 12. That's because this is the age at which the vaccine produces the best immune response in the body, and because it's important to protect girls well before the onset of sexual activity. In the U.S., about 6 million people, including teens, become infected with HPV each year, and 4,000 women die from cervical cancer. This is a life-saving vaccine that can protect girls from cervical cancer. (Marion Burton, "AAP Statement on HPV Vaccine," American Academy of Pediatrics, September 13, 2011, https://www.aap.org/en-us/about-the-aap/aap-press-room/pages/AAP-Statement-on-HPV-Vaccine.aspx?nfstatus=401&nftoken=00000000-0000-0000-0000-000000000000&nfstatusdescription=ERROR:+No+local+token, accessed July 7, 2016)

I do not wish to defend Bachmann's claims, which come from a far-right position that is wedded to a host of antiscientific stances, and that in this context also has to be seen in relation to the regressive far-right positions on sexual and reproductive freedom for women. I just wish to suggest that the unequivocal manner in which the question of the HPV vaccine was deemed to be settled by those advocating a rational, progressive position in the United States sits uneasily with some of the questions that were being asked of the vaccine in India—indeed, at the very same time, since the firestorm around Bachmann's comments in the United States was occurring exactly when active mobilization against unethical clinical trials, using the HPV issue as a focal point, was occurring in India.

61. Population-wide prevalence of HPV infection among women ages fourteen to fifty-nine in the United States, in contrast, has been estimated at nearly 27 percent (Dunne et al. 2007, 8).

62. Normally, cervical cancer screening is done by Pap smear, which does require laboratory infrastructure and technically trained human resources. The low-cost alternative is visualization by acetic acid, which involves applying vinegar to the cervix and looking for abnormal tissue that temporarily turns white when contacted by the vinegar.

63. In defense of this argument, Tsu and LaMontagne cited what was then a forthcoming piece in the *Bulletin of the World Health Organization*, on which LaMontagne was the first author, which used data from the Phase 2 demonstration studies that were shut down in India (LaMontagne et al. 2011). That article created much controversy among civil society groups who had questioned the HPV vaccine studies, who could not understand how data could be cited from a study that had been shut down due to ethical violations. The obvious implications were either that data were being used from an incomplete study, or that data collection had continued even after ICMR

had shut the study down. There was absolutely no mention in the *Bulletin* piece about the ethical controversies that the study had been embroiled in.

64. This is not to suggest that vaccines, drugs, and other kinds of biomedical artifacts cannot provide extremely efficient public health interventions. In some cases the lack of overall health infrastructure might even make these artifacts more important than they otherwise might be. My argument here is with a public health imaginary that decontextualizes the vaccine from health policy and therefore circumscribes the problem of public health to a problem of manufacturing and delivering artifacts. I am grateful to Satyajit Rath for conversations about public health interventions as driven by artifacts as opposed to by policies. An example that Rath provided me in distinguishing between the two modalities is as follows. In an artifact-driven modality, solving the problem of tuberculosis would involve investing in resources to develop a new or better anti-TB drug. A policy-driven modality would begin with the question of TB as a social problem, generating information about reasons, contexts, indicators, and prevalence for the disease, and working forward from that point. The latter could well involve drug development as part of its strategy, but this would be part of an overall policy context, and not the technocratic driver that would claim to conjure a comprehensive approach to the disease in its wake.

65. For an analysis of the state as such an ambivalent site in the context of women's issues and feminist politics in India, see R. Sunder Rajan (2003). Sunder Rajan frames this problematic precisely in terms of a scandal of the state, and I draw upon this in framing my own analysis here.

66. Letter from Brinda Karat, Member of Parliament, Rajya Sabha, to Ghulam Nabi Azad, Union Minister for Health and Family Welfare, Government of India, March 22, 2010. While Karat has been tireless in bringing the HPV studies into political focus, it must be acknowledged that she too operates within a terrain of representative politics, and there might well have been motivations having to do with causing embarrassment to the ruling United Progressive Alliance government in India. This is not to cast aspersions on Karat's motives—on the contrary, Karat's advocacy on women's issues within arenas of representative politics in India over the past three decades has been consistent. An adequate ethnographic understanding of debates, however, requires situating them within the multiplicity of locations, perspectives, and motivations from which they emanate and within which they are embedded. In this regard, the political contexts of these interventions cannot be ignored. An identically worded letter from a civil society group such as Sama, for instance, would have come from a different place and would have to be situated differently.

67. Letter from Brinda Karat, Member of Parliament, Rajya Sabha, to Ghulam Nabi Azad, Union Minister for Health and Family Welfare, Government of India, February 17, 2011. Emphasis in original (including the statement "emphasis added," which is added by Karat while quoting from the government report).

68. Letter from Brinda Karat, Member of Parliament, Rajya Sabha, to Ghulam Nabi Azad, Union Minister for Health and Family Welfare, Government of India, May 9, 2011.

69. It is worth remembering here that one of the major drivers of global harmonization of clinical trials is multinational pharmaceutical companies, since the need

to conduct separate clinical trials of equivalent scale in multiple countries in order to get regulatory approval in each country would make drug development more expensive many times over. Attempts at global harmonization of clinical trials have been made through the ICH, and Japan has always provided the strongest resistance to harmonization. Wen-Hua Kuo (2005, 2012) has studied how harmonization played out in comparative context, situating the case of Japan next to those of Taiwan and Singapore.

70. "Calling attention to HPV vaccine programme by PATH in certain states of India and Government's Policy on introduction of such vaccines," motion in Rajya Sabha, April 22, 2010 (henceforth "HPV Parliamentary Debates").

71. In fact, 176 had been given the vaccine, and 178 placebos.

72. Parliament of India, Rajya Sabha, Department Related Parliamentary Standing Committee, Seventy-Second Report on Alleged Irregularities in the Conduct of Studies Using Human Papilloma Virus (HPV) Vaccine by PATH in India, Department of Health Research, Ministry of Health and Family Welfare, presented to the Rajya Sabha on August 30, 2013 (henceforth "HPV Parliamentary Report").

73. HPV Parliamentary Report, 1, 4, 5.

74. HPV Parliamentary Report, 5. The initial memorandum of understanding between PATH and ICMR was signed in 2006, at which point the only vaccine under consideration was Gardasil. Cervarix was only approved for marketing by the U.S. Food and Drug Administration in 2009.

75. HPV Parliamentary Report, 6–7.

76. Gazette Notification G.S.R. 53 (E), Ministry of Health and Family Welfare, Department of Health Notification, January 30, 2013. Drugs and Cosmetics (First Amendment) Rules, 2013 (henceforth "2013 Schedule Y revisions").

77. This is based on conversations with members of MSF; at their request, I do not provide further details.

78. Minutes of the 63rd DTAB meeting of the Drugs Technical Advisory Board held on May 16, 2013, New Delhi (henceforth "DTAB minutes").

79. In addition to these parliamentary and regulatory trajectories, the HPV scandals also followed a subsequent judicial trajectory, as two public interest litigations were filed in the Supreme Court of India in 2014 that questioned the conduct of the studies. Since these are still sub judice and have not been resolved at the time of writing this account, I do not provide a further account of them here. I recognize that by the time this book is published, further developments might have occurred on this score; I encourage readers to look these up. However, the politics of the HPV vaccine were fully developed in other representative arenas through the route of public scandal before they came to be judicialized. This is a different trajectory from that followed in the politics around intellectual property and access to medicines, which were immediately judicialized, as discussed in chapter 3.

80. See Sama (2011) for more about both of these scandals. Also see the introduction for a brief account of the Bhopal scandal. I conducted some interviews in Bhopal in the aftermath of the scandal. I do not elaborate upon this situation as much as about HPV because the latter has been the issue around which representative politics

in relation to unethical clinical trials in India have most fully developed. The Bhopal scandal attached to the politics of unethical clinical trials, but also folded back into the larger scandal of Bhopal itself, concerning the lack of adequate health care and justice for victims of the gas disaster for over three decades. Meanwhile, the Indore scandal developed its own controversial trajectories. Anand Rai, who brought various unethical clinical research practices at MGM Medical College Indore to light, was removed from service at the hospital and acquired the status of a heroic whistleblower exposing unethical clinical practices, especially garnering enormous foreign media publicity. But questions subsequently emerged over Rai himself. See for instance "Madadgaar doctor hi nikla chor" [The helpful doctor himself turns out to be the crook], *News Today*, May 25, 2012. (*News Today* is an Indore-based Hindi language newspaper.) This article alleged that Rai had helped a foreign agency make a film about the Indore scandal in exchange for payment of 50,000 euros, a reminder that scandal sells, and that brokerage economies operate not just in clinical research but in the mediation of scandal that allows for a voyeuristic exposure of the exploitation of vulnerable populations as guinea pigs to global audiences. Some civil society advocates against unethical clinical trials in India have distanced themselves from espousing Rai's cause or sharing a platform with him.

81. "Government Plans to Reintroduce HPV Vaccine," *Asian Age*, July 28, 2015. According to the article, the government has asked the National Technical Advisory Group to conduct a feasibility study regarding the introduction of the vaccine in the immunization program.

82. This speaks to the two registers of representation, as proxy and as portrait, which Gayatri Spivak (1988) insists is vital to stay attentive to while discussing political subjectivity.

83. See the Belmont Report, which is the normative framework under which human subjects research in the United States operates (National Commission for the Protection of Human Subjects of Biomedical and Behavioral Research 1978). Similar principles had been earlier enshrined in the 1964 Helsinki Declaration of the World Medical Association (WMA 2013), which has since been updated seven times. This declaration developed principles for ethical experimentation that were propounded in the 1947 Nuremberg Code, passed to prevent the kinds of experimental atrocities committed by the Nazi regime (available at https://history.nih.gov/research /downloads/nuremberg.pdf, last accessed July 9, 2016).

84. See Scocozza (1989) for an articulation of this ethical value system.

85. Folayan herself has been actively involved in advocacy against unethical trials and for access to medicines in Nigeria, and I have benefited greatly from her work and insights, for which many thanks.

86. At a national consultation on unethical clinical trials in India that Sama organized in 2011, I suggested that we think about Folayan and Allman's proposal and wondered what would happen if advocacy demands were reframed from a position that understood experimental subjects as laborers rather than volunteers. Not surprisingly, the provocation generated divergent responses, the Marxists in the room the most supportive but many others resistant or outright opposed to such reframing.

One sees similar divisions in feminist debates around prostitution and sex work, as Rajeswari Sunder Rajan (2003, 117–146) has explored.

87. See especially appendix 12 of 2013 Schedule Y revisions.

88. "Formula to Determine the Quantum of Compensation in the Cases of Clinical Trial Related Serious Adverse Events (SAES) or Deaths Occurring during Clinical Trials," report prepared by expert committee constituted by the Drug Controller General of India, March 14, 2013 (henceforth "Compensation formula").

89. The ways in which particular kinds of experimental subjectivity, rendered ethical by way of "voluntary" contract, come to be retroactively figured at the moment of pain or death has parallels to the ways in which the subject of widow immolation (sati) has been figured, as Rajeswari Sunder Rajan (1993, 15–39) has shown. Tanika Sarkar (2012) had argued that the widow who had to immolate herself in colonial Bengal in the early to mid-nineteenth century was the bearer of "something like rights," as the regulation of sati by the British colonial state saw a gradual transmutation of the idea of consent. Far from framing it as a "traditional" practice that was antithetical to the modern liberal law that the colonial state was instituting, Sarkar shows how in fact the British regime allowed for a continuation of the practice, as long as it could be rendered lawful, which itself was based (in the early colonial state in Bengal) in the formal institutionalization of the widow's consent to be immolated: what was deemed proper consent. In the process, Sarkar argues that the colonial state gave consent an importance that did not exist earlier. Just as it is worth dislocating experimental subjectivity as voluntary activity in a gift economy by attending to the actually prevalent, deeply capitalized political economies in which it increasingly operates today, so too is it worth recognizing that the normative ideals of consent that give sanction to these fictions of voluntarism have roots not just in twentieth-century liberal ethics as instituted in Euro-American contexts, but in much longer colonial legal histories of regulating traditional patriarchal practices which themselves have postcolonial echoes and continuities. See also Pedersen (1991), whose arguments about the early twentieth-century British colonial regulation of clitoridectomy in Kenya show considerable parallels with Sarkar's account of the nineteenth-century regulation of sati in Bengal.

90. A similar discursive structure is also reflected in portrayals of the organ trade, such as Manjula Padmanabhan's (2003) dystopic play *Harvest*.

91. For instance, the HPV vaccine studies could legitimately be seen as Western exploitation of Indian bodies; given that a number of the experimental subjects were tribal girls, it could equally be seen as yet another extractive biomedical enterprise performed upon indigenous populations, layered onto the enormous amount of resource extraction of land populated by indigenous people ongoing in areas such as Chattisgarh. For indigenous and First Nations critiques of biocolonialism, see especially Maori author Patricia Grace's (1998) stunning novel *Baby No-Eyes*. It is also important here to note the complex racialized histories of biomedical research in the United States, for which see note 17.

92. In this regard, see especially Sarah Franklin's (2006) exploration of what she calls "the spaces of transbiology" in her account of embryo transfer.

93. For biosociality, see Rabinow (1992, 2007); for biological citizenship, see Petryna (2002), Novas and Rose (2005), Rose (2006).

94. See Sheila Jasanoff's (2011) development of the idea of constitutional moment in relation to the life sciences in terms of what she calls bioconstitutionalism. I expand upon this term in greater detail in chapter 3. See introduction for the salience of constitutionalism to understanding pharmocracy.

95. In chapter 3, I elaborate upon this argument for the importance of situating cancer in contexts that are distinct and dispersed from Euro-American centers of research and development. As with Gleevec, India was a site where safety and efficacy trials for HPV vaccines had not been conducted; but this did not prevent India from becoming a critical site of public health intervention and capital accumulation from these vaccines. It is worth reading Lochlann Jain's (2013) *Malignant*, which theorizes cancer largely out of American contexts, alongside Julie Livingston's (2012) *Improvising Medicine*, an ethnographic account of Botswana's solitary oncology ward. Both are extraordinary narratives, and their juxtaposition suggests that situating cancer involves something more than just imagining Euro-America as a site of plenty and the Third World as one of lack. Rather, the very configurations of both biomedicine and disease come to be at stake.

96. Again, one can see an identical structure of ethical publicity in feminist debates around the regulation of prostitution, between abolitionists who see prostitution as fundamentally exploitative, and liberals who see it as potentially a volitional and contractual act that needs only to be regulated so that its violent and violating aspects are curtailed (R. Sunder Rajan 2003, 117–146). As Rajeswari Sunder Rajan points out, these positions tend to elide the structural political economies of poverty and debt that operate in the lives of most (especially Third World) prostitutes, which in fact render exploitation a more complicated sociological phenomenon than the agential transaction of money for sex, and that render claims to volition hollow. This is not to say that an acknowledgment of these political economies is entirely absent in feminist debate; just that the framing of the problem in terms of ethics alone has no space for it. Neither ethical solution in itself would actually intervene in the structuring of the conditions that render these normative binaries as solutions in the first place. Similarly, Cohen points to the political economy of indebtedness that almost without exception led the kidney sellers he interviewed (who were invariably women) to sell their kidneys. These sellers would again fall back into debt, but now they would only have one kidney left to sell.

97. See Bateson et al. (1956) and Bateson (1972, 271–278), for elaborations of the notion of the double bind, and Fortun (2001) for its use in studying the political economy of global technoscience.

CHAPTER THREE. **Constitutional Values**

1. Paragraphs 4–6 of the Doha Declaration are especially pertinent here:

4. The TRIPS Agreement does not and should not prevent Members from taking measures to protect public health. Accordingly, while reiterating our

commitment to the TRIPS Agreement, we affirm that the Agreement can and should be interpreted and implemented in a manner supportive of WTO Members' right to protect public health and, in particular, to promote access to medicines for all. In this connection, we reaffirm the right of WTO Members to use, to the full, the provisions in the TRIPS Agreement, which provide flexibility for this purpose.

5. Accordingly and in the light of paragraph 4 above, while maintaining our commitments in the TRIPS Agreement, we recognize that these flexibilities include:

(a) In applying the customary rules of interpretation of public international law, each provision of the TRIPS Agreement shall be read in the light of the object and purpose of the Agreement as expressed, in particular, in its objectives and principles.

(b) Each Member has the right to grant compulsory licenses and the freedom to determine the grounds upon which such licenses are granted.

(c) Each Member has the right to determine what constitutes a national emergency or other circumstances of extreme urgency, it being understood that public health crises, including those relating to HIV/AIDS, tuberculosis, malaria and other epidemics, can represent a national emergency or other circumstances of extreme urgency.

(d) The effect of the provisions in the TRIPS Agreement that are relevant to the exhaustion of intellectual property rights is to leave each Member free to establish its own regime for such exhaustion without challenge, subject to the MFN and national treatment provisions of Articles 3 and 4.

6. We recognize that WTO Members with insufficient or no manufacturing capacities in the pharmaceutical sector could face difficulties in making effective use of compulsory licensing under the TRIPS Agreement. We instruct the Council for TRIPS to find an expeditious solution to this problem and to report to the General Council before the end of 2002.

See World Trade Organization, Ministerial Declaration of November 14, 2001, WT/MIN(01)/DEC/2, 41 I.L.M. 746 (2002).

2. Examples include the 2010 revocation of Roche's patent on its antiviral drug Valcyte, which is used as part of HIV-AIDS treatment regimens; the dismissal, early in 2012, by the Delhi High Court of a patent infringement suit filed by Hoffmann-La Roche against Cipla, relating to its anticancer drug Tarceva; the issuance of India's first compulsory license in March 2012 on Bayer's anticancer drug Nexavar, which allowed the Hyderabad-based Natco Pharmaceuticals to manufacture generic versions of the drug; the revocation of Pfizer's patent for its anticancer drug Sutent in October 2012, which was a reversal by the Patent Controller of India of a 2007 patent that had been granted on this drug, following adjudication of an opposition filed by the Indian company Cipla to the granting of the patent; and the revocation of Hoffman-La Roche's 2006 patent for its anti–hepatitis C drug Pegasys in November 2012 by India's IPAB, following an appeal by the Indian company Wockhardt and the civil society group Sankalp Rehabilitation Trust.

3. A significant interlude that set the stage for the Supreme Court hearing was a ruling by a newly constituted tribunal, the IPAB, which upheld the Madras High Court verdict. The Supreme Court however largely disregarded the IPAB verdict and considered the case more or less afresh. Hence, while I allude to the IPAB verdict in this chapter, I do not enter a detailed account or discussion of it.

4. *Novartis AG v. Cipla Ltd.*, http://saffron.pharmabiz.com/red.asp?fn=/services/docs/PatAct1970-06.asp, accessed July 10, 2016, emphasis added.

5. The parallels between Indian and Brazilian state strategies in such pushing back in the arena of pharmaceuticals are essential to think through in comparative perspective. In addition to Biehl and Petryna (2011), see Biehl (2013) for accounts of judicialization of pharmaceutical politics in Brazil; see also Cassier (2012) for important accounts of contemporary pharmaceutical politics in Brazil that are more centrally concerned with capitalist logics.

6. *Novartis AG and Another v. Union of India and Others*, 4 MLJ 1153 (2007), emphasis added.

7. *Diamond v. Chakrabarty*, 447 U.S. 303 (1980).

8. Of course, the sacrality of property in the United States, especially as it pertains to intellectual property rights, has always been contested. The U.S. Constitution says that patents and copyrights are intended to make knowledge and invention available for public good and not for monopoly ownership rights. It is just that the pendulum has swung far from this. This is why a constitutional analysis can never be concerned just with what is stated in an authoritative constitutional text but has to see constitution as a process, which resolves differently in the context of different judicial and political cultures. See for instance Jasanoff (2012), who shows how the patent application for the transgenic Oncomouse followed different trajectories in the United States (where it was granted) and in Canada (where it was subsequently denied). Even today, there is friction over the unquestioned sanctity of intellectual property rights in biotechnology in the United States. The seminal verdict denying a patent on the *brca* genes to Myriad Genetics, *Association for Molecular Pathology v. Myriad Genetics, Inc.* (U.S. 12-398, 2013), which held that isolated human genes cannot be patented, is an important example of such friction. However, it is the case that while the United States has seen contention around gene patents, it has not done so in any significant manner around the question of drug patents as instruments of corporate monopoly, a value system that has become progressively naturalized.

9. For an elaboration of the notion of technoscientic imaginaries, see Marcus (1995) and Jasanoff and Kim (2015) (who refer to "socio-technical imaginaries").

10. Special Leave Petition (Civil) of 2009, between Novartis AG and (1) Union of India (2) the Controller General of Patents and Designs (3) Assistant Controller of Patents and Designs (4) M/s Cancer Patients Aid Association (5) Natco Pharma Ltd (6) Cipla Ltd (7) Ranbaxy Laboratories Ltd (8) Hetero Drugs Ltd (henceforth "Novartis Supreme Court SLP"). In between the High Court verdict and the Supreme Court appeal, the matter of the technical adjudication of the patentability of Gleevec had passed through a newly constituted tribunal, the IPAB. Hence, this was, strictly speaking, an appeal against the IPAB verdict, which itself had a number of interesting

and significant aspects. Briefly, while the Patent Office had initially denied the Gleevec patent on three grounds—utility, nonobviousness (the criteria by which the molecule would have been deemed inventive), and Section 3(d)—the IPAB upheld the denial only on the grounds of Section 3(d), stating that in fact the drug was useful and nonobvious. Therefore, the CPAA and Natco Pharmaceuticals filed their own petitions to the Supreme Court, challenging those aspects of the IPAB verdict that supported Novartis's claims of invention and nonobviousness. All these petitions were heard together, and a single verdict given by the court. In the process, the court chose to largely disregard the IPAB verdict and considered all aspects of the case afresh. Because the IPAB verdict did not impact the Supreme Court judgment, I do not discuss it in detail here. However, the IPAB would subsequently become an important appellate tribunal in its own right, deciding further cases that would have an impact on the interpretive landscape of intellectual property law. See for instance the IPAB's upholding of a compulsory license that had been issued on Bayer's anticancer drug Nexavar in September 2012, and its revocation of Hoffman-La Roche's 2006 patent for its anti-hepatitis C drug Pegasys in November 2012 following an appeal by the Indian company Wockhardt and the civil society group Sankalp Rehabilitation Trust. For the former, see Intellectual Property Appellate Board, 2012, *Bayer Corporation v. Union of India and Others*, Chennai, 14 September, M.P. Nos. 74 to 76 of 2012 & 108 of 2012 in OA/35/2012/PT/MUM, Order number 223 of 2012. For the latter, see Intellectual Property Appellate Board, 2012, *Sankalp Rehabilitation Trust v. F. Hoffmann La Roche AG and Another*, 2 November, OA/8/2009/PT/CH and M.P. Nos. 85 & 111 of 2012 In OA/8/2009/PT/CH, Order number 250 of 2012.

11. Recall that one saw this in the initial High Court verdict regarding Section 3(d)'s constitutionality as well, which saw the court insisting upon the objective that the amended section sought to achieve, the ensurance of good health for Indian citizens.

12. Supreme Court of India, Civil Appellate Jurisdiction, Civil Appeal Nos. 2706–2716 of 2013 (arising out of SLP (C) Nos. 20539–20549 of 2009), *Novartis AG v. Union or India and Others*, with Civil Appeal No. 2728 of 2013 (arising out of SLP (C) No. 32706 of 2009), *Natco Pharma Ltd. v. Union of India and Others*, and Civil Appeal Nos. 2717–2727 of 2013 (arising out of SLP (C) Nos. 12984–12994 of 2013), SLP (C). . . . /2011 CC Nos. 6667–6677, *M/s Cancer Patients Aid Association v. Union of India and Others*. The two-member bench was constituted by Justice Aftab Alam and Justice Ranjana Prakash Desai. Justice Alam wrote the verdict for the court, which was delivered on April 1, 2013. (Henceforth referred to as "Supreme Court verdict.")

13. 3 SCC 279 (1987), cited in Supreme Court verdict, 15.

14. 1 SCC 424 (1987), cited in Supreme Court verdict, 15. Both of the verdicts read as methodological precedent for judicial interpretation were delivered by Justice Chinnappa Reddy, who was a bold supporter of democratic freedoms during the state of Emergency imposed by Indira Gandhi from 1975–77. Justice Reddy died on April 20, 2013, less than three weeks after the verdict on Gleevec was delivered using his teachings on legislative interpretation. It is important to be attentive to the generational dynamics of judicial cultures in India.

15. This is not to say that legal history does not matter in American judicial cultures. It is one of the fundamental things that has to be outlined in the briefing of a case and is important in the writing of decisions in the United States as well. What I wish to emphasize here is the naturalized purification of the authority of the patent claim in the United States in a manner that the Indian courts have refused, a refusal that is exemplified in the mode of reasoning employed by the Indian Supreme Court, as I describe here.

16. The schematic outline provided below is based on that found in the Supreme Court verdict. For a more detailed analysis of the history of Indian patent law and its impact on the Indian pharmaceutical industry, see Chaudhuri (2005).

17. See especially Section 83(b): "that [patents] are not granted merely to enable patentees to enjoy a monopoly for the importation of the patented article"; (c) "that the protection and enforcement of patent rights contribute to the promotion of technological innovation and to the transfer and dissemination of technology, to the mutual advantage of producers and users of technological knowledge and in a manner conducive to social and economic welfare"; (d) "that patents granted do not impede protection of public health and nutrition and should act as an instrument to promote public interest"; and (g) "that patents are granted to make the benefit of the patented invention available at reasonably affordable prices to the public."

18. Letter from Jim Yong Kim, HIV/AIDS director of the World Health Organization, to A. Ramadoss, minister for health and family welfare, Government of India, December 17, 2004, http://www.cptech.org/ip/health/c/india/who12172004.html; letter from Achmat Dangor, director of advocacy, communication and leadership, UNAIDS, to Kamal Nath, minister for commerce and industry, Government of India, February 23, 2005, http://www.cptech.org/ip/health/c/india/unaids02232005.html.

19. Section 2(1)(j) defined invention in the following terms: "a new product or process involving an inventive step and capable of industrial application." *Inventive step* was further defined in Section 2(1)(j(a)) as "a feature of an invention that involves technical advance as compared to the existing knowledge or having economic significance or both and that makes the invention not obvious to a person skilled in the art."

20. Recall that the question of whether Gleevec was an invention was a matter for adjudication for the court in spite of the IPAB's decision that it was, because of CPAA's and Natco's petitions before the court that challenged those elements of the IPAB verdict that were in Novartis's favor. Hence, the court reconsidered the questions of whether the conversion of imatinib to β-imatinib mesylate constituted a nonobvious invention, alongside a consideration of whether the latter showed enhanced efficacy in order to meet the requirements of 3(d). During the hearing of the case, Justice Alam declared that "the IPAB order, with due respect, is a strange mishmash. We will come to our own findings, [and] are not at all satisfied with the findings of the IPAB" (author's field notes taken at Supreme Court hearings, October 31, 2012).

21. See Pottage and Sherman (2012), who develop this argument with reference to the history of the figure of invention in liberal Western patent law.

22. Recall that the patent application for β-imatinib mesylate in India was filed in 1998. This was subsequent to the 1997 filing of a patent application in Switzerland, not the United States.

23. The NDA is the basis upon which all drugs are evaluated and approved for market by the FDA. As stated by the FDA, "The documentation required in an NDA is supposed to tell the drug's whole story, including what happened during the clinical tests, what the ingredients of the drug are, the results of the animal studies, how the drug behaves in the body, and how it is manufactured, processed and packaged" (U.S. Food and Drug Administration 2016).

24. NDA #21-335.

25. As cited in Supreme Court verdict, 65. A package insert is the document provided along with a prescription medication when it is marketed, and provides the formal regulatory description of the drug as approved for market. In the United States, it must be approved by the FDA.

26. Author's field notes taken at Supreme Court hearings, October 31, 2012.

27. This means that the drafting of the patent claim, and the forms that it takes, is a complex strategic exercise that embodies what Pottage and Sherman (2012) call the "figure of invention." See their argument in *Figures of Invention* for a historical elaboration of these forms and their role in the history of the legal constitution of invention.

28. The focus of my analysis in chapter 4 is GIPAP. I do not discuss it further here because the court did not deem it relevant in its own judgment of the patentability of Gleevec. Indeed, counsel for Novartis tried repeatedly to bring GIPAP to the attention of the court during its hearings, until Justice Alam finally admonished them by stating that he did not want to hear mention of its charitable program any more since it did not have bearing on the case at hand. While rendered irrelevant to the legal interpretation of India's new patent laws, initiatives such as GIPAP are central to the broader political terrain of pharmaceutical monopoly, pricing, and access.

29. "A patent relating to a particular area of technology which prevents another patent from being used because the other patent relies on technology covered by the first," as defined at Wiktionary, http://en.wiktionary.org/wiki/blocking_patent, accessed February 18, 2014.

30. Written submissions on behalf of the intervenor, in the matter of *Novartis AG v. Union of India and Others*, Shamnad Basheer, intervenor (henceforth "Basheer intervention"). Basheer has been a leading voice in matters relating to intellectual property rights and their interpretation in India over the past decade. At the time of the Supreme Court case, Basheer was a professor of law at the National University of Juridical Sciences, Kolkata.

31. The ODA was passed in 1983 to facilitate the development and commercialization of drugs for diseases with small markets by providing incentives in terms of tax breaks and market monopolies to the developers of such drugs.

32. Of course, if one considers the appropriation of health by capital as described in chapter 1, one could argue that it is increasingly the case that the purpose of medicines is not to cure disease but to grow markets. Hence, the court here is insisting

upon a definition of health that has not been appropriated into logics of surplus value generation.

33. The original quote is from Mofitt (1979), cited in Basheer intervention, 18, and subsequently in Supreme Court verdict, 94.

34. *Economic and Political Weekly*, 48, no. 32, August 10, 2013.

35. This politics played out in the case of Herceptin in the early 1990s, and was deeply influenced by the politics of HIV-AIDS patient groups such as ACT-UP in the United States in the late 1980s and early 1990s. See Epstein (1996) for an account of the latter.

36. For key articles that describe some of these developments, see Witte et al. (1978), Witte, Dasgupta, and Baltimore (1980), de Klein et al. (1982), Heisterkamp et al. (1982, 1985), and Fainstein et al. (1987). Also see Mukherjee (2011, 430–431), and Keating and Cambrosio (2012, 323–330); also Wapner (2014) for a longer history of research into the Philadelphia chromosome.

37. It is worth pointing out that both Mukherjee and Keating and Cambrosio only ever refer to Gleevec as imatinib.

38. See for instance Dutfield (2013).

39. My account of the trials is a summary of Keating and Cambrosio's (2012, 316–323) more detailed account.

40. For an elaboration of this initial reluctance, and the institutional politics involved in Druker's push to conduct trials, see his own account (Druker 2007b).

41. Keating and Cambrosio do mention the (political and judicial, not clinical) trials of Gleevec in India in their account, by devoting a paragraph to how Gleevec's "success story has been partly clouded" by Indian generic competition and a "series of setbacks in the Indian courts" (2012, 319–320). The fact that Gleevec has had a checkered history in India is acknowledged in their account, but almost parenthetically; it is in no way deemed central to either the history of the development of the drug, or even to the notion of oncopolitics as developed by the authors in relation to that history. My attempt here is to provide a differently situated perspective on the history of Gleevec, one that does not similarly reproduce center-periphery dichotomies where politics elsewhere is acknowledged only to be bracketed and then dismissed.

42. I am indebted to conversations with a number of key actors on the left who have been involved with these debates as activists, interlocutors, and policy makers over the past three decades. They could be placed in four broad and sometimes overlapping categories and include (1) Members of Parliament of leftist parties, especially the Communist Party of India (Marxist) (CPI-M), who have been important legislative voices in these debates; (2) members of CPI-M affiliated trade unions, especially medical representatives' unions; (3) members of the Peoples Science Movement, founded in Kerala in the late 1970s (for accounts of which, see Kannan 1976, 1978, 1990; Varma 2001; and (4) members of the National Working Group on Patent Laws (NWGPL), founded in the late 1980s. Unlike the other three, NWGPL is not formally affiliated with the Communist Parties of India, but has had a major role in providing policy-based opposition and alternatives to global intellectual property regimes throughout and since the Uruguay Round negotiations (see Sengupta 2010, 2013). I am especially grateful to Nilotpal Basu and Brinda Karat (CPI-M Members of Parliament), Amitava

Guha (CPI-M trade union activist), Amit Sengupta of the Peoples Science Movement, and Dinesh Abrol of NWGPL for insights and material on the history of the politics around intellectual property rights issues in India since the mid-1980s. I draw upon perspectives gleaned from them individually over the years in my account here, but especially from an interview with Basu, who was actively involved in interparty and parliamentary negotiations around Section 3(d).

43. In the United States, medical representatives are usually known as sales representatives. Unlike those in the United States, medical representatives in India are strongly unionized.

44. These and subsequent quotes in this section, unless otherwise specified, are from Nilotpal Basu, CPI-M Member of Parliament, interview with the author, November 30, 2011 (henceforth "Basu interview").

45. The Congress-led coalition government under Prime Minister Manmohan Singh that passed the 2005 Patent Act came to power in May 2004, with the leftist parties as coalition members. Prior to this, the Bharatiya Janata Party (BJP) headed two separate coalition governments from 1998 to 2004. The first two amendments to the 1970 Patent Act, in 1999 (initiating provisions for mailbox applications and exclusive marketing rights) and 2002 (broadening the definition of invention) had been enacted by this government. The 2005 Amendment was the third amendment. The BJP itself was in a contradictory position with relation to multinational corporate capital. On the one hand, its ideological wing, the Rashtriya Swayamsevak Sangh, has always adopted a nationalist aversion to multinational capital in the interests of protecting domestic industry; on the other hand, the BJP as a political party has always tended to be pro-business of any kind, domestic or multinational. On the whole, in spite of internal contradictions, the BJP coalition did not indicate any significant opposition to TRIPS while in power.

46. While the Congress gave in to leftist demands in the case of 2005 Patent Act flexibilities, similar negotiations between the two parties would break down in 2008 around a proposed nuclear deal between India and the United States, which the Left strongly opposed, leading to their leaving the coalition.

47. This ambivalence is reflected, for instance, in a note circulated by the Prime Minister's Office to the Ministry of Health and Family Welfare, Department of Industrial Policy and Promotion, the Department of Legal Affairs, and the Department of Pharmaceuticals on July 16, 2010. The note records discussions held by the Prime Minister's Office with the Organization of Pharmaceutical Producers of India, which is the major lobbying group for the multinational pharmaceutical industry in India. CEOs of the Indian divisions of Novartis, Pfizer, Bristol-Myers Squibb, and Sanofi-Aventis were reportedly at this meeting. A copy of this note was obtained by civil society groups fighting for access to essential medicines. The note requests feedback on the adoption of monopolistic intellectual property measures that go far beyond the requirements of the TRIPS agreement, including the dilution of Section 3(d). L. K. Latheeq, Prime Minister's Office, South Block, note to Secretary, Ministry of Health and Family Welfare; Secretary, Department of Industrial Policy and Promotion; Secretary, Department of Legal Affairs; and Secretary, Department of Pharmaceuticals, July 16, 2010.

48. I recognize that the question of what constitutes the southern world is a complex one, given emergent economies throughout the former Third World; the becoming global of many southern cities; increasing inequalities within northern countries; and demographic transformations through postcolonial migrations that constitute postcolonies within the First World (for which, see especially Balibar [2004] regarding Europe). At the same time, long shadows of colonial geopolitical histories persist, and take new and continuing imperialist forms. In the context of this discussion, I use *southern* simply to extend the Gleevec story beyond the Euro-American focus of Keating and Cambrosio's account. Global geopolitical configurations in the pharmaceutical political economies are more fully considered in chapter 5.

49. The account of Gleevec's history in Korea that I provide here is summarized from interviews I conducted there in 2009 with leukemia patient activists, pharmacists, lawyers, and doctors. I am grateful to Ahn Gi Jong, Mi-Ran Kwon, Chul Won Jung, Hee Seob Nam, and Seoc-Kyun Woo for their conversations and insights on this history; to Sang-Hyun Kim and Youngyung Paik for facilitating introductions with key actors involved with Gleevec there, and for providing me with historical context of Korean social movements around health; and to Youngyung Paik and Seo-Young Park for acting as translators as I conducted my interviews.

50. For an elaboration of the notion of monopsony and its relationship to global pharmaceutical pricing strategies, see chapter 1.

51. It is worth bearing in mind that Euro-America is not a singular entity either, and there are huge differences in both health care structures and state relationships with the pharmaceutical industry within Europe and between Europe and the United States.

52. A wonderful moment in the Supreme Court hearings came when Justice Alam was attempting to understand some complicated chemistry relating to imatinib and its crystalline salts, and counsel for Natco Pharmaceuticals (who happened to be one of the only female lawyers arguing the case of either side) explained it to him. Justice Alam paused and said, "That is remarkable. You know the law and you know chemistry. Our country needs more young women like you." Author's field notes taken at Supreme Court hearings, October 31, 2012.

53. While India has well-developed infrastructure for drug manufacture (its local pharmaceutical industry) and distribution (a thriving pharmacy market), these often raise acute problems in other national contexts where such infrastructures are weaker. See especially Kristin Peterson's (2014b) account of the political economy of drug access in Nigeria. Peterson shows that the lack of infrastructure in the country is itself a function of global economic logics that saw capital flight after the oil bust in the late 1970s and the subsequent evisceration of drug manufacture and distribution under World Bank–imposed structural adjustment programs in the 1980s. Also see chapter 4 for an account of strategic maneuvering around provision of drugs, as I discuss Novartis's drug donation program for Gleevec, GIPAP.

54. More than in the Gleevec patent case, one can see this is an earlier case brought before the Supreme Court around exclusive marketing rights that had been granted for the drug in 2002. I discuss this in chapter 4.

55. Justice Prabha Sridevan, interview with the author, October 29, 2012.

56. See Derrida (1992) for a philosophical development of the place of law in relation to what he calls "the promise of justice." The law itself, as a formal instrument of adjudication and governance, too often is inadequate to justice—too instrumental, too reductive, and appropriable by powerful interests. And yet the law provides an opening to justice, which itself is not something teleological, capable of being posited or defined in advance. Rather it is a promissory horizon, always deferred and itself a site of politics. Crucially for Derrida, the very possibility of democracy depends upon the promise of justice, just as the work of deconstruction is that of keeping this promise open (see also Derrida 1994).

57. See Chakrabarty (2000) for the absolute importance of understanding European philosophical inheritance for any adequate conceptualization of postcolonial politics.

58. In this regard, Gayatri Spivak distinguishes a mid-twentieth-century postcolonial constitution such as India's from the American Constitution. While the latter is also strictly speaking a postcolonial constitution, a particular kind of origin story— one signifying a clean slate upon which to make a fresh start—could only be secured "because the colonists encountered a sparsely populated, thoroughly pre-capitalist social formation that could be managed by pre-political maneuvers" (Spivak 1990, 136). Comaroff and Comaroff (2006) further distinguish mid-twentieth-century constitutions from the slew of constitutions (over a hundred) that have come to be drafted since 1989, ones that have emerged in a conjuncture of neoliberalism.

59. Compare this to the form of normative legitimation that biomedical ethics underlying good clinical practice operates through, as discussed in the conclusion to chapter 2. In contrast to the paralogical legitimation employed by the Indian courts, what one sees there is rather a procedural legitimation, one that narrows and closes down possibilities for normative questioning and innovation and therefore at its worst becomes nothing more than a ritual that is appropriate to capital expansion, one whose breaches are not adequately held accountable.

60. He outlines these as follows: "(i) the text adopted in 1950; (ii) the Nehruvian constitution, demanding a compelling respect by the [Supreme Court of India] for parliamentary sovereignty; (iii) the 1973 *Kesavananda Bharati* constitution, a decision that confers constitutional power on the [Supreme Court of India]; (iv) the state Finance Capitalist constitution presaged by the Indira Nehru Gandhi constitution, via the nationalization of banks and insurance industries and the abolition of the privy purses; (v) the Emergency constitution of 1975–77; (vi) the post-Emergency constitution which marks both judicial populism as well as the emergence of expansive judicial activism; and (vii) the Neo-liberal constitution which redefines India as a vast global market" (Baxi 2010).

61. *Novartis AG and Another v. Union of India and Others*, 4 MLJ 1153 (2007), emphasis added.

62. In this regard, see John Kelly and Martha Kaplan's (2001) theorization of the nation as a "represented community."

63. For an analysis of intellectual property in this broader framework of the politics of technology in the American context, see Hilgartner (2009).

64. I have discussed this ideological role of innovation discourse in the context of the Gleevec Supreme Court case in an op-ed in the *Indian Express* (see K. Sunder Rajan 2012).

65. See Jasanoff (2013) for a broader consideration of the relationship between science and public reason.

66. In 2007, the Philippines passed legislation inspired by and similar to India's Section 3(d); the Supreme Court verdict provides strength and legitimacy to such policies. This is recognized by the multinational pharmaceutical lobby and the American government, as evidenced in TRIPS-plus frameworks that are being pushed which restrict such flexibilities (see chapter 5).

67. *Citizens United v. Federal Election Commission*, No. 08-205, 558 U.S. 310 (2010).

68. Public interest litigation is a form of litigation that seeks to advance the interests of disadvantaged groups. It has been a major mechanism by which social policy issues have come to be judicialized in India since the late 1970s. See Deva (2009) for a broader critique of public interest litigation in India. It is worth remembering that while this has become a common route to judicialization, the Gleevec case was one of a corporation suing the government, and was not therefore itself public interest litigation.

69. In 2009, the Delhi High Court had deemed Section 377 unconstitutional, but the Supreme Court overturned this in December 2013, just months after the Gleevec verdict (see Supreme Court of India, Civil Appeal No. 10972 of 2013 (Arising Out of SLP (C) No. 15436 of 2009, December 11, 2013, http://judis.nic.in/supremecourt/imgs1 .aspx?filename=41070). Hence, even within the same time horizon, one sees radically divergent verdicts from the perspective of social justice. See R. Sunder Rajan (2003) (especially the introduction) for an elaboration of the tenuous nature of the law in relation to questions of feminism; Sunder Rajan nonetheless insists that the law's own checkered history is not enough cause to abandon it as a site for articulating progressive political demands.

70. Latha Jishnu's reportage has been invaluable and relentless in exposing such moves to sensitize judges to intellectual property (see for instance Jishnu 2010b). See also her article regarding the role of George Washington University's India Project in such sensitization (Jishnu 2010a). I am grateful to Jishnu for conversations that have helped me understand the processes by which such sensitization occurs.

71. I use "common sense" in the sense that Gramsci does, as a set of naturalized background assumptions that provide the basis for hegemonic interpretations of situations at particular places and times. Given that the Indian judiciary has been crucial in interrupting multinational corporate hegemony, changing its common sense becomes a crucial site of politics.

CHAPTER FOUR. **Philanthropic Values**

1. Even though Novartis counsel did not answer this question, there are some obvious structural reasons why, for which see chapter 1.

2. See also Peterson (2014a), who discusses pharmaceutical monopoly in Nigeria, and Ecks (2008), who discusses this point in relation to Gleevec in India.

3. Letter from Sipho Mthathi, General Secretary, Treatment Action Campaign, to Prime Minister of India Manmohan Singh, January 23, 2007, http://www.tac.org.za /community/node/2172 (accessed March 7, 2014); letter from Henry Waxman, Chairman of the House Committee on Oversight and Government Reform, U.S. House of Representatives, to Daniel Vasella, CEO, Novartis Pharmaceuticals, February 13, 2007; letter from German Members of Parliament Jella Teuchner, Wolfgang Wodarg, Ute Koczy, Monika Knoche, Frank Spieth, Herta Daubler-Gmelin, Sascha Raabe, Martina Bunge, Ilja Seifert, Christel Riemann-Hanewinckel, and Harald Terpe to Prime Minister of India Manmohan Singh, March 22, 2007; letter from Julian Reinhard, Campaign Director, Berne Declaration, to Daniel Vasella, CEO Novartis, October 10, 2006.

4. Max Foundation, "About the Max Foundation," http://www.themaxfoundation .org/aboutus/default.aspx (accessed March 7, 2014). Information about GIPAP is available on the Max Foundation website, and also on the Novartis website at https:// www.novartis.com/about-us/corporate-responsibility/expanding-access-healthcare /oncology-patient-assistance-programs (accessed July 11, 2016).

5. All quotes here, unless otherwise mentioned, from the Writ petition filed in the Supreme Court of India in its original civil jurisdiction and in its jurisdiction under Article 32 of the Constitution of India in the matter of *Cancer Patients Aid Association and Another (Petitioners) v. Union of India and Others (Respondents)*, 2004 (henceforth "CPAA writ petition").

6. It is worth emphasizing the importance of these battles in setting the stage for the parliamentary debates around the 2005 Patent Act that would lead to the amendment of Section 3(d) to prevent evergreening, as described in chapter 3.

7. I have discussed how the Indian Supreme Court drew upon Section 83 in its verdict on the Gleevec case in chapter 3 (see chapter 3, note 17).

8. Conversion rate at the time would have been approximately Rs. 40–45 per U.S. dollar.

9. CPAA writ petition, emphasis added.

10. There is also, parenthetically, an interesting conflation of *health* here with *cure*, as therapy almost stands in for health in this framing.

11. Writ petition (civil) no. 340 in the Supreme Court of India (Civil Original Jurisdiction) in the matter of *Cancer Patients Aid Association and Another (Petititioners) v. Union of India and Others (Responder)*, Counteraffidavit of Respondents No. 4 & 5 to the Petition (2004) (henceforth "Novartis counterpetition").

12. Novartis counterpetition.

13. Novartis counterpetition. As I subsequently describe, this is in fact an untrue statement.

14. As I show in the next section, actual access to the medicine for many patients depended upon companies providing the drug at less than the stated price point. And so market entities, including generic companies, did in fact make the drug accessible in certain actual instances; but CPAA's argument highlighted the fact that neither monopoly nor free market capitalism necessarily does so.

15. Novartis counterpetition.

16. See Patricia Williams's (1992) *Alchemy of Race and Rights* for an important political and conceptual engagement with the issue of needs versus rights in the context of race relations. Williams persuasively argues that rights-based interventions lead to more solid gains from the perspective of minority rights and social justice.

17. See Max Foundation, https://themaxfoundation.org/GIPAP (accessed July 11, 2016; emphasis added).

18. All quotes in this section (unless otherwise specified) from Raghunada Rao, interview with the author, July 29, 2010.

19. While Rao himself did not make much of this requirement to report casualties, it opened up a controversial aspect of GIPAP that I discuss in the next section.

20. Affidavit of Dr. P. M. Parikh in the High Court of Judicature of Madras, Special Original Jurisdiction, Writ Petition Nos. 24759 of 2006, in the matter of *Novartis AG, Switzerland v. Union of India and Others* (henceforth "Parikh affidavit"). I discuss this affidavit at greater length in the next section.

21. Parikh affidavit, point 14.

22. Indeed, Rao suggested that GIPAP has been implemented far more effectively than the drug donation program for the next-generation drug for the treatment of CML, Bristol-Myers Squibb's dasatinib (brand name Sprycel). Over a period of time, some patients on Gleevec have been shown to develop resistance to the drug. Sprycel and Novartis's second-generation drug Tasigna (nilotinib) are the two drugs currently used for such patients, but both are patented medications that are even more expensive than Gleevec. In the Indian context, being post-1995 drugs, both are eligible for and under product patent. While Tasigna is now also a part of GIPAP, Bristol-Myers Squibb has its own drug donation program for Sprycel, which Rao himself has been unhappy with: "Dasatinib is unbelievably more expensive, and of course it's no longer available on a support program. There is a support program for dasatinib, but by and large it is 'avoid the phone call' type of support program. So he will record that this phone call comes from this department or the staff members or students here, and a patient is wanting to go on to the program. So he will do his utmost to . . . so, there's a disparity in their recommendation and offer versus the implementation of the program. So it is almost impossible to put patients on dasatinib in this country for free."

23. Parikh affidavit, point 15.

24. Parikh affidavit, point 21.

25. Parikh affidavit, note 11.

26. Parikh affidavit, point 12.

27. Parikh affidavit, point 16.

28. Parikh affidavit, point 18, point 19, point 20.

29. Juzgadonacional de Primera Instancia en lo Criminal de Instruccion no. 8, Dra Yamile Susana Bernal Secretario Dr. Gutierrez [First instance in criminal prosecution no. 8, Dr. Yamile Susana Bernal and Secretary Dr. Gutierrez], *Zulma Pilar Labrana v. The Max Foundation Argentina and Others*. The quote above comes from a case summary provided by MSF's Access to Treatment and Medicines Group, personal communication (see also García 2006).

30. Most of these involved drugs for communicable diseases, and were donations either to developing country public health programs, or to global health programs such as those of the World Health Organization. In this regard, GIPAP is unusual in terms of being an early drug donation program for an anticancer drug, and for being perhaps the first direct-to-patient donation program mediated through another private entity.

31. See chapter 1 for an elaboration of some of these value logics, and Ecks (2008) for an account of how GIPAP has protected Novartis's Western market interests. This strongly monopolistic model is not seamless or even necessarily sustainable, in part because of the resistance and legal defeats encountered by companies such as Novartis in India.

32. For a manifesto that instructs corporations to behave ethically in this win-win fashion, see Edward Grefe and Martin Linsky (1995), *The New Corporate Activism*.

CHAPTER FIVE. **Postcolonial Values**

1. See the introduction for my discussion of the conjunctural and the organic.

2. *Little Magazine* 4, nos. 5–6 (2003): 50–51.

3. *Positive Nation*, no. 91 (June 2003): 96. This would often contrast with articles about the Euro-American pharmaceutical industry as one that was "trading in death" (Hamied 2003).

4. Cipla was founded in 1935 by Yusuf Hamied's father, K. A. Hamied, who ran the company until his death in 1972. Hence, even though a publicly traded company, Cipla's ethos is largely that of a family business. This is not unusual for Indian pharmaceutical companies.

5. Having said this, the Euro-American R&D-driven pharmaceutical industry itself often recombines existing molecules and claims the result as a new and therefore innovative molecule, by virtue of applying for a product patent on the recombined molecule. Product patents on such combinations have been disallowed under one of the public health flexibilities in the 2005 Indian Patent Act, Section 3(e), but they are commonly granted in the United States and Europe.

6. See Nguyen (2010) for an account of (a) how the AIDS crisis in Africa opened the possibilities for global biomedical, political, and market interventions in Africa; (b) the emergence of Africa as a biomedical and political epicenter of AIDS in the 1990s; and (c) the development of problems of drug resistance in resource-poor environments in West Africa where access to the triple therapy cocktail was often difficult or impossible, but where sporadic treatment with less ideal or compliant regimens would nonetheless take place.

7. The quotes from Hamied in this chapter, unless otherwise stated, are from two interviews that I conducted with him, on August 28, 2008, and January 11, 2009 (henceforth "Hamied interviews"). Therefore, this is at a post-WTO moment, when Gleevec had been denied a patent and Novartis had lost its case in the Madras High Court, but the Supreme Court case had not begun. Pharmaceutical politics in India, however, were already judicialized, and at the time of these conversations Cipla was

in litigation with Hoffmann-La Roche over a patent concerning Roche's drug erlotinib, a treatment for lung cancer (the brand name of the patented medication was Tarceva; *F. Hoffmann-La Roche Ltd. and Others v. Cipla Ltd.*, cs (os) No. 89, 2008, henceforth "Tarceva High Court verdict"). Roche had been granted a patent on the drug, which Cipla felt was not valid. It filed a postgrant opposition, but even before that could be adjudicated started manufacturing generic erlotinib under its brand name, Erlocip. Roche took Cipla to the Delhi High Court. The court made an initial decision to allow Cipla to continue manufacturing the generic while the case was sub judice on the grounds of public interest and access to essential medicines. In 2012, Roche went on to lose the case. While not discussed in detail in this book, the Tarceva verdict is a further important one in establishing the interpretive terrain of post-TRIPS patent regimes in India.

In these interviews, I engaged Hamied in conversation about (a) contemporary patent-related controversies such as those concerning Gleevec and Tarceva; (b) broader historical trajectories of the Indian pharmaceutical industry in relation to national patent regimes and international trade regimes; and (c) his own biographical trajectories. As with the case of my interviews with Raghunada Rao in chapter 4, the purpose of including quotes from our conversations is not to provide the reality of what happened around any of these cases, as much as it is to provide an embodied and situated account of the stakes of these battles from the perspective of the Indian generic industry. The question of whether and how representative Hamied's point of view is of the Indian industry's is itself a complex empirical question that I discuss through the course of this chapter.

8. Daniel Pearl and Alix Freedman (2001) undertook an in-depth analysis of these logics in the *Wall Street Journal*. I draw extensively on their interpretation of Cipla's actions here.

9. The WHO prequalification program evaluates and lists essential medicines of quality for the treatment of HIV-AIDS, tuberculosis, and malaria. Therefore it is significant in directing governments and aid agencies involved in medicinal procurement for these disease toward therapeutic options that it deems beneficial from both a medical and policy perspective. For more on the program, see World Health Organization, "Prequalification Programme," http://apps.who.int/prequal/ (accessed February 14, 2015).

10. Ironically, Pearl and Freedman (2001) point out that Cipla struggled to sell its AIDS therapies in India in the 1990s, and in fact nearly abandoned its antiretroviral program altogether. It persisted largely because of the insistence of A. V. Rama Rao, an academic researcher at the Indian Institute of Chemical Technology, Hyderabad, and a longtime friend of Hamied's. This parallels Novartis's reluctance to pursue the development of Gleevec, which only proceeded at the insistence of academic researcher Brian Druker (see chapter 3). Yet neither Cipla nor Novartis has been shy about taking moral credit for their therapeutic developments once they proved successful and revolutionary.

11. For Bush's speech, see George W. Bush, "2003 State of the Union Address," C-SPAN, January 28, 2003, http://www.c-span.org/video/?174799-2/2003-state-union. This was the speech in which Bush announced his President's Emergency Plan for

AIDS Relief (PEPFAR) program. I am grateful to conversations with Kristin Peterson regarding PEPFAR as simultaneously a biomedical, humanitarian, and geopolitical initiative.

12. The Gujral Committee was established under the aegis of the Parliamentary Standing Committee on Commerce. In Indian parliamentary procedure, much of the research into specific legislation is conducted in committees, which are broadly of two types. Ad hoc committees are established for specific purposes and dissolved as soon as the purpose is served. Standing committees exist over longer terms and may appoint specific committees under their purview to investigate particular items of legislative importance. Ironically, the chairman of this committee report, I. K. Gujral, would subsequently become the prime minister of India in 1997. He therefore would come to have the executive task of implementing India's adherence to an agreement that he himself had recommended against. "Final Recommendation of Gujral Committee (Draft Dunkel Proposals presented on 14-12-1993) to the Rajya Sabha Department Related Parliamentary Standing Committee on Commerce (1993–94)" (henceforth "Gujral Committee Report").

13. This last constraint would be eased in 2001 under the Doha Declaration of TRIPS, which allowed national governments to issue compulsory licenses and introduce other public health flexibilities into their patent legislation in situations of public health emergency. It is the Doha Declaration that provided the leeway for India to incorporate public health flexibilities such as Section 3(d) into its 2005 Patent Act (see chapter 3).

14. Gujral Committee Report, 4.

15. Parliament of India, Rajya Sabha, Department Related Parliamentary Standing Committee on Commerce (1993–94), Third Report Draft of Dunkel Proposals, Evidence (henceforth "Evidence before Gujral Committee"), 288.

16. Evidence before Gujral Committee, 299.

17. Evidence before Gujral Committee, 299. The focus of Nanjundaswamy's attack was on the impact the Dunkel Draft would have on agriculture and food security.

18. Evidence before Gujral Committee, 288.

19. Evidence before Gujral Committee, 289.

20. Hamied interviews. In 1992, Canada endorsed the Dunkel Draft, and by 1993 had changed its patent regime to be compliant with TRIPS (and with intellectual property provisions of the North American Free Trade Agreement, which were similar to those of TRIPS), thereby also moving to a monopolistic product patent regime.

21. An amendment to the Indian Patent Act in 1999 introduced EMR (see chapters 3 and 4).

22. This refers to the then ongoing Delhi High Court case on Tarceva (see note 7).

23. For the full text of the Doha Declaration, see WTO (2001).

24. I return to discussing the role of the American state in upholding monopolistic pharmaceutical interests subsequently, while discussing the Trans-Pacific Partnership Agreement and TRIPS-plus free trade strategies.

25. It is worth remembering that the negotiation Hamied is describing here was happening at the same time that the Bush administration was rolling out PEPFAR

and being hailed as the savior of the African continent because of its humanitarian initiative. I thank Kristin Peterson for conversations about the ways in which PEPFAR has been integrally tied in to monopolistic corporate interests (see also Peterson [2014b] for a broader political economic situation of such understandings). Peterson is currently studying the articulations between humanitarian, monopolistic, military-security, and oil economies in West Africa.

26. This is why, while not in disagreement with the neoliberalism literature, I tend to use the term myself in very limited fashion, because I do not think it does justice to explaining the specificities of state action that are at stake and in need of conceptualization (see introduction, note 48).

27. In 2011, Hamied was listed by *Forbes* magazine as the thirtieth richest person in India. This indicates one effect of economic liberalization, in relation to the loosening of regulations for individual wealth accumulation (http://www.forbes.com/lists/2011 /77/india-billionaires-11_Yusuf-Hamied_ITUQ.html, accessed February 17, 2015).

28. See Brotherton (2008, 2012) for how the socialist Cuban state acts occasionally in capitalist interests, and even more often as if capitalist.

29. Report of the Committee on Drugs and Pharmaceutical Industry (Hathi Committee Report), Ministry of Petroleum and Chemicals, Govt. of India, April 1975 (henceforth "Hathi Committee Report").

30. It is important to situate the story I am telling in this section in relation especially to the Alma Ata Declaration of the WHO and the kinds of international public health imaginaries that were being articulated there. This declaration was adopted at the International Conference on Primary Health Care, Alma Ata, Kazhakstan, in 1978, emphasizing the importance of a concerted, state-driven, internationalist agenda toward ensuring primary health care for all. This imagination of an internationalist public health, one that significantly represents Third World interests, gets replaced by its neoliberal avatar, global health, by the start of the twenty-first century (Gaudilliere 2014). I am grateful to Jean-Paul Gaudilliere for conversations about this transition.

31. Direct-to-consumer advertising was subsequently disallowed in India.

32. Hathi Committee Report, 16.

33. In addition to the report, see Indian Drug Manufacturers Association (1981) and Hamied (2005) for further accounts of the history of the development of the Indian pharmaceutical industry.

34. Accounts of K. A. Hamied's life story are drawn from his own autobiography, *A Life to Remember* (K. A. Hamied 1972), and also from published memorial solicitations given by a number of people after his passing (Cipla 1973). While Hamied had always desired to return to India, his move was precipitated by the rise of Nazi power in Germany. Hamied's biography was as cosmopolitan as it was diasporic, as while in Berlin he had met and married a Polish Jewish communist, Luba. This cosmopolitanism reflects in the elite nationalist ethos of Yusuf Hamied, one that he inherited from his upbringing but which also reflects the essence of Bombay, as a certain kind of cosmopolitan city in which such an ethos flourished. This is the Bombay of Salman Rushdie's *Midnight's Children*, and it is one that has an integral place in a Nehruvian idea of India (Rushdie 1980; Khilnani 1999). Both Rushdie's Bombay and Nehru's

India constitute a vanishing presence, especially since the strong rise of Hindu nationalism, which existed in the city since the 1960s but became a particularly salient national political force by the early 1990s.

35. The period from 1919 to 1922 was in some ways the high noon of India's freedom struggle, a time that saw a transition from more modest demands for representation in colonial governance by the ruling nationalist elite to a full-fledged demand for swaraj or home rule. This period also saw Gandhi's rise to prominence in the nationalist struggle through his strategy of noncooperation. Factors that influenced this included the passage of the draconian Rowlatt Act in 1919, which prevented gatherings for peaceful demonstrations; the horrific Jallianwala Bagh massacre in Amritsar in April 1919, when General Dyer ordered the shooting of peaceful protesters in the enclosed gardens where they had gathered, leading to the death of hundreds of unarmed civilians, including women and children; Gandhi's making of common cause with Turkish opposition to British rule through an alliance with the Ali brothers, Maulana and Shaukat Ali, through the Khilafat movement (which also had a significant impact in cementing Hindu-Muslim unity and providing a pan-national consciousness that transcended religious affiliation); and in 1921, his call for nationwide noncooperation toward the British, including a boycott of British goods and institutions. The noncooperation movement was called off at its height in 1922 when it turned violent in the town of Chauri Chaura, Bihar, much to the chagrin of many nationalist leaders. For an important subaltern history of the Chauri Chaura uprising, see Amin (1995).

36. "Here" refers to the building where we were having our conversation, as Cipla's headquarters have remained at the same place since it was founded.

37. Hindustan Antibiotics Ltd. was established in 1954 in Pimpri, and Indian Drugs and Pharmaceuticals Ltd. in 1961 in Hyderabad (with a focus on manufacturing synthetic drugs) and Rishikesh (focusing on antibiotic production).

38. This situation came to be completely reversed subsequently through industrial policy that would facilitate domestic bulk drug manufacture. Today, the Indian industry is not just self-sufficient: it is the major supplier of APIs worldwide to the pharmaceutical industry, including to the Euro-American, R&D-driven industry.

39. This pattern continues in relation to the post-1980s R&D focus of the multinational industry, which (from an Indian perspective) is still mostly R&D elsewhere. For instance, Novartis did not undertake any of its R&D activity for Gleevec in India (see chapter 4). An aspect of drug development that did start moving to India after 2005 of course was clinical trials, which are largely outsourced to CROs (see chapter 2). The notable exception to this pattern is AstraZeneca, which has established a major research facility in Bangalore.

40. Hathi Committee Report, 96.

41. Hathi Committee Report, 54. In contrast, see chapter 4 for my discussion of how MSF sees the long-term solution to the problem of access to medicines in the 2000s as coming from the generics industry. This suggests how the horizons of social solutions have shifted over three decades, to a point when an imaginary of drug access that is not tied to private market interests comes to be virtually unthinkable, the political terrain now being constituted simply as a battle between different forms of

capitalism. While it is currently appropriate to speak of the Indian industry as a ge-nerics industry, this nomenclature would have been less accurate in the early 1970s or before. As Cori Hayden (2011) has pointed out, "the generic" itself is a relational term that only has valence in relation to the patent, which established itself as a dominant reference point relatively recently. In India, it was only with the abolition of product patents in 1970 that the patent, ironically, came to have valence, because it is only then that the function of the patent in preventing the establishment of certain kinds of free market competition in drugs became evident. In the United States, which always had a product patent regime, the generic only came to be an important category in the 1980s subsequent to legislative measures that were explicitly aimed at stimulating generic production in monopolistic environments; the Hatch-Waxman Act of 1984 is especially important in this regard (Greene 2014). Europe and Canada never had the consistent product patent environments of the United States, and different countries introduced such environments at different times in piecemeal fashion. Therefore much of the industrialized world (bar the United States) in fact had thriving econo-mies in pharmaceutical copies for much of the twentieth century. The idea that the patented molecule is the norm to which outliers such as India must harmonize—the idea propagated and naturalized under TRIPS—therefore does not reflect the extent to which the product patent is both utterly exceptional and peculiarly American in the history of twentieth-century pharmaceutical development.

42. Hathi Committee Report, 54. It is not necessarily the case that simply abolishing brands would lead to a thriving public sector. Hayden (2007) points out that both the Mexican and Argentinian governments passed legislation that prevented physicians from prescribing branded drugs (in 1998 and 2002 respectively), but this still led to the consolidation of private players in complex and differentiated ways. There are many modalities by which private players can establish themselves even in relatively socialized markets; the political question then is less one of purely socialized market alternatives than of the extent to which (a) alternatives to the market are part of policy imaginaries of the spectrum of possibilities that exist, and (b) private players operate in markets that allow therapeutics to be more or less accessible. It is also worth re-membering that what is at stake is the construction of terrains of pharmaceuticaliza-tion, which do not necessarily or in any straightforward manner translate into better public health. The committee did recognize this even as it emphasized the importance of building capacity for drug manufacture, stating that "the firms have reduced life to a disease to be cured" (Hathi Committee Report, 95).

43. That kind of expertise was embodied more by Manmohan Singh, the first Indian finance minister to hold a doctorate in economics (from Oxford), after which he held a series of bureaucratic positions himself. Indian bureaucrats at the time tended to have great admiration for Singh, contrasting his economic knowledge and expertise to the more commonly encountered minister, who was simply a politician.

44. It is worth noting that this is a conjuncture at which a whole series of politi-cal transformations were happening in India. In 1989, Rajiv Gandhi, who had been elected with a massive mandate in 1984, was voted out of office on the back of corrup-tion charges, bringing a non-Congress coalition government led by Janata Dal's V. P.

Singh to power, supported from the outside by both the Right (the Hindu nationalist Bharatiya Janata Party, BJP) and the Left (the various communist parties of India). The Janata Dal government immediately embarked upon an ambitious caste-based affirmative action program that generated tremendous backlash from upper-caste Hindus, eventually leading to the BJP's withdrawal of support from the government. It also coincided with the heightening of the BJP's own aggressive Hindu nationalist politics, orchestrated around a demand to build a Ram Temple at the site of the Babri Masjid mosque in Ayodhya. The early 1990s would see repeated caste- and religion-based conflagrations, and also witnessed Rajiv Gandhi's assassination by a Sri Lankan Tamil suicide bomber. See Menon and Nigam (2007) for a sense of how this moment was a transformative one in postcolonial Indian history. The economic liberalization programs initiated by the Narasimha Rao–led Congress government in 1991, implemented in large measure by Manmohan Singh, must be situated in this historical moment.

45. See Jack Kloppenburg's ([1988] 2005) *First the Seed* for a comprehensive political economic account of agricultural biotechnology in the context of the United States.

46. Such an imaginary of rural India as untapped market was pioneered by Proctor and Gamble. See for instance the writings of Gurcharan Das (2001), who spearheaded Proctor and Gamble's rural marketing offensive and has been an articulate cheerleader of India's neoliberal reforms over the past two decades.

47. Remember that Nanjundaswamy's position was from the perspective of agricultural interests.

48. I base this largely on Raghavan's (1990) description of the GATT negotiations and their implications for the Third World. Raghavan was a journalist who closely followed the years of negotiation leading up to and including the Uruguay Round. At the time, these were largely esoteric trade negotiations whose implications were not widely acknowledged or anticipated—though by the time TRIPS came into effect in 1995, it had become a hugely political issue in many Third World nations. Raghavan's account, *Recolonization*, was a seminal work in helping to publicize the intricacies and stakes of these negotiations.

49. Most notable in this regard were the series of Third World dialogues among newly decolonized nations in the 1950s that led to the Bandung conference of 1955 and the formation of the nonaligned movement. While in many ways Bandung represented a failed promise, it also represented the possibility of imagining globalization Otherwise, as a world where globalization actually represented the possibility of the consolidation of postcolonial power against existing Euro-American global hegemony. Perhaps the most poignant account of the promises and failures of Bandung is to be found in Richard Wright's ([1956] 1995) *The Color Curtain*. For a collection of essays dealing with "the Bandung Moment," see Christopher Lee's (2010) *Making a World after Empire*.

50. I use Third World rather than Global South since this was the appropriate terminology of the time. While the latter is the currently politically correct usage, both are problematic enough that I do not automatically default to Global South rather

than Third World. Raghavan himself uses Third World through *Recolonization*, writing as he had before Global South became the fashionably appropriate parlance.

51. Following Raghavan, who uses the term consistently, I use northern to refer to U.S.-Europe-Japanese interests.

52. The OPEC actions refer to the quadrupling of oil prices by the world's major oil producers between October 1973 and January 1974. This was the culmination of years of acrimony between oil producers and the American government, of which a signature event was Richard Nixon's decision in 1971 to suspend the convertibility of dollars into gold. This was a response to America's balance of payments crisis, and ended the regime of fixed exchange rates that had been established at the Bretton Woods conference of 1944. For an argument regarding the importance of the breakdown of Bretton Woods for understanding the politics of late twentieth-century global capitalism, see Eric Hobsbawm's (1994) *The Age of Extremes*.

53. Cooper diagnoses this as neoliberalism; Raghavan as recolonization. It is worth considering whether these different diagnoses are simply semantic or whether they reflect different understandings of political economic structure. Certainly both authors are concerned with pharmaceutical imperialism. Raghavan (1990) is well aware that the Uruguay Round would have huge implications for the pharmaceutical sector and for access to medicines worldwide, and Cooper (2008) discusses the impacts of TRIPS, especially on access to antiretrovirals in Africa, in her chapter "Pharmaceutical Empire" in *Life as Surplus*.

54. The impact of the real and perceived threat of Japan to American economic hegemony cannot be underestimated. As William Lazonick (2010) has argued, this was a major factor that led to the restructuring and increased financialization of the American corporation, a point I discuss in chapter 1. It is worth marking the simultaneous financialization of the corporation (a speculative internal restructuring) with its geopolitical investments in a global economic restructuring, both supported and driven by the sympathetic Reagan-era American state and undergirded by ideologies of innovation.

55. Indeed, the Philippines enacted Section 3(d)-like legislation in 2007, inspired by the Indian curtailment of pharmaceutical evergreening. Therefore the threat of India serving as a model to the so-called Global South is real.

56. Examples of FTAs signed by the United States over the past decade, all of which have more stringent intellectual property provisions than TRIPS, include the 2004 U.S.-Singapore FTA, the 2004 U.S.-Chile FTA, the 2005 U.S.-Australia FTA, the 2006 U.S.-Peru FTA, and the 2007 U.S.–South Korea FTA. The EU and India launched FTA negotiations that are, at the time of writing, still ongoing, and contain intellectual property-related issues that have provoked intense political opposition in India.

57. These have been posted on the website of the civil society advocacy group Knowledge Ecology International, which has been at the forefront of advocacy against the TPP. See "Trans-Pacific Partnership Intellectual Property Rights Chapter," Draft, February 10, 2011, http://keionline.org/sites/default/files/tpp-10feb2011-us-text-ipr -chapter.pdf for the February 2011 draft (henceforth "TPP Feb. 2011 IPR draft"), and "Trans-Pacific Partnership Intellectual Property Rights Chapter (Selected Provisions),"

September 2011, http://www.citizenstrade.org/ctc/wp-content/uploads/2011/10
/TransPacificIP1.pdf for the September 2011 draft (henceforth "TPP Sept. 2011 IPR
draft"). Unless otherwise mentioned, I draw upon these two drafts in my description
of the TPP intellectual property provisions in this section. An updated version of this
chapter was released by WikiLeaks on October 26, 2014, but this did not show significant changes in the IPR chapter. See "Secret Trans-Pacific Partnership Agreement
(TPP), IP Chapter," November 13, 2013, http://wikileaks.org/tpp/ (henceforth "TPP
Oct. 2014 IPR draft"). The summary of the TPPA as negotiated is available at Office of
the United States Trade Representative (2015). The agreement's intellectual property
provisions are substantially similar to those that were being proposed in the leaked
drafts. Since the leaked drafts were the versions available to my interlocutors at the
time of writing this chapter, I refer to those in my discussion here.

58. Data exclusivity and patent linkage are instruments used to articulate patent
approvals structures and processes with those for market approvals for drugs. In the
process, they explicitly link intellectual property to clinical trials, while suggesting the
limits of the patent itself as a monopolistic instrument. Data exclusivity is a form of
data monopoly. It means that clinical trials data submitted to regulatory authorities as
part of a process of market approval for a drug remains the property of the company
that has submitted the data. If a generic manufacturer wanted regulatory approval for
its version of the drug subsequent to patent expiration, or in another territory where
the patent was not valid, regulators would not be allowed to look at clinical trial data
that has already been evaluated in order to approve the patented version for market. This means either that the generic cannot be approved for the duration of data
exclusivity (typically three to five years after patent expiration, thereby extending the
effective patent life of a drug from twenty years to as much as twenty-five), or that the
generic manufacturer would have to duplicate clinical trials on a drug earlier proven
safe and efficacious. This raises the bar for generic entry into the market while opening up ethical questions around the conduct of human subject experiments for drugs
already on the market. Data exclusivity is routinely granted in the United States and
Europe, but is not a required provision under TRIPS, and many countries do not have
data exclusivity provisions in their patent legislation. Patent linkage provisions seek to
couple the processes of patenting a drug and obtaining regulatory approval (which are
normally kept independent), placing a burden upon regulatory authorities to ensure
that a generic drug they approve for market does not violate existing patents. This
also raises the bar on generic entry into the market while increasing the burden on
regulators. While a common intellectual property norm in the United States (with the
U.S. Food and Drug Administration maintaining an online database of pharmaceutical products under patent, commonly known as the "Orange Book"), patent linkage is
unusual even in most European countries. The TPP provisions seek to impose patent
linkage as a requirement rather than just as a norm.

59. There has been considerable civil society opposition to these provisions, and
those seeking greater detail can refer to statements outlining concerns about it.
See, for instance, a Doctors without Borders/MSF Campaign for Access to Essential
Medicines "TPP Issue Brief," September 2011, https://www.msfaccess.org/sites/default

/files/MSF_assets/Access/Docs/Access_Briefing_TPP_ENG_2011.pdf; "Civil Society Comments on the Trans-Pacific Partnership Agreement," drafted by Doctors without Borders/MSF, Health Action International—Global, Health GAP, Knowledge Ecology International, Oxfam America, Public Citizen, Universities Allied for Essential Medicines, and (in part, relating to sections covering pharmaceutical pricing provisions) the National Legislative Association on Prescription Drug Price, http://keionline.org /sites/default/files/TPPApunchlist_18may2011.pdf (henceforth "Civil Society Comments"); briefing memo put out by Public Citizen, Health Gap Global Access Project, I-MAK, and Third World Network, "Analysis of the Leaked U.S. Paper on Eliminating Patent Pre-Grant Opposition," July 7, 2011, http://www.citizen.org/analysis-of-leaked -US-paper-on-eliminating-patent-pre-grant-opposition; and Program on Information Justice and Intellectual Property, American University, Washington College of Law, "Public Interest Analysis of the US TPP Proposal for an IP Chapter," Draft Version 1.3, December 6, 2011, http://digitalcommons.wcl.american.edu/cgi/viewcontent.cgi ?article=1023&context=research. See also a letter from MSF to U.S. president Barack Obama, July 15, 2013, outlining concerns over TPP provisions under negotiation, available at http://www.doctorswithoutborders.org/sites/usa/files/130715_TPP%20 Open%20Letter_USA.pdf.

60. The classification guidance for the TPP was issued on March 4, 2010, and the draft proposals are classified under category 1.4(b). This is a category of the U.S. government classification system, concerning "foreign government information." According to this guidance, these documents could be declassified "four years from entry into force of the TPP agreement or, if no agreement enters into force, four years from the close of the negotiations" (TPP Feb. 2011 IPR draft; TPP Sept. 2011 IPR draft).

61. Office of the United States Trade Representative, "Advisory Committees," https:// ustr.gov/about-us/advisory-committees, accessed November 1, 2013.

62. Civil Society comments.

63. USTR, "Transparency and the Trans-Pacific Partnership," June 2012, http:// www.ustr.gov/about-us/press-office/fact-sheets/2012/june/transparency-and-the-tpp (henceforth "Transparency Fact Sheet"). For a broader conceptual consideration of transparency and its relationship to democracy in the context of technoscience, see Sperling (2013), especially chapter 3, "Transparent Fictions."

64. Transparency Fact Sheet.

65. Transparency Fact Sheet.

66. What this suggests is that a final version of an agreement would be made public for comments before signing, but not the various inputs—such as the U.S. draft provisions—that went into drafting that final version.

67. For a consideration of this question in relation to the history of the Cold War and post–Cold War American security state, see Masco (2010).

68. See "Six-Nation TPP Bloc Rallies against US," *Sunday Star Times*, July 28, 2013, which describes the emergence of consolidated opposition to the United States in TPP negotiations from Australia, New Zealand, Canada, Malaysia, and two other nations in the eighteenth round of negotiations held in Malaysia. *Sunday Star Times* is a New

Zealand paper published out of Auckland. See also a leaked memorandum showing New Zealand's opposition to the American position (Public Citizen 2010). Malaysia's strong oppositional role in the negotiations has been described to me by civil society activists who have been following the negotiations.

69. See Sloterdijk (1988) for a philosophical elaboration and critique of cynical reason.

70. In this regard, see *An Unfinished Agenda*, the autobiography of K. Anji Reddy (2015), the founder of another major Indian company, Dr. Reddy's Laboratories, which reflects an ethos similar to Hamied's. Reddy passed away in 2013 and the book was posthumously completed and published by Raghu Cidambi. I thank Cidambi for providing insights on the Indian generic industry and especially on Dr. Reddy's Laboratories as I was researching Cipla's history.

71. Veblen wrote this treatise in October 1918 as a document intended for Woodrow Wilson prior to the post–World War I negotiations in Versailles. While about corporate interests, this is a work that is intensely, intimately, and immediately about a geopolitical conjuncture, written in the aftermath of the greatest sustained tragedy the world had known. My reading of Veblen has benefited greatly from discussions with John Kelly, for which many thanks.

72. This is the point at which Veblen departs from a political economy in the tradition of Adam Smith (which includes Marx), which assumed the primacy of industrial production as the generator of value (Smith [1776] 2014). Marx ([1894] 1974) himself comes to realize by volume 3 of *Capital* that this is not the case: far from leading to the dissolution of capitalist relations of production, the contradictions of industrial capitalism that he had traced in his prior work were leading to the consolidation of more and more corporate forms. While diagnosing this, Marx was not able to develop an adequate analytics—the tone of the analysis in volume 3 is one that approaches moral outrage. My own analysis of the financialization of the (especially American) R&D-driven pharmaceutical industry over the past three decades, undertaken in chapter 1, must be situated in the context of a prior trajectory that sees the progressive uncoupling of business enterprise and the corporate form from industrial production and the factory, and then the subsequent financialization of this increasingly autonomous corporate form.

73. Evidence before Gujral Committee, 289–290.

74. For the full speech, see Nehru (1947). For a description of the idea of India that Nehru articulated, see Khilnani (1999). Perhaps the most masterful articulation of the Nehruvian vision and its embodiment in the lives of the generation that inherited independent India—one that weaves together postcolonial history with individual life history and psychobiography through the genre of magical realism—is Salman Rushdie's (1980) *Midnight's Children*. Rajeswari Sunder Rajan (2008) has argued that this responsibility articulates through a sense of noblesse oblige.

75. Ritu Birla's (2009) *Stages of Capital* is an important history of cultures of kin-based mercantile capitalism in colonial India.

76. *Time* magazine's cover story in its August 18, 1952, issue is a typical portrayal of Merck and his repeated emphasis on "people over profits."

CONCLUSION

1. Patent application No. 537/DEL/1996, filed on March 13, 1996.

2. *F. Hoffmann-La Roche Ltd and OSI Pharmaceuticals Ltd vs. Cipla Ltd*, High Court of New Delhi, CS (OS) No. 89/2008 (henceforth "Tarceva judgment").

3. Parliament of India Rajya Sabha, Department-Related Parliamentary Standing Committee on Health and Family Welfare, Fifty-Ninth Report on the Functioning of the Central Drugs Standards Control Organisation (CDSCO), May 8, 2012, 2 (henceforth "CDSCO Report").

4. CDSCO Report, 19.

5. Some genotypes of hepatitis C require a twenty-four-week treatment course, doubling the cost. In October 2014, a newer-generation drug to treat the disease, Harvoni, also developed by Gilead, was approved for market by the FDA. It is claimed to be an even better drug than Sovaldi and its price is $94,500 for a full course, which would typically be eight weeks.

6. Differential pricing, while still the exception, does have precedent. Nonetheless, the possibility of Sovaldi's differential pricing was particularly newsworthy given the novelty of the drug, its exceedingly high price, and its superiority over existing standards of care. The significance of such a high-profile drug as Sovaldi being differentially priced even as its pricing in Europe and the United States was generating controversy cannot be underestimated.

7. This move was initially undercut by the Indian Patent Office, which denied Gilead a patent on Sovaldi in January 2015 based on pregrant oppositions filed by Natco Pharmaceuticals and the nonprofit Initiative for Medicines, Access and Knowledge, potentially allowing Indian companies to manufacture generic versions of the drug ("Gilead Denied Sovaldi Patent" 2015). In May 2016, India reversed course, as the deputy controller of patents and designs decided to issue Gilead a patent on the drug after all.

8. Sean Brotherton's (2012) work on socialized medicine in Cuba beautifully illustrates how complexly interrelated these apparent binaries between capitalism and socialism, in fact, can be in practice.

9. See Cori Hayden's (2010) account of "the politics of the copy" for an elaboration of this argument.

10. I am grateful to Satyajit Rath, an immunologist based in Delhi, for helping me think through some of these issues through his insistence on the difference between what he calls "incremental" and "transformative" innovations (personal conversations). Rath insists that left to itself, market incentives lead private industry toward incremental innovations, and that transformative biomedical innovations have always required public investment. In the United States (and to a significant but lesser extent in Europe), early-stage drug discovery tended to be driven by fundamental research in universities and publicly funded laboratories through much of the second half of the twentieth century, with the U.S. National Institutes of Health playing a particularly important role. In this regard, the move toward more corporatized models of public research funding that demand short-term, visible forms of return on investment either monetarily or in terms of products is particularly consequential, and can

be seen throughout the world (certainly in the United States and Europe with the prioritization of translational research over basic research, and also more recently in India, based on early indications of scientific research funding and policy under the Narendra Modi government). I explore some of these issues concerning translational research and the changing nature of biomedical research universities and institutions in another book that I am currently working on.

11. See Gopakumar (2013), who emphasizes this point and insists on recognizing its importance as indicating the limits of the victory achieved through the Gleevec verdict.

12. Letter from Union for Affordable Cancer Treatment to Ambassador Michael Froman, USTR, October 29, 2014, http://cancerunion.org/files/UACT-Froman-Oct292014-dasatinib.pdf.

13. See chapter 4, note 22, for the opinion of the physician Raghunada Rao on Bristol-Myers Squibb's drug donation program for dasatinib, which he called an "avoid-the-phone-call type of program." This emphasizes the limits of corporate social responsibility as a mechanism to ensure drug access under monopoly regimes except at the will of the holder of monopoly.

14. In this regard, see Žižek (2006) on the "vileness" of capitalist philanthropy, precisely because it projects not just the inherent strength of capitalist regimes but also their inherent goodness in ways that obviate the need for any conversation about structural transformation (see chapter 4). See also McGoey (2015) on the functioning of the Gates Foundation in relation to the capitalization of global health, which substantiates such a claim through an account of the institution that is arguably becoming among the most powerful in setting public health agendas in the developing world today. One of my interlocutors (kept anonymous at her request) could have read Žižek as she explained to me in conversation the "evil" of the Clinton Foundation. In her rendering, this is an organization that does very little to build institutional capacity on the ground (in the manner that an earlier generation of philanthropic organizations such as the Rockefeller Foundation, while still resolutely in the business of protecting capitalist and American geopolitical interests, nonetheless did; see Smith [2009]). Instead, it uses its influence in corridors of power across many countries in the Global South to act as a broker for pharmaceutical interests by suggesting that it can help negotiate therapeutic and public health needs with the industry for these governments, and thus dissuades them from using sovereign policy instruments that would structurally curtail corporate interests. Here, one sees brokerage economies using the language of ethics and responsibility along with philanthropic instruments to preserve monopolistic corporate hegemony.

15. The "promise of justice" is Derrida's (1992, 1994) term. This does not refer to justice in the narrow or instrumental sense of the application of the law, but in the broader sense of the horizon of the political—the promise of justice is a promise that is in practice endlessly deferred, but that precisely through its deferral constitutes an expansive horizon for imagining praxis.

16. I am grateful for a discussion between Etienne Balibar and Susan Buck-Morss (Columbia University, October 22, 2014) for helping me think through the question of democratic politics in relation to "seizing the state."

17. Article 32 of the Indian Constitution provides for this tool that articulates the interests of the public to the roles and responsibility of the judiciary. This allows any member of the public to take a matter of public interest to the courts *suo moto*. The politics of access to medicines has for the most part not followed this route, since it is invariably multinational pharmaceutical interests who have approached the courts disputing denied or violated patents. But this route has been followed in relation to clinical trials and the filing of a PIL investigating the HPV vaccine studies. See the Postcript to chapter 3 for a consideration of the limits of public interest–based judicialization for progressive and democratic politics.

18. My account in this section is inspired significantly by deliberations at a national consultation organized in New Delhi in September 2011 concerning the regulation of unethical drug trials. This was the first such consultation to be held at such a scale, and it provided the platform for further conversations that have continued in years since. The 2011 consultation was organized by Sama, the Delhi-based women's health advocacy group that was responsible in large measure for bringing the HPV vaccine studies to public attention (see chapter 2). Other organizers of the consultation included the Centre for Studies in Ethics and Rights Mumbai; Locost (Low Cost Standard Therapeutics) Baroda; All Indian Peoples' Science Network; and Drug Action Forum, Karnataka, a member of the All India Drug Action Network. This brought together groups that had shared but distinct commitments—bioethicists, groups involved with fighting for access to medicines, peoples' science and peoples' health movements, and feminist groups—who did not always speak with a single voice. My purpose here is not to describe the discussions or outcomes at the consultation and beyond, which are complex and have their own trajectories. It is rather to point to the spectrum of political imaginaries contained within such a conversation, and the possibilities and constraints that exist in relation to these.

19. See Rajeswari Sunder Rajan's (2003) *Scandal of the State* for a consideration of the ambivalent place of the state in relation to feminist political imaginaries and praxis in India. R. Sunder Rajan (2010) nonetheless calls for an agonistic politics toward the state. This does not preclude critique; on the contrary. It just insists upon critique in relation to the specific political terrains that it is responding to. It is not just the case that the state, under certain conditions, has the potential to be leveraged in politically accountable (and perhaps even progressive) ways; it is also that the state remains a primary bulwark against entrenched power structures such as those of capital or patriarchy. This agonistic political sentiment also animates a number of other teachers whose praxis has inspired my own, including Sheila Jasanoff (1997, 2005, 2011, 2013), whose investments in science and technology studies involve opening up spaces in both law and science policy for critical thinking that could open the possibility of more reflexive engagements between the state and society around issues of governance and regulation of science and technology; Michael Fischer's (2003) investment in the function of ethnography as creating "third spaces" that could facilitate the development of reflexive social institutions; or Etienne Balibar's (2004) careful reading of Western philosophy in order to make agonistic interventions into contemporary political debates, such as around the question of secularism in France, or

that of Europe. (For an account of the value of Balibar's agonistic philosophy relative to what he calls the more theological alternatives provided by well-known contemporaries such as Slavoj Žižek and Alain Badiou, see Robbins [2013]).

20. See Pathak and R. Sunder Rajan (1989) for how discourses of vulnerability that emerged in relation to the Shahbano case, which had to do with the scope of Muslim personal law, often operated in the cause of both patriarchal and majoritarian agendas.

21. There are many examples of such work, but for three important representative examples that are quite distinct in their empirical and conceptual trajectories but nonetheless are invested in the link between politics and life itself, see Biehl (2005, 2009), Franklin (2000), and Rose (2006).

22. Or to put it less politely: thinking of such politics in terms of life itself feels altogether too Euro-American in its location and Christian in its ontotheology to adequately capture what is at stake in this analysis.

23. See chapter 3 for a brief account of the Korean controversy around Gleevec. My observations here are based on conversations and interviews with concerned actors in Korea in 2009, and follow-up conversations in subsequent years.

Accenture Life Sciences. 2012. "Beyond the Patent Cliff: Signs of Recovery in Bio-pharma's New Normal." https://www.accenture.com/t20150523T060659__w__/us -en/_acnmedia/Accenture/Conversion-Assets/Microsites/Documents2/Accenture -Life-Sciences-Beyond-The-Patent-Cliff-Signs-Of-Recovery-in-Biopharmas-New -Normal.pdf.

Access Campaign. 2014. "Novartis, Drop the Case!" Medicins sans Frontieres. Accessed March 7. http://www.msfaccess.org/novartis-drop-the-case.

Ackerman, Bruce A. 1991. We the People. Cambridge, MA: Belknap.

Althusser, Louis, and Etienne Balibar. (1970) 2009. Reading Capital. London: Verso.

American Academy of Pediatrics. 2012. "AAP Recommends HPV Vaccines for Both Males and Females." February 27. https://www.aap.org/en-us/about-the-aap/aap -press-room/pages/AAP-Recommends-HPV-Vaccines-For-Both-Males-and -Females.aspx.

Amin, Shahid. 1995. Event, Metaphor, Memory: Chauri Chaura, 1922–1992. Berkeley: University of California Press.

Appadurai, Arjun. 2011. "The Ghost in the Financial Machine." Public Culture 23 (3): 517–539.

———. 2013. The Future as Cultural Fact: Essays on the Global Condition. London: Verso.

Austin, Granville. 1967. The Indian Constitution: Cornerstone of a Nation. Delhi: Oxford University Press.

Balibar, Etienne. 1995. The Philosophy of Marx. London: Verso.

———. 2004. We, the People of Europe? Reflections on Transnational Citizenship. Princeton, NJ: Princeton University Press.

Bateson, Gregory. (1936) 1958. Naven: A Survey of the Problems Suggested by a Composite Picture of the Culture of a New Guinea Tribe Drawn from Three Points of View. Stanford, CA: Stanford University Press.

———. 1972. Steps to an Ecology of Mind. Chicago: University of Chicago Press.

Bateson, Gregory, Don Jackson, Jay Haley, and John Weakland. 1956. "Towards a Theory of Schizophrenia." Behavioral Science 1 (4): 251–254.

Baxi, Upendra. 2010. "The Judiciary as a Resource for Indian Democracy." Seminar 615, November. http://www.india-seminar.com/2010/615/615_upendra_baxi.htm.

Bhan, Gautam. 2009. "Evictions, the Urban Poor, and the Right to the City in Millennial Delhi." *Environment and Urbanisation* 21 (1): 127–142.

Biehl, João. 2005. *Vita: Life in a Zone of Social Abandonment*. Princeton, NJ: Princeton University Press.

———. 2009. *Will to Live: AIDS Therapies and the Politics of Survival*. Princeton, NJ: Princeton University Press.

———. 2013. "The Judicialization of Biopolitics: Claiming the Right to Pharmaceuticals in Brazilian Courts." *American Ethnologist* 40 (3): 419–436.

Biehl, João, and Adriana Petryna. 2011. "Bodies of Rights and Therapeutic Markets." *Social Research* 78 (2): 359–386.

Birla, Ritu. 2009. *Stages of Capital: Law, Culture and Market Governance in Late Colonial India*. Durham, NC: Duke University Press.

Brenner, Neil, Jamie Peck, and Nik Theodore. 2010. "Variegated Neoliberalization: Geographies, Modalities, Pathways." *Global Networks* 10 (2): 182–222.

Brotherton, P. Sean. 2008. "'We Have to Think Like Capitalists but Continue Being Socialists': Medicalized Subjectivities, Emergent Capital, and Socialist Entrepreneurs in Post-Soviet Cuba." *American Ethnologist* 35 (2): 259–274.

———. 2012. *Revolutionary Medicine: Health and Body in Post-Soviet Cuba*. Durham, NC: Duke University Press.

Brown, Wendy. 2015. *Undoing the Demos: Neoliberalism's Stealth Revolution*. Cambridge, MA: Zone.

Buchdunger, Elizabeth, Jürg Zimmermann, Helmut Mett, Thomas Meyer, Marcel Müller, Brian J. Druker, and Nicholas B. Lydon. 1996. "Inhibition of the Abl Protein-Tyrosine Kinase In Vitro and In Vivo by a 2-Phenylaminopyrimidine Derivative." *Cancer Research* 56 (1): 100–104.

Callon, Michel. 1986. "Some Elements of a Sociology of Translation: Domestication of the Scallops and the Fishermen of St. Brieuc Bay." In *Power, Action, Belief: A New Sociology of Knowledge?*, edited by John Law, 196–223. London: Routledge.

———. 1998. *The Laws of the Markets*. Hoboken, NJ: Wiley-Blackwell.

Callon, Michel, Yuvan Millo, and Fabian Muniesa, eds. 2007. *Market Devices*. Hoboken, NJ: Wiley-Blackwell.

Carroll, John. 2013. "NIH Confirms It Is Shelving India Drug Trials in Wake of New Regs." Fierce Biotech, July 17. http://www.fiercebiotech.com/r-d/nih-confirms-it-shelving-india-drug-trials-wake-of-new-regs.

Cassier, Maurice. 2005. "Appropriation and Commercialization of the Pasteur Anthrax Vaccine." *Studies in History and Philosophy of Science Part C* 36 (4): 722–742.

———. 2012. "Pharmaceutical Patent Law in-the-Making: Opposition and Legal Action by States, Citizens and Generics Laboratories in Brazil and India." In *Ways of Regulating Drugs in the 19th and 20th Centuries*, edited by Jean-Paul Gaudilliere and Volker Hess. London: Routledge-Palgrave.

Centers for Disease Control and Prevention. 2014. "What Can I Do to Reduce My Risk of Cervical Cancer?" http://www.cdc.gov/cancer/cervical/basic_info/prevention.htm.

Chakrabarty, Dipesh. 2000. *Provincializing Europe: Postcolonial Thought and Historical Difference*. Princeton: Princeton University Press.

Chatterjee, Partha. 2004. *The Politics of the Governed: Reflections on Popular Politics in Most of the World*. New York: Columbia University Press.

———. 2008. "Democracy and Economic Transformation," debate, Kafila, June 13. http://kafila.org/2008/06/13/democracy-and-economic-transformation-partha -chatterjee/.

———. 2011. *Lineages of Political Society: Studies in Postcolonial Democracy*. New York: Columbia University Press.

Chaudhuri, Sudip. 2005. *The WTO and India's Pharmaceutical Industry: Patent Protection, TRIPS, and Developing Countries*. Delhi: Oxford University Press.

Cipla. 1973. *Cipla News*, 8 (1, April).

Clarke, Adele. 1998. *Disciplining Reproduction: Modernity, American Life Sciences, and the Problems of Sex*. Berkeley: University of California Press.

Cohen, Lawrence. 1999. "Where It Hurts: Indian Material for an Ethics of Organ Transplantation." *Daedelus* 128 (4): 135–165.

Comaroff, Jean, and John Comaroff. 2006. "Law and Disorder in the Postcolony: An Introduction." In *Law and Disorder in the Postcolony*, edited by Jean Comaroff and John Comaroff, 1–56. Chicago: University of Chicago Press.

Cooper, Melinda. 2008. *Life as Surplus: Biotechnology and Capitalism in the Neoliberal Era*. Seattle: University of Washington Press.

Cooper, Melinda, and Catherine Waldby. 2014. *Clinical Labor: Tissue Donors and Research Subjects in the Global Bioeconomy*. Durham, NC: Duke University Press.

Cruickshank, Carol. 2009. "Make Your Move: Taking Clinical Trials to the Best Location." A. T. Kearney. http://www.atkearney.com/en_GB/health/ideas-insights/article /-/asset_publisher/LCcgOeS4t85g/content/make-your-move/10192.

Das, Gurcharan. 2001. *India Unbound*. New York: Anchor.

Das, Veena. 2006. *Life and Words: Violence and the Descent into the Ordinary*. Berkeley: University of California Press.

———. 2011. "State, Citizenship, and the Urban Poor." *Citizenship Studies* 3–4: 319–333.

———. 2015. *Affliction: Health, Disease, Poverty*. New York: Fordham University Press.

Das, Veena, and Ranendra K. Das. 2006. "Pharmaceuticals in Urban Ecologies." In *Global Pharmaceuticals: Ethics, Markets, Practices*. Durham, NC: Duke University Press.

Davies, Gail. 2012a. "Caring for the Multiple and the Multitude: Assembling Animal Welfare and Enabling Ethical Critique." *Environment and Planning D: Society and Space* 30: 623–638.

———. 2012b. "What Is a Humanized Mouse? Remaking the Species and Spaces of Translational Medicine." *Body and Society* 18: 126–155.

———. 2013a. "Arguably Big Biology: Sociology, Spatiality and the Knockout Mouse Project." *Biosocieties* 4 (8): 417–431.

———. 2013b. "Mobilizing Experimental Life: Spaces of Becoming with Mutant Mice." *Theory, Culture and Society: Explorations in Critical Social Science* 30: 129–153.

De Klein, A., A. H. Geurts van Kessel, G. Grosveld, C. R. Bartram, N. K. Spurr, N. Heisterkamp, J. Groffen, and J. R. Stephenson. 1982. "A Cellular Oncogene is Translocated to the Philadelphia Chromosome in Chronic Myelocytic Leukemia." *Nature* 300: 765–767.

Deloitte. 2008. "The Future of the Life Sciences Industries: Transformation amongst Rising Risks." https://www.biocity.co.uk/file-manager/Group/reports2009/2009 -futurels-transformationrisk-final2.pdf.

———. 2009. "Acquisitions versus Product Development: An Emerging Trend in Life Sciences." https://www.scribd.com/document/56792814/Acquisitions-Versus -Product-Development.

Department of Anthropology. 2012. "Trans-Science Conference Schedule." University of Chicago. http://anthropology.uchicago.edu/resources/trans_science_conference _schedule/.

Derrida, Jacques. 1992. "Force of Law: The 'Mystical Foundation of Authority.' " *Cardozo Law Review* 11: 920–1045.

———. 1994. *Specters of Marx: The State of the Debt, the Work of Mourning, and the New International.* Abingdon, UK: Psychology Press.

Deva, Surya. 2009. "Public Interest Litigation in India: A Critical Review." *Civil Justice Quarterly* 28 (1): 19–40.

Dhar, Aarti. 2010. "Centre Halts HPV Vaccine Project." *Hindu*, April 8. http://www .thehindu.com/todays-paper/centre-halts-hpv-vaccine-project/article746151.ece.

DiMasi, Joseph A., R. W. Hansen, H. G. Grabowski, and L. Lasagna. 1991. "Cost of Innovation in the Pharmaceutical Industry." *Journal of Health Economics* July: 107–142.

Doyal, Imogen Pennell Lesley. 1979. *The Political Economy of Health.* Boston: Pluto.

Drews, Jurgen, and Stefan Ryser. 1996. "Innovation Deficit in the Pharmaceutical Industry." *Drug Information Journal* 30: 97–108.

"Drugs Firms Must Not Prey on Poverty." 2011. *Independent*, November 14. http:// www.independent.co.uk/voices/editorials/leading-article-drugs-firms-must-not -prey-on-poverty-6261959.html.

Druker, Brian. 2007a. "Don't Abuse Patents: Scientists." *Live Mint*, August 15. http:// www.livemint.com/Opinion/26rbSkGiTxNYKobbO568kL/Don8217t-abuse-patents -scientists.html.

———. 2007b. "Targeting Hope When Nobody Believes in You: Dr. Brian Druker's OHSU Commencement Speech." *Oregonian*, June 7. http://blog.oregonlive.com /oregonianextra/2007/06/dr_brian_drukers_ohsu_commence.html.

Druker, Brian, Moshe Talpaz, Debra Resta, Bin Peng, Elisabeth Buchdunger, John Ford, Nicholas Lydon, Hagop Kantarjian, Renaud Capdeville, Sayuri Ohno-Jones, and Charles Sawyers. 2001. "Efficacy and Safety of a Specific Inhibitor of the bcr-abl Tyrosine Kinase in Chronic Myeloid Leukemia." *New England Journal of Medicine* 344 (14, April 5): 1031–1037.

Druker, Brian, S. Tamura, E. Buchdunger, S. Ohno, G. M. Segal, S. Fanning, J. Zimmerman, and N. B. Lydon. 1996. "Effects of a Selective Inhibitor of Abl Tyrosine Kinase on the Growth of Bcr-abl Positive Cells." *Nature Medicine* 2: 561–566.

Dumit, Joseph. 2012a. *Drugs for Life: How Pharmaceutical Companies Define Our Health*. Durham, NC: Duke University Press.

———. 2012b. "Prescription Maximization and the Accumulation of Surplus Health in the Pharmaceutical Industry: The_BioMarx_Experiment." In *Lively Capital: Biotechnologies, Ethics and Governance in Global Markets*, edited by Kaushik Sunder Rajan, 45–92. Durham, NC: Duke University Press.

Dunne, Eileen F., Elizabeth R. Unger, Maya Sternberg, Geraldine McQuillan, David C. Swan, Sonya S. Patel, and Lauri E. Markowitz. 2007. "Prevalence of HPV Infection among Females in the United States." *JAMA* 297 (8): 813–819.

Duster, Troy. 2006. "Lessons from History: Why Race and Ethnicity Have Played a Major Role in Biomedical Research." *Journal of Law, Medicine and Ethics* 34 (3): 487–496.

Dutfield, Graham. 2013. "Who Invented Glivec? Does It Matter Anyway?" *Economic and Political Weekly* 48 (32): 41–42.

Ecks, Stefan. 2008. "Global Pharmaceutical Markets and Corporate Citizenship: The Case of Novartis' Anti-cancer Drug Glivec." *Biosocieties* 3: 165–181.

Edmonds, Alexander, and Emilia Sanabria. 2014. "Medical Borderlands: Engineering the Body with Medical Hormones and Plastic Surgery in Brazil." *Anthropology and Medicine* 21 (2): 202–216.

Epstein, Steven. 1996. *Impure Science: AIDS, Activism, and the Politics of Knowledge*. Berkeley: University of California Press.

———. 2007. *Inclusion: The Politics of Difference in Medical Research*. Chicago: University of Chicago Press.

Express Scripts. 2014. "Harvoni: Orphan-Drug Pricing for a Non-Orphan Drug." October 23. http://lab.express-scripts.com/lab/insights/specialty-medications/harvoni-orphan-drug-pricing-for-a-nonorphan-drug.

Fainstein, E., C. Marcelle, A. Rosner, E. Canaani, R. P. Gale, O. Dreazen, S. D. Smith, and C. M. Croce. 1987. "A New Fused Transcript in Philadelphia Chromosome Positive Acute Lymphocytic Leukemia." *Nature* 330 (6146): 386–388.

Farquhar, Judith, and Lili Lai. 2014. "Information and Its Practical Other: Crafting Zhuang Nationality Medicine." *East Asian Science and Technology Studies* 8: 417–437.

Fernandez, Jose-Maria, Roger Stein, and Andrew Lo. 2012. "Commercializing Biomedical Research through Securitization Techniques." *Nature Biotechnology* 30: 964–975.

Fischer, Michael M. J. 1980. *Iran: From Religious Dispute to Revolution*. Madison: University of Wisconsin Press.

———. 2003. *Emergent Forms of Life and the Anthropological Voice*. Durham, NC: Duke University Press.

———. 2009. *Anthropological Futures*. Durham, NC: Duke University Press.

———. 2013. "The Peopling of Technologies." In *When People Come First: Critical Studies in Global Health*, edited by João Biehl and Adriana Petryna, 347–374. Princeton, NJ: Princeton University Press.

———. 2014. "The Lightness of Existence and the Origami of 'French' Anthropology: Latour, Descola, Viveiros de Castro, Meillassoux, and Their So-Called Ontological Turn." *Hau: Journal of Ethnographic Theory* 4 (1): 331–355.

Fischer, Michael M. J., and Mehdi Abedi. 1990. *Debating Muslims: Cultural Dialogues in Postmodernity and Tradition*. Madison: University of Wisconsin Press.

Fisher, Jill A. 2008. *Medical Research for Hire: The Political Economy of Pharmaceutical Clinical Trials*. New Brunswick, NJ: Rutgers University Press.

Fleck, Ludwik. (1927) 1986. "Some Specific Features of the Medical Way of Thinking." In *Cognition and Fact: Materials on Ludwik Fleck*, edited by R. S. Cohen and T. Schnelle, 39–46. Dordrecht: D. Reidel.

Folayan, Morenike, and Dan Allman. 2011. "Clinical Trials as an Industry and an Employer of Labour." *Journal of Cultural Economy* 4 (1): 97–104.

Fortun, Kim. 2001. *Advocacy after Bhopal: Environmentalism, Disaster, New Global Orders*. Chicago: University of Chicago Press.

———. 2012. "Ethnography in Late Industrialism." *Cultural Anthropology* 27 (3): 446–464.

———. 2014. "From Latour to Late Industrialism." *Hau: Journal of Ethnographic Theory* 4 (1): 309–329.

———. 2016. "Making Environmental Sense." Unpublished manuscript.

Foucault, Michel. (1970) 1994. *The Order of Things*. New York: Vintage.

———. (1973) 2003. *The Birth of the Clinic*. New York: Routledge.

———. (1976) 1990. *The History of Sexuality*, vol. 1: *An Introduction*. New York: Vintage.

———. 1980. *Power/Knowledge: Selected Interviews and Other Writings*. New York: Vintage.

———. 2008. *The Birth of Biopolitics: Lectures at the College de France, 1978–1979*. London: Picador.

Fox, Renee, and Judith Swayze. 1992. *Spare Parts: Organ Replacement in American Society*. Oxford: Oxford University Press.

Franklin, Sarah. 2000. "Life Itself: Global Nature and the Genetic Imaginary." In *Global Nature, Global Culture*, edited by Sarah Franklin, Celia Lury, and Jackie Stacey, 188–227. Thousand Oaks, CA: Sage.

———. 2006. "The Cyborg Embryo: Our Path to Transbiology." *Theory, Culture and Society* 23 (7–8): 167–187.

———. 2013. *Biological Relatives: IVF, Stem Cells, and the Future of Kinship*. Durham, NC: Duke University Press.

Froud, Julie, and Johal Sukhdev. 2006. *Financialization and Strategy: Narrative and Numbers*. London: Routledge.

Fukuyama, Francis. (1991) 2006. *The End of History and the Last Man*. New York: Free Press.

Ganesan, A. V. 1994. *The GATT Uruguay Round Agreement: Opportunities and Challenges*. New Delhi: Rajiv Gandhi Foundation.

García, Silvia. 2006. "Argentina: El Peor de los Engaños: Fraude del Laboratorio Novartis y la Fundación Max a Pacientes Con Cáncer." *Revista El Médico* (Argentina), June 15. http://www.saludyfarmacos.org/lang/es/boletin-farmacos/boletines/sep2006/etica-y-medicamentos/#Argentina:_El_peor_de_los_enga%C3%B1os._Fraude_del_laboratorio_Novartis_y_la_Fundaci%C3%B3n_Max_a_pacientes_con_c%C3%A1ncer.

Gaudilliere, Jean-Paul. 2014. "De la santé publique internationale à la santé globale. L'OMS, la Banque mondiale et le gouvernement des thérapies chimiques." In *Le Gouvernment des Technosciences: Gouverner le Progres et ses Degat depuis 1945*, edited by Domonique Pestre, 65–96. Paris: La Decouverte.

"Gilead Denied Sovaldi Patent Protection in India, Paving Way for Generics." 2015. *FDAnews Drug Daily Bulletin*, January 22. http://www.fdanews.com/articles/169652 -gilead-denied-sovaldi-patent-protection-in-india-paving-way-for-generics.

Ginsburg, Faye, and Rayna Rapp. 1995. *Conceiving the New World Order: The Global Politics of Reproduction*. Berkeley: University of California Press.

Good, Mary-Jo DelVecchio, Byron Good, C. Schaffer, and S. E. Lind. 1990. "American Oncology and the Discourse on Hope." *Culture, Medicine and Psychiatry* 14: 59–79.

Gopakumar, K. M. 2013. "The Need to Curb Patents on Known Substances." *Economic and Political Weekly* 48 (32): 55–57.

Grace, Patricia. 1998. *Baby No-Eyes*. Honolulu: University of Hawaii Press.

Gramsci, Antonio. (1926) 2000. "Some Aspects of the Southern Question." In *The Antonio Gramsci Reader: Selected Writings 1916–1935*, edited by David Forgacs, 171–185. New York: NYU Press.

———. 2000. *The Antonio Gramsci Reader: Selected Writings 1916–1935*, edited by David Forgacs. New York: NYU Press.

Greene, Jeremy. 2014. *Generic: The Unbranding of Modern Medicine*. Baltimore, MD: Johns Hopkins University Press.

Grefe, Edward A., and Martin Linsky. 1995. *The New Corporate Activism: Harnessing the Power of Grassroots Tactics for Your Organization*. New York: McGraw-Hill.

Guilloux, Allain, and Sureie Moon. 2001. "Hidden Price-Tags: Disease-Specific Drug Donations: Costs and Alternatives." MSF/DND Working Group paper.

"Gujarat Launches Cervical Cancer Vaccine." 2009. *Press Trust of India*, August 13.

Gulhati, Chandra. 2010. "Bhopal Gas Victims Used as Guinea Pigs." *Monthly Index of Medical Specialties*, June.

———. 2011. "Chronic Clinical Investigators: New Breed of Body Hunters." *Monthly Index of Medical Specialties*, May.

Habermas, Jürgen. 1984. *Theory of Communicative Action*, vol. 1: *Reason and the Rationalization of Society*. Translated by Thomas McCarthy. Boston: Beacon.

———. 1985. *Theory of Communicative Action*, vol. 2: *Lifeworld and System: A Critique of Functionalist Reason*. Translated by Thomas McCarthy. Boston: Beacon.

Hacking, Ian. 1990. *The Taming of Chance*. Cambridge: Cambridge University Press.

Hamied, Khwaja A. 1972. *An Autobiography: A Life to Remember*. Bombay: Lalvani.

Hamied, Yusuf. 2003. "Trading in Death." *Little Magazine* 5 (4–5): 44–51.

———. 2005. "Indian Pharma Industry: Decades of Struggle and Achievements." Presentation on the occasion of Dr. A. V. Rama Rao's 70th birthday, Hyderabad, April 2.

Hanna, Bridget. 2006. "The Circle of Poison Continues." International Campaign for Justice in Bhopal, December 5. http://www.bhopal.net/the-circle-of-poison -continues/.

Haraway, Donna. 1991. *Simians, Cyborgs and Women: The Reinvention of Nature*. London: Free Association.

———. 2007. *When Species Meet*. Minneapolis: University of Minnesota Press.

Hart, Keith. 2000. *The Memory Bank: Money in an Unequal World*. London: Profile.

Harvey, David. 2003. *The New Imperialism*. Oxford: Oxford University Press.

———. 2007. *A Brief History of Neoliberalism*. Oxford: Oxford University Press.

Hayden, Cori. 2007. "A Generic Solution? Pharmaceuticals and the Politics of the Similar in Mexico." *Current Anthropology* 48 (4): 475–495.

———. 2010. "The Proper Copy: The Insides and Outsides of Domains Made Public." *Journal of Cultural Economy* 3 (1): 85–102.

———. 2011. "No Patent, No Generic: Pharmaceutical Access and the Politics of the Copy." In *Making and Unmaking Intellectual Property: Creative Production in Legal and Cultural Perspective*, edited by Mario Biogioli, Peter Jaszi, and Martha Woodmansee, 285–304. Chicago: University of Chicago Press.

Heisterkamp, Nora, John Groffen, John Stephenson, N. K. Spurr, P. N. Goodfellow, E. Solomon, B. Carritt, and W. F. Bodmer. 1982. "Chromosomal Localization of Human Cellular Homologues of Two Viral Oncogenes." *Nature* 299 (5885): 747–749.

Heisterkamp, Nora, K. Stam, John Groffen, A. de Klein, and G. Grosveld. 1985. "Structural Organization of the Bcr Gene and Its Role in the Ph' Translocation." *Nature* 315 (6022): 758–761.

Helfand, Carly. 2014a. "Gilead to Offer Cheap Sovaldi to 80 Countries." Fierce Pharma, September 5. http://www.fiercepharma.com/sales-and-marketing/gilead-to-offer-cheap-sovaldi-to-80-countries.

———. 2014b. "Mylan, Ranbaxy, Others to Bring Cheap Sovaldi to 91 Markets." Fierce Pharma, September 15. http://www.fiercepharma.com/sales-and-marketing/mylan-ranbaxy-others-to-bring-cheap-sovaldi-to-91-markets.

Helmreich, Stefan. 2008. "Species of Biocapital." *Science as Culture* 17 (4): 463–478.

Hilgartner, Stephen. 2009. "Intellectual Property and the Politics of Emerging Technology: Inventors, Citizens, and Powers to Shape the Future." *Chicago-Kent Law Review* 84 (1): 197–224.

Ho, Karen. 2009. *Liquidated: An Ethnography of Wall Street*. Durham, NC: Duke University Press.

Hoare, Quintin, and Geoffrey Nowell-Smith. 1971. *Selections from the Prison Notebooks of Antonio Gramsci*. New York: International.

Hobsbawm, Eric. 1994. *The Age of Extremes: A History of the World, 1914–1991*. New York: Vintage.

Honig, Bonnie. 2009. *Emergency Politics: Paradox, Law, Democracy*. Princeton, NJ: Princeton University Press.

Howlett, Peter, and Mary Morgan, eds. 2010. *How Well Do Facts Travel? The Dissemination of Reliable Knowledge*. Cambridge: Cambridge University Press.

ICMR. 2010. *Final Report of the Committee Appointed by the Govt of India (vide Notification No. V. 25011/160/2010-HR*. New Delhi: Indian Council of Medical Research.

Indian Drug Manufacturers Association. 1981. "A Report on the Indian Drug Industry, 1980–2000 A.D." April 15.

Jain, S. Lochlann. 2013. *Malignant: How Cancer Becomes Us*. Berkeley: University of California Press.

Jan Swasthya Abhiyan. 2011. "Memorandum of Concerns Regarding the Interim Report of the Committee Appointed by the Government of India to Enquire into 'Alleged Irregularities in the Conduct of Studies Using Human Papilloma Virus (HPV) Vaccine.'" *Sama: Resource Group for Women and Health*, April 23. https://samawomenshealth.wordpress.com/2011/04/23/memorandum-of-concerns -regarding-the-interim-report-of-the-committee-appointed-by-the-government -of-india-to-enquire-into-"alleged-irregularities-in-the-conduct-of-studies-using -human-papillom/.

Jasanoff, Sheila. 1997. *Science at the Bar: Law, Science and Technology in America.* Cambridge, MA: Harvard University Press.

———. 2003. "In a Constitutional Moment: Science and Social Order at the Millunnium." *Sociology of Science Yearbook* 23 (2): 155–180.

———. 2004. *States of Knowledge: The Co-production of Science and the Social Order.* New York: Routledge.

———. 2005. *Designs on Nature: Science and Democracy in Europe and the United States.* Princeton, NJ: Princeton University Press.

———. 2011. *Reframing Rights: Bioconstitutionalism in the Genetic Age.* Cambridge, MA: MIT Press.

———. 2012. "Taking Life: Private Rights in Public Nature." In *Lively Capital: Biotechnologies, Ethics and Governance in Global Markets*, edited by Kaushik Sunder Rajan, 155–183. Durham, NC: Duke University Press.

———. 2013. *Science and Public Reason.* New York: Routledge.

———. 2015. "Serviceable Truths: Science for Action in Law and Policy." *Texas Law Review* 93: 1722–1749.

Jasanoff, Sheila, and Sanghyun Kim, eds. 2015. *Dreamscapes of Modernity: Sociotechnical Imaginaries and the Fabrication of Power.* Chicago: University of Chicago Press.

Jishnu, Latha. 2010a. "Insidious India Project." *Business Standard*, March 4. http://www.business-standard.com/article/opinion/latha-jishnu-insidious-india-project -110030400053_1.html.

———. 2010b. "Why Do Judges Need to Be 'Sensitised'?" *Down to Earth*, July 26. http://www.downtoearth.org.in/blog/why-do-judges-need-to-be-sensitised-1617.

Jones, James Howard, and Tuskegee Institute. 1981. *Bad Blood: The Tuskegee Syphilis Experiment.* New York: Free Press.

Jones, Jennifer, and Alan Zuckerman. 2007. "Clinical Research Trials: Creating Competitive and Financial Advantages." *Managing the Margin Newsletter.* www.hfma .org. Accessed May 1, 2007.

Kahn, Jonathan. 2014. *Race in a Bottle: The Story of BiDil and Racialized Medicine in a Post-genomic Age.* New York: Columbia University Press.

Kannan, K. P. 1976. "Science for Social Revolution." *Economic and Political Weekly* 11 (26): 943–944.

———. 1978. "Science for the People." *Economic and Political Weekly* 13 (40): 1691–1692.

———. 1990. "Secularism and People's Science Movement in India." *Economic and Political Weekly* 25 (6): 311–313.

Kaviraj, Sudipta. 1989. *Our Government, How It Functions: A Textbook in Civics for Class X*. New Delhi: National Council for Educational Research and Training.
———. 1997. *Politics in India*. New Delhi: Oxford University Press.
———. 2010. *The Imaginary Institution of India: Politics and Ideas*. New York: Columbia University Press.
Keating, Peter, and Alberto Cambrosio. 2012. *Cancer on Trial: Oncology as a New Style of Practice*. Chicago: University of Chicago Press.
Kelly, John, and Martha Kaplan. 2001. *Represented Communities: Fiji and World Decolonization*. Chicago: University of Chicago Press.
Khilnani, Sunil. 1999. *The Idea of India*. New York: Farrar, Straus and Giroux.
Kloppenburg, Jack. (1988) 2005. *First the Seed: The Political Economy of Plant Biotechnology*. Madison: University of Wisconsin Press.
Knight, Frank. 1921. *Risk, Uncertainty and Profit*. Boston: Hart, Schaffner and Marx.
Knorr Cetina, Karin, and Alex Preda, eds. 2005. *The Sociology of Financial Markets*. Oxford: Oxford University Press.
———. 2007. "The Temporalization of Financial Markets: From Network to Flow." *Theory, Culture and Society* 24 (7–8): 116–138.
———, eds. 2013. *The Oxford Handbook of the Sociology of Finance*. Oxford: Oxford University Press.
Kosek, Jake. Forthcoming. *Homo Apians: A Critical Natural History of the Modern Honeybee*.
Kosselleck, Reinhart, and Michaela Richter. 2006. "Crisis." *Journal of the History of Ideas* 67 (2): 357–400.
Kotiswaran, Prabha. 2011. *Dangerous Sex, Invisible Labor: Sex Work and the Law in India*. Princeton, NJ: Princeton University Press.
Krishna, R. Jai, and Jeanne Whalen. 2013. "Novartis Loses Glivec Patent Battle in India." *Wall Street Journal*, April 1. http://online.wsj.com/news/articles/SB10001424127887323296504578395672582230106.
Krishnan, Vidya, and Jacob P. Koshy. 2013. "US Agency NIH Scraps Nearly 40 Clinical Trials in India." Live Mint, July 11. http://www.livemint.com/Politics/zwG7cCA7nFYFdpzYLXcCVM/US-agency-NIH-cancels-nearly-40-ongoing-clinical-trials-in-I.html.
Kuo, Wen-Hua. 2005. "Japan and Taiwan in the Wake of Bio-globalization: Drugs, Race and Standards." PhD dissertation, Program in Science, Technology and Society, Massachusetts Institute of Technology.
———. 2012. "Transforming States in the Era of Global Pharmaceuticals: Visioning Clinical Research in Japan, Taiwan and Singapore." In *Lively Capital: Biotechnologies, Ethics and Governance in Global Markets*, edited by Kaushik Sunder Rajan, 279–305. Durham, NC: Duke University Press.
Lakshmi, Rama. 2012. "India's Drug Trials Fuel Controversy." *Washington Post*, January 1. http://www.washingtonpost.com/world/asia_pacific/indias-drug-trials-fuel-controversy/2011/12/01/gIQAAcCrUP_story.html.
LaMontagne, Scott, Sandhya Barge, Nga Thi Le, Emmanuel Mugisha, Mary E. Penny, Sanjay Gandhi, Amynah Janmohamed, Edward Kumakech, N. Rocio Mosqueira,

Nghi Quy Nguyen, Proma Paul, Yuxiao Tang, Tran Hung Minh, Bella Patel Uttekar, and Aisha O. Jumaan. 2011. "Human Papillomavirus Vaccine Delivery Strategies That Achieved High Coverage in Low- and Middle-Income Countries." *Bulletin of the World Health Organization* 89: 821–830.

Latour, Bruno. 1987. *Science in Action: How to Follow Scientists and Engineers through Society.* Cambridge, MA: Harvard University Press.

———. 1988. *The Pasteurization of France.* Cambridge, MA: Harvard University Press.

———. 1993. *We Have Never Been Modern.* Cambridge, MA: Harvard University Press.

———. 2004. *Politics of Nature.* Cambridge, MA: Harvard University Press.

———. 2005. *Reassembling the Social: An Introduction to Actor-Network Theory.* Oxford: Oxford University Press.

Lazonick, William. 2010. "Innovative Business Models and Varieties of Capitalism: Financialization of the U.S. Corporation." *Business History Review* 84 (4): 675–702.

le Carré, John. 2001. *The Constant Gardener.* London: Hodder and Stoughton.

Lee, Christopher. 2010. *Making a World after Empire: The Bandung Moment and Its Political Afterlives.* Athens: Ohio University Press.

Leonelli, Sabina. 2016. *Data-Centric Biology: A Philosophical Study.* Chicago: University of Chicago Press.

Lewis, Michael. 2010. *The Big Short: Inside the Doomsday Machine.* New York: Norton.

Lewis, Tracy R., Jerome H. Reichman, and Anthony D. So. 2007. "The Case for Public Funding and Public Oversight of Clinical Trials." *Economists' Voice* 4 (1).

LiPuma, Edward, and Benjamin Lee. 2004. *Financial Derivatives and the Globalization of Risk.* Durham, NC: Duke University Press.

Livingston, Julie. 2012. *Improvising Medicine: An African Oncology Ward in an Emerging Cancer Epidemic.* Durham, NC: Duke University Press.

Love, James. 2003. "Novartis Outlays on R&D R&D for Glivec: Evidence Suggests Outlays Are Substantially Below Average Costs Estimated by Tufts University Study." Consumer Project on Technology, September 22. http://www.cptech.org/ip/health/gleevec/.

Lyotard, Jean-François. 1984. *The Postmodern Condition: A Report on Knowledge.* Minneapolis: University of Minnesota Press.

Mackenzie, Donald. 2006. *An Engine, Not a Camera: How Financial Models Shape the Markets.* Cambridge, MA: MIT Press.

Mahajan, Manjari. 2008. "Designing Epidemics: Models, Policymaking, and Global Foreknowledge in India's AIDS Epidemic." *Science and Public Policy* 35 (8): 585–596.

———. Forthcoming. *The Anatomy of Humanitarian Emergencies.*

Maine, Deborah, Sarah Hurlburt, and Dana Greeson. 2011. "Cervical Cancer Prevention in the 21st Century: Cost Is Not the Only Issue." *American Journal of Public Health* 101 (9): 1549–1555. doi:10.2105/AJPH.2011.300204.

Mallikarjun, Y. 2010. "Vaccine Programme in A.P. Only after Centre's Clearance." *Hindu,* April 8. http://www.thehindu.com/news/national/vaccine-programme-in-ap-only-after-centres-clearance/article392163.ece.

Marcus, George, ed. 1995. *Technoscientific Imaginaries: Conversations, Profiles, Memoirs.* Chicago: University of Chicago Press.

Marks, Harry M. 2000. *The Progress of Experiment: Science and Therapeutic Reform in the United States, 1900–1990*. Cambridge: Cambridge University Press.

Martin, Emily. 1998. "Anthropology and the Cultural Study of Science." *Science, Technology and Human Values* 23 (1): 24–44.

Marx, Karl. (1852) 1977. *The Eighteenth Brumaire of Louis Bonaparte*. Moscow: Progress.

———. (1857) 1993. *Grundrisse: Foundations of a Critique of Political Economy*. Translated by Martin Nicolaus. London: Penguin.

———. (1867) 1976. *Capital: A Critique of Political Economy*. London: Penguin.

———. (1871) 2009. *The Civil War in France*. Gloucester, UK: Dodo.

———. (1894) 1974. *Capital: A Critique of Political Economy*, vol. 3, edited by Frederick Engels. Moscow: Progress.

Masco, Joseph. 2010. "Sensitive but Unclassified: Secrecy and the Counterterrorist State." *Public Culture* 22 (3): 433–463.

———. 2014. *The Theater of Operations: National Security Affect from the Cold War to the War on Terror*. Durham, NC: Duke University Press.

Mattheij, I., A. M. Pollock, and P. Brhlikova. 2012. "Do Cervical Cancer Data Justify HPV Vaccination in India? Epidemiological Data Sources and Comprehensiveness." *Journal of the Royal Society of Medicine* 105 (6): 250–262.

Maurer, Bill. 2002. "Repressed Futures: Financial Derivatives Theological Unconscious". *Economy and Society* 31 (1): 15–36.

———. 2012. "Finance." *Cultural Anthropology*, May 1. http://culanth.org/fieldsights/333-finance.

Maxmen, Amy. 2012. "Trade Deal to Curb Generic-Drug Use." *Nature* 489: 16–17.

McGoey, Linsey. 2015. *No Such Thing as a Free Gift: The Gates Foundation and the Price of Philanthropy*. London: Verso.

Meadows, Donella H., Dennis L. Meadows, Jorgen Randers, and William W. Behrens. 1972. *The Limits to Growth: A Report on the Club of Rome's Project for the Predicament of Mankind*. London: Pan Books.

Meister, Bob. 2011. "Debt and Taxes: Can the Financial Industry Save Public Universities?" *Representations* 116: 128–155.

Menon, Nivedita, and Aditya Nigam. 2007. *Power and Contestation: India since 1989*. London: Zed.

Mezzadra, Sandro, and Brett Neilson. 2013. *Border as Method: Or, the Multiplication of Labor*. Durham, NC: Duke University Press.

Mezzadra, Sandro, Julian Reed, and Ranabir Samaddar. 2013. *The Biopolitics of Development: Reading Michel Foucault in the Postcolonial Present*. New York: Springer.

Miranda, Debora. 2011. "WHO: Screening Still the 'Best Buy' for Tackling Cervical Cancer." *Bulletin of the World Health Organization* 89: 828–829.

Miyazaki, Hirokazu. 2007. "Between Arbitrage and Speculation: An Economy of Belief and Doubt." *Economy and Society* 36 (3): 397–416.

———. 2013. *Arbitraging Japan: Dreams of Capitalism at the End of Finance*. Berkeley: University of California Press.

"Modi's Chief Economic Adviser Arvind Subramanian Had Opposed India on IPR till Recently." 2014. *Times of India*, October 25. http://timesofindia.indiatimes.com

/india/Modis-chief-economic-adviser-Arvind-Subramanian-had-opposed-India
-on-IPR-till-recently/articleshow/44929094.cms.

Mofitt, Jane. 1979. "Appropriateness of Bioavailability and Bioequivalency as Pre-market Clearance Considerations." *Food, Drug and Cosmetic Law Journal* 34: 640.

Montoya, Michael. 2011. *Making the Mexican Diabetic: Race, Science, and the Genetics of Inequality.* Berkeley: University of California Press.

Mukherjee, Siddhartha. 2011. *The Emperor of All Maladies: A Biography of Cancer.* New York: Scribner.

Murphy, Michelle. 2012. *Seizing the Means of Reproduction: Entanglements of Feminism, Health, and Technoscience.* Durham, NC: Duke University Press.

———. 2017. *The Economization of Life.* Durham, NC: Duke University Press.

NASSCOM. 2002. *NASSCOM-McKinsey Report, 2002: Strategies to Achieve the Indian IT Industry's Aspiration.* New Delhi: National Association of Software and Service Companies.

National Commission for the Protection of Human Subjects of Biomedical and Behavioral Research. 1978. *The Belmont Report: Ethical Principles and Guidelines for the Protection of Human Subjects of Research.* ERIC Clearinghouse.

Navarro, Vicente. 1976. *Medicine under Capitalism.* New York: Prodist.

Negri, Antonio. (1973) 1992. *Marx beyond Marx: Lessons on the Grundrisse.* Boston: Pluto.

Nehru, Jawaharlal. 1947. "Tryst with Destiny." Speech delivered in the Constituent Assembly, New Delhi, August 14. http://www.wwnorton.com/college/english/nael/noa/pdf/27636_20th_U04_Nehru-1.pdf.

Nguyen, Vinh-Kim. 2010. *The Republic of Therapy: Triage and Sovereignty in West Africa's Time of AIDS.* Durham, NC: Duke University Press.

Norton, Ronald. 2001. "Clinical Pharmacogenomics: Applications in Pharmaceutical R & D." *Drug Discovery Today* 6 (4): 180–185.

Novas, Carlos, and Nikolas Rose. 2005. "Biological Citizenship." In *Global Assemblages: Technology, Politics, and Ethics as Anthropological Problems,* edited by Aihwa Ong and Stephen Collier, 439–463. Oxford: Blackwell.

Nowell, Peter, and David Hungerford. 1960. "A Minute Chromosome in Human Chronic Granulocytic Leukemia." *Science* 132: 1497–1501.

Nundy, Samiran, and Chandra M. Gulhati. 2005. "A New Colonialism? Conducting Clinical Trials in India." *New England Journal of Medicine* 352 (16): 1633–1636. doi:10.1056/NEJMp048361.

Office of the USTR. 2009. "USTR NEWS: Kirk Comments on Trans-Pacific Partnership." November. https://ustr.gov/about-us/policy-offices/press-office/press-releases/2009/november/ustr-news-kirk-comments-trans-pacific-partnership.

———. 2013. "Transparency and the Trans-Pacific Partnership." June. https://ustr.gov/about-us/policy-offices/press-office/fact-sheets/2012/june/transparency-and-the-tpp.

———. 2015. "Summary of the Trans-Pacific Partnership Agreement." October. https://ustr.gov/about-us/policy-offices/press-office/press-releases/2015/october/summary-trans-pacific-partnership.

Ong, Aihwa, and Stephen Collier. 2005. *Global Assemblages: Technology, Politics, and Ethics as Anthropological Problems.* Oxford: Blackwell.

Outterson, Kevin. 2005. "Pharmaceutical Arbitrage: Balancing Access and Innovation in International Prescription Drug Markets." *Yale Journal of Health Policy Law and Ethics* 193: 262–265.

Padmanabhan, Manjula. 2003. *Harvest*. London: Aurora Metro.

Parliament of India Rajya Sabha. 2012. "Fifty-Ninth Report on the Functioning of the Central Drugs Standards Control Organisation (CDSCO)." Department-Related Parliamentary Standing Committee on Health and Family Welfare, May 8.

PATH. 2009. *Shaping a Strategy to Introduce HPV Vaccines in India—Formative Research Results from the HPV Vaccines: Evidence for Impact Project*. Vaccine Resource Library. http://www.path.org/vaccineresources/details.php?i=1361.

Pathak, Zakia, and Rajeswari Sunder Rajan. 1989. "Shahbano." *Signs*, 558–582.

Pearl, Daniel, and Alix Freedman. 2001. "Altruism, Politics and Bottom Line Intersect at Indian Generics Firm." *Wall Street Journal*, March 12.

Pedersen, Susan. 1991. "National Bodies, Unspeakable Acts: The Sexual Politics of Colonial Policy-Making." *Journal of Modern History* 63 (4): 647–680.

Peterson, Kristin. 2014a. "On the Monopoly: Speculation, Pharmaceutical Markets, and Intellectual Property Law in Nigeria." *American Ethnologist* 41 (1): 128–142.

———. 2014b. *Speculative Markets: Drug Circuits and Derivative Life in Nigeria*. Durham, NC: Duke University Press.

Petryna, Adriana. 2002. *Life Exposed: Biological Citizens after Chernobyl*. Princeton, NJ: Princeton University Press.

———. 2005. "Ethical Variability: Drug Development and Globalizing Clinical Trials." *American Ethnologist* 32 (2): 183–197. doi:10.1525/ae.2005.32.2.183.

———. 2009. *When Experiments Travel: Clinical Trials and the Global Search for Human Subjects*. Princeton, NJ: Princeton University Press.

"Pilot Programme for Vaccination against Cervical Cancer Launched." 2009. *Hindu*, July 10. http://www.thehindu.com/todays-paper/tp-national/tp-andhrapradesh/pilot-programme-for-vaccination-against-cervical-cancer-launched/article226126.ece.

Pordie, Laurent, and Jean-Paul Gaudilliere. 2014. "The Reformulation Regime in Drug Discovery: Revisiting Polyherbals and Property Rights in the Ayurvedic Industry." *East Asian Science, Technology and Society* 8 (1): 57–79.

Porter, Natalie. 2013. "Bird Flu Biopower: Strategies for Multispecies Coexistence in Vietnam." *American Ethnologist* 40 (1): 132–148.

———. 2015. "Ferreting Things Out: Biosecurity, Pandemic Flu, and the Transformation of Experimental Systems." *BioSocieties* 11: 22–45. doi: 10.1057/biosoc.2015.4.

Postone, Moishe. 1993. *Time, Labor and Social Domination: A Reinterpretation of Marx's Critical Theory*. Cambridge: Cambridge University Press.

———. 2012. "Thinking the Global Crisis." *South Atlantic Quarterly* 111 (2): 227–249.

Pottage, Alain, and Brad Sherman. 2012. *Figures of Invention: A History of Modern Patent Law*. Oxford: Oxford University Press.

Proctor, Robert. 2012. *Golden Holocaust: Origins of the Cigarette Catastrophe and the Case for Abolition*. Berkeley: University of California Press.

Proctor, Robert, and Londa Schiebinger. 2008. *Agnotology: The Making and Unmaking of Ignorance*. Stanford, CA: Stanford University Press.

Public Citizen. 2010. "Leaked New Zealand Paper Challenges Past U.S. FTA Models in Trans-Pacific Trade Negotiations." December 4. http://www.citizen.org/documents/MemoonTPPleakedNZpaperandaccesstomedicines.pdf.

Rabinow, Paul. 1992. "Artificiality and Enlightenment: From Sociobiology to Biosociality." In *Incorporations*. New York: Zone.

———. 2003. *Anthropos Today: Reflections on Modern Equipment*. Princeton, NJ: Princeton University Press.

———. 2007. "Afterword: Concept Work." In *Biosocialities, Genetics, and the Social Sciences: Making Biological Identities*, edited by Sahra Gibbon and Carlos Novas. London: Routledge.

Raghavan, Chakravarthi. 1990. *Recolonization: GATT, the Uruguay Round, and the Third World*. London: Zed.

Rahman, Zia Haider. 2014. *In the Light of What We Know*. London: Picador.

Rapp, Rayna. 2000. *Testing Women, Testing the Fetus: The Social Impact of Amniocentesis in America*. New York: Routledge.

Reddy, K. Anji. 2015. *An Unfinished Agenda: My Life in the Pharmaceuticals Industry*. New York: Penguin.

Redfield, Peter. 2013. *Life in Crisis: The Ethical Journey of Doctors without Borders*. Berkeley: University of California Press.

Reverby, Susan. 2000. *Tuskegee's Truths: Rethinking the Tuskegee Syphilis Study*. Chapel Hill: University of North Carolina Press.

Riles, Annelise. 2004. "Real Time: Unwinding Technocratic and Anthropological Knowledge." *American Ethnologist* 31 (3): 1–14.

———. 2011. *Collateral Knowledge: Legal Reasoning in the Global Financial Markets*. Chicago: University of Chicago Press.

Robbins, Bruce. 2013. "Balibarism!" *n+1*, no. 16. https://nplusonemag.com/issue-16/reviews/balibarism/.

Roitman, Janet. 2013. *Anti-crisis*. Durham, NC: Duke University Press.

Rose, Nikolas. 2006. *The Politics of Life Itself: Biomedicine, Power, and Subjectivity in the Twenty-First Century*. Princeton, NJ: Princeton University Press.

Rowley, Janet. 1973. "A New Consistent Chromosomal Abnormality in Chronic Myelogenous Leukemia." *Nature* 243: 290–293.

Rushdie, Salman. 1980. *Midnight's Children*. New York: Modern Library.

Sahlins, Marshall. 1988. "Cosmologies of Capitalism: The Trans-Pacific Sector of the World System." *Proceedings of the British Academy* 74: 1–51.

———. 2013. "On the Culture of Material Value and the Cosmography of Riches." *HAU: Journal of Ethnographic Theory* 3 (2): 161–195.

Said, Edward. 1976. *Orientalism*. New York: Vintage.

Sama. 2010. *Constructing Conceptions: The Mapping of Assisted Reproductive Technologies in India*. CommunityHealth.in. http://www.communityhealth.in/~commun26/wiki/images/0/0f/Sama_Constructing_Conceptions.pdf.

———. 2011. *National Consultation on Regulation of Drug Trials: A Report by Sama–Resource Group for Women and Health*. Delhi: Sama–Resource Group for Women and Health.

Sanabria, Emilia. 2016. *Plastic Bodies: Sex Hormones and Menstrual Suppression in Brazil*. Durham, NC: Duke University Press.

Sandler, Tim. 2012. "In India, Oversight Lacking in Outsourced Drug Trials." *NBC News*, March 4. http://investigations.nbcnews.com/_news/2012/03/04/10562883-in -india-oversight-lacking-in-outsourced-drug-trials.

Sarkar, Tanika. 2012. "Something Like Rights? Faith, Law, and Widow Immolation Debates in Colonial Bengal." *Indian Economic Social History Review* 49: 295–320.

Sarojini, N. B., S. Anjali, and S. Ashalata. 2010. "Findings from a Visit to Bhadracha- lam: HPV Vaccine 'Demonstration Project' Site in Andhra Pradesh." New Delhi: Sama Women's Health, March 27–30.

Schoonveld, Ed. 2011. *The Price of Global Health: Drug Pricing Strategies to Balance Patient Access and the Funding of Innovation*. Aldershot, UK: Gower.

Schumpeter, Joseph. 1942. *Capitalism, Socialism, and Democracy*. Harper and Brothers.

Scocozza, Lone. 1989. "Ethics and Medical Science: On Voluntary Participation in Biomedical Experimentation." *Acta Sociologica* 32 (3): 283–293.

Sell, Susan. 2003. *Private Power, Public Law: The Globalization of Intellectual Property Rights*. Cambridge: Cambridge University Press.

Sengupta, Amit. 2010. "B.K. Keayla: A Personal Reminiscence." *Economic and Political Weekly* 45 (51): 25–26.

———. 2013. "Two Decades of Struggle." *Economic and Political Weekly* 48 (32): 43–45.

Sharma, Sanchita. 2010. "Cancer Vaccine Study in a Spot." *Hindustan Times*, April 10. http://www.hindustantimes.com/delhi/cancer-vaccine-study-in-a-spot/story -W8gpXAjUWbpCWx7JpXwmDM.html.

Silverman, Chloe. 2011. *Understanding Autism: Parents, Doctors, and the History of a Disorder*. Princeton, NJ: Princeton University Press.

Silverman, Ed. 2010. "One More Reason That Lilly Must Do a Deal, Fast." *Pharmalot*, October 21. http://seekingalpha.com/article/231297-one-more-reason-lilly-must-do -a-deal-fast. Accessed July 7, 2016.

Silverman, Milton, and Philip R. Lee. 1974. *Pills, Profits and Politics*. Berkeley: Univer- sity of California Press.

Singh, Mahim Pratap. 2012. "Drug Trials Claimed 30 Lives in January This Year." *Hindu*, July 13. http://www.thehindu.com/sci-tech/health/medicine-and-research /drug-trials-claimed-30-lives-in-january-this-year/article3635756.ece.

Sloterdijk, Peter. 1988. *Critique of Cynical Reason*. Minneapolis: University of Min- nesota Press.

Smith, Adam. (1776) 2014. *The Wealth of Nations*. CreateSpace.

Smith, Elta. 2009. "Imaginaries of Development: The Rockefeller Foundation and Rice Research." *Science as Culture* 18 (4): 461–482.

Spivak, Gayatri Chakravorty. 1985. "Scattered Speculations on the Question of Value." *Diacritics* 15 (4): 73–93.

———. 1988. "Can the Subaltern Speak?" In *Marxism and the Interpretation of Cul- tures*, edited by Cary Nelson and Lawrence Grossberg, 271–313. Basingstoke, UK: Macmillan Education.

———. 1990. "Constitutions and Culture Studies." *Yale Journal of Law and the Humanities* 2 (1): 133–147.

———. 1998. *A Critique of Postcolonial Reason: Toward a History of the Vanishing Present*. Cambridge, MA: Harvard University Press.

———. 2014. "Postcolonial Theory and the Specter of Capital." *Cambridge Review of International Affairs* 27 (1): 184–98. doi:10.1080/09557571.2014.877262.

Staton, Tracy. 2014. "Sovaldi May Be Cost-Effective, but the U.K. Can't Afford It, Documents Say." Fierce Pharma, October 7. http://www.fiercepharma.com/story /sovaldi-may-be-cost-effective-uk-cant-afford-it-documents-say/2014-10-07.

Subramanian, Sreenivasan, ed. 2001. *Measurement of Inequality and Poverty*. New Delhi: Oxford University Press.

Sunder Rajan, Kaushik. 2005. "Subjects of Speculation: Emergent Life Sciences and Market Logics in the U.S. and India." *American Anthropologist* 107 (1): 19–30.

———. 2006. *Biocapital: The Constitution of Postgenomic Life*. Durham, NC: Duke University Press.

———. 2007. "Experimental Values—Indian Clinical Trials and Surplus Health." *New Left Review*, no. 45: 67.

———. 2008. "Making the Medicine Go Down" [Editorial]. *Indian Express*, October 28.

———. 2012. "A Bitter Pill." *Indian Express*, September 24.

Sunder Rajan, Kaushik, and Sabina Leonelli. 2013. "Introduction: Biomedical Transactions, Postgenomics, and Knowledge/Value." *Public Culture* 25 (3): 463–476.

Sunder Rajan, Rajeswari. 1993. *Real and Imagined Women: Gender, Culture, Postcolonialism*. London: Routledge.

———. 2003. *The Scandal of the State: Women, Law, and Citizenship in Postcolonial India*. Durham, NC: Duke University Press.

———. 2008. "Refusing Benevolence: Gandhi, Nehru, and the Ethics of Postcolonial Relations." In *Burden or Benefit: Imperial Benevolence and Its Legacies*, edited by Helen Gilbert and Chris Tiffin. Bloomington: Indiana University Press.

———. 2010. "From Antagonism to Agonism: Shifting Paradigms of Women's Opposition to the State." *Comparative Studies of South Asia, Africa and the Middle East* 30 (2): 164–78. doi:10.1215/1089201X-2010-002.

Taussig, Michael T. 1980. "Reification and the Consciousness of the Patient." *Social Science and Medicine, Part B: Medical Anthropology* 14 (1): 3–13.

"10 Die per Week in Drug Trials in India." 2012. *Indian Express*, July 9. http://archive .indianexpress.com/news/10-die-per-week-in-drug-trials-in-india/971963/1.

Tett, Gillian. 2009. *Fool's Gold: The Inside Story of J. P. Morgan and How Wall Street Greed Corrupted Its Bold Dream and Created a Financial Catastrophe*. New York: Free Press.

Thacker, Teena. 2010. "Ministry Admits to Lapses in HPV Vaccine Trial." *Indian Express*, April 29. http://archive.indianexpress.com/news/ministry-admits-lapses-in -hpv-vaccine-trial/612823/.

Thompson, Charis. 2006. *Making Parents: The Ontological Choreography of Reproductive Technologies*. Cambridge, MA: MIT Press.

———. 2013. *Good Science: The Ethical Choreography of Stem Cell Research*. Cambridge, MA: MIT Press.

Timmermans, Stefan, and Marc Berg. 2003. *The Gold Standard: The Challenge of Evidence-Based Medicine and Standardization in Health Care*. Philadelphia: Temple University Press.

Tsu, Vivien Davis, and D. Scott LaMontagne. 2012. "Human Papillomavirus Vaccine Inaccuracies." *American Journal of Public Health* 102 (3): 389–390. doi:10.2105/AJPH.2011.300474.

Tufts University. 2014. "Cost to Develop and Win Marketing Approval for a New Drug Is $2.6 Billion." Tufts Center for the Study of Drug Development. November 18. http://csdd.tufts.edu/news/complete_story/pr_tufts_csdd_2014_cost_study.

U.S. Food and Drug Administration. 2016. "New Drug Application (NDA)." http://www.fda.gov/Drugs/DevelopmentApprovalProcess/HowDrugsareDevelopedandApproved/ApprovalApplications/NewDrugApplicationNDA/.

Varma, Roli. 2001. "People's Science Movements and Science Wars?" *Economic and Political Weekly* 36 (52): 4796–4802.

Vasella, Daniel. 2003. *Magic Cancer Bullet: How a Tiny Orange Pill Is Rewriting Medical History*. New York: Harper Business.

Veblen, Thorstein. (1904) 1978. *The Theory of Business Enterprise*. Piscataway, NJ: Transaction.

———. (1919) 2005. *The Vested Interests and the Common Man*. New York: Cosimo Classics.

Venkatesan, J. 2012. "Centre Must Take Corrective Steps on Illegal Clinical Trials: Supreme Court." *Hindu*, March 27. http://www.thehindu.com/todays-paper/tp-national/centre-must-take-corrective-steps-on-illegal-clinical-trials-supreme-court/article3248953.ece.

Wailoo, Keith, Julie Livingston, Steven Epstein, and Robert Aronowitz. 2010. *Three Shots at Prevention: The HPV Vaccine and the Politics of Medicine's Simple Solutions*. Baltimore, MD: Johns Hopkins University Press.

Waldby, Catherine, and Melinda Cooper. 2008. "The Biopolitics of Reproduction: Post-Fordist Biotechnology and Women's Clinical Labor." *Australian Feminist Studies* 23 (55): 57–73.

Wapner, Jessica. 2014. *The Philadelphia Chromosome: A Genetic Mystery, a Lethal Cancer, and the Improbable Invention of a Life-Saving Treatment*. New York: Experiment.

Weber, Max. (1922) 1978. *Economy and Society*, vol. 1. Berkeley: University of California Press.

Williams, Patricia. 1992. *Alchemy of Race and Rights: The Diary of a Law Professor*. Cambridge, MA: Harvard University Press.

Williams, Raymond. 1978. *Marxism and Literature*. Oxford: Oxford University Press.

Witte, O. N., A. Dasgupta, and D. Baltimore. 1980. "Abelson Murine Leukemia Virus Is Phosphorylated In Vitro to Form Phosphotyrosine." *Nature* 283: 826–831.

Witte, O. N., N. Rosenberg, M. Paskind, A. Shields, and D. Baltimore. 1978. "Identification of an Abelson Murine Leukemia Virus-Encoded Protein Present in Transformed Fibroblast and Lymphoid Cells." *Proceedings of the National Academy of Sciences* 75: 2488–2492.

Wittgenstein, Ludwig. 1972. *On Certainty*. New York: Harper and Row.

WMA. 2013. "WMA Declaration of Helsinki: Ethical Principles for Medical Research Involving Human Subjects." Last amended October 2013. http://www.wma.net/en/30publications/10policies/b3/index.html.

Wright, Richard. (1956) 1995. *The Color Curtain*. Jackson: University Press of Mississippi.

WTO. 2001. "Declaration on the TRIPS Agreement and Public Health." WT/MIN(01)/DEC/2, November 20. https://www.wto.org/english/thewto_e/minist_e/min01_e/mindecl_trips_e.htm.

Zaloom, Caitlin. 2006. *Out of the Pits: Traders and Technology from Chicago to London*. Chicago: University of Chicago Press.

Žižek, Slavoj. 2004. "The Ongoing 'Soft Revolution.'" *Critical Inquiry* 30 (2): 292–323.

———. 2006. "Nobody Has to Be Vile." *London Review of Books* 28 (7). http://www.lrb.co.uk/v28/n07/slavoj-zizek/nobody-has-to-be-vile.

brokerage economy(ies), 15, 63, 69–70, 100, 108, 236, 271n80, 298n14

bulk and drug manufacture, 210–11, 290n38

Burrill and Co., 1, 4

business model(s), 39–40, 46–47, 53, 257n6

Cancer Patients Aid Association (CPAA), 15, 117, 119, 161, 275n10, 276n12, 284n5

Central Drugs Standard Control Organisation of India (CDSCO), 2

Central Government Health Scheme (CGHS), 49, 243

Cervarix, 13, 72, 85, 90, 270n74

cervical cancer, 13, 27, 71–74, 76, 89–93, 102–3, 110, 183, 265n25, 268n60

Chattisgarh, 71, 75, 265n20, 272n91

chronic myelogenous leukemia (CML), 12–13, 258n11

chronic myeloid leukemia. See chronic myelogenous leukemia

Ciba-Geigy, 115, 140–41, 159

Cipla, 3, 29–30, 146, 189, 193–97, 200, 205, 207–11, 216, 223–24, 226, 230, 274n2, 286n4, 287nn7–8, 287n10, 290n36, 296n70, 297n2

civil society, 5, 23, 25, 28–29, 35, 68, 80, 100, 101, 103, 109–11, 114, 138, 146, 148, 158, 165, 188–89, 205, 221, 231, 236, 241, 242, 248n18, 251n30, 253n34 263n12, 268n63, 269n66, 271n80, 274n2, 276n10, 280n47, 293n57, 294n59, 296n68; global, 15, 17, 25, 30, 153, 193–95, 220, 223

clinical labor, 104, 251n27, 264n12

clinical research organization (CRO), 9, 32, 34, 63–67, 69, 75, 88, 101, 231–32, 247n9, 262n4, 263nn8–9, 290n39

Club of Rome, 218

Commerce Ministry of India. See Indian Ministry of Commerce

communicative action, 25

Communist Party of India (Marxist) (CPI-M), 15, 279n42, 280n44

compulsory license, 128, 163, 198, 235, 274nn1–2, 276n10, 278n13

Congress Party, 32–33, 264n18

conjuncture, 31–32, 37, 151, 193–94, 197, 206–7, 212–13, 223, 233, 236, 249n20, 255n45, 282n58, 291n44, 296n71

constitution(alism), 17, 24–25, 28, 76, 107, 114, 121–24, 130, 144, 150–53, 156, 162–63, 169, 192, 229–30, 239–41, 250n26, 273n94, 275n8, 276n11, 282n58, 283n69, 299n17

Constitution of India. See Indian Constitution

coproduction, 18, 26–27, 123, 127, 130, 152

corporate social responsibility (CSR), 29, 165, 168–69, 188, 191–92, 212, 238–39, 265n28, 298n13

crisis, 37–43, 52–53, 56–57, 59–61, 153, 189, 195, 203–4, 217–18, 256n1, 260n21, 262n31, 286n6

Daiichi Sankyo, 74

Dana-Farber Cancer Institute, 141

dasatinib, 235, 285n22, 298n13

data exclusivity, 220, 294n58

decolonization, 217–18

deconstruction, 256n1, 282n56

Delhi High Court, 229–30, 274n2, 283n69, 287n7, 288n22

deliberative, 241, 252n33

demonstration studies, 13, 71, 88, 90, 99–100, 268n63

Derrida, Jacques, 238–39, 256n1, 282n56, 298n15

differential pricing, 49, 60, 167, 232, 259n15, 259n18, 297n6

directive principles, 152, 212

direct-to-consumer advertising, 39, 208, 289n31

discursive gap(s), 34, 256n50

distributive justice, 28, 123, 153, 234

division of labor, 21, 105, 210

Doha Declaration, 113, 128, 145, 203–4, 219, 273n1, 288n13

double bind, 109, 164, 273n97

Drop the Case campaign, 158, 188, 248n18

Dr. Reddy's Laboratories, 208, 296n70

Drug Controller General of India (DCGI), 95, 105, 272n88, 275n2, 275n10

drug development, 6, 8–9, 18, 26, 38–39, 42, 44, 52–55, 58, 60, 69, 113, 115, 139–140, 147–49, 158–59, 195, 234–35, 237, 257n5, 259n14, 261n29, 269n64, 270n69, 278n39, 279n41, 290n39

drug discovery, 9, 18, 26, 38, 40, 53, 55, 118, 140, 158–59, 257n11, 259n18

Intellectual Property Appellate Board (IPAB), 113, 117, 122, 124–25, 130–34, 235, 274n2, 275n3, 276n10, 277n20

International Agency for Research on Cancer (IARC), 92

International Conference on Harmonisation of Technical Requirements for Registration of Pharmaceuticals for Human Use (ICH), 5, 9, 63, 248n10

International Trade Organization (ITO), 217

investor-state, 222, 225, 242

Jamia Millia Islamia University, 209

Johnson and Johnson, 56

judicial cultures, 127, 151, 153, 227, 251n30, 275n8, 276n14, 277n15

judicialization, 11, 13–14, 16–17, 29–30, 107, 114, 148, 150–55, 189, 204, 237, 240–41, 248n12, 248–49n18, 249n19, 283n68

Karat, Brinda, 94–95, 97–99, 279n42

Karnataka Rajya Raitha Sangha (KRRS), 199

Keynes, John Maynard, 217, 256n2

knowledge/value, 102, 253n36

labor theory of value, 19, 21, 249n22, 252n32

Lambda, 64

Lawyers Collective, 15, 251n30

legislative intent, 126–30, 136, 143, 146, 230, 236

Lydon, Nicholas, 139, 141–42

Madras High Court, 14, 114, 117–18, 121–24, 127, 134, 137, 150, 152, 158, 161, 175, 180, 183, 191, 229, 248n18, 251n30, 275n3, 286n7

manufacturing capital(ism). See industrial capital(ism)

market: growth, 44; risk, 9; value, 9, 22. See also emerging markets; financial markets; free markets

Marx, Karl, 18, 20, 58, 60, 249n22, 249n23, 250n26, 252n32, 254n41, 261n31, 296n72

Max Foundation, 160, 169–71, 174, 177, 184–87

Médecins Sans Frontières (MSF), 15, 31, 158, 188, 190, 195, 239, 248n18, 254n44, 256n2, 270n77, 285n29, 290n41

megafund, 53–55, 60

Merck, 13, 15, 44, 56, 68, 78, 86, 93, 227, 296n76

mergers and acquisitions (M&A), 41–42, 60

monopoly(ies), 6, 10–11, 17, 21, 29–30, 40–41, 43, 46–52, 60, 99–100, 113–14, 118, 128–31, 133, 135–36, 138, 148–69, 173, 188–204, 207, 210, 219–27, 230, 232, 234–38, 246, 247n5, 249n18, 250n26, 259n18, 275n8, 277n17, 278n28, 278n31, 280n47, 283n2, 284n14, 288n20, 289n25, 291n41, 294n58, 298n13

monopsony, 49–50, 281n50

Monsanto, 159

mortgage-backed securities, 55

multinational companies. See multinational corporations

multinational corporations, 3, 22–23, 66, 95, 98, 165, 189–90, 195, 201, 211, 216–17, 227, 262n4

multiplication of labor, 21, 105, 251n27

Myriad Genetics, 276n8

Nanjundaswamy, M. D., 199, 207, 214–16, 292n47

Narasimha Rao government, 213, 292n44

Narendra Modi government, 234, 298n10

Natco Pharmaceuticals, 51, 131, 274n2, 275–76n10, 281n52, 297n7

National Aids Research Institute (NARI), Pune, 90, 265n22

National Cancer Registry Programme (NCRP), 92

national health insurance, 147

national immunization program (Indian), 13, 27, 71, 86, 89, 93, 97, 99, 149, 271n81

National Institutes of Health (NIH), 101, 297n1

National Rural Health Mission (NRHM), 33, 255n49

Nehru, Jawaharlal, 213, 227, 289n34

neoliberal(ism), 33, 69, 169, 205–7, 218, 237, 239, 248n9, 252n32, 255n47, 255n48, 256n2, 282n58, 289n26, 292n46, 293n53

Nexavar, 235, 274n2, 276n10

Nicholas Piramal India Limited, 47, 64

nilotinib, 285n22

nonknowledge, 222–23

Novartis, 12–15, 21, 29, 49–51, 60, 113–14, 117–22, 124–25, 127, 129–39, 141–42, 144, 146–49, 157–90, 196, 232, 238, 246, 248n14, 248n18, 251n30, 258n11, 259n18, 276n10, 277n20, 278n28, 278n30, 280n47, 283n1, 285n22, 286n31, 287n10, 290n39

Nuremberg Code, 271n83

off-label use, 39, 44, 61, 257n6

Onconova, 182

oncopolitics, 142–43, 148, 279n41

OPEC, 218, 293n52

Oregon Health and Science University, 139, 141, 158–59

Organization of Pharmaceutical Producers of India (OPPI), 280n47

OSI Pharmaceuticals, 229–30

out-licensing, 42

outsourcing, 11, 44, 48, 58, 63–64, 100, 105, 106

parliamentary debate(s), 98–99, 126, 129–30, 143–44, 270n70, 284n6

patent(ed/s): adjudication, 17, 40, 47, 66, 100, 120–24, 125, 152, 165, 274n2, 275n10, 277n20; agreements, 38; claim, 22, 120–37, 141, 143, 148–49, 153, 277n15, 278n27; cliff, 40–42, 53–54, 64; denial, 14, 21, 27, 113–14, 117–18, 121–22, 126, 132, 138, 158, 276n10; drug, 9; disputes, 12, 114, 120–22, 161, 230, 235; expiration, 41, 294n58; history, 113–15, 124, 126–29, 131–35, 141, 143, 277n16; law, 5, 10, 18, 112–18, 125–28, 135, 148–49, 164–65, 173, 197, 199, 203–4, 207, 210, 277n16, 278n28; legislation, 14, 112, 118, 135, 145, 229, 235, 288n13, 294n58; medication, 4, 10–11, 38, 51, 118; process, 10, 32, 44, 46, 112, 115, 172, 194, 198–99, 210, 235; product, 10, 14, 21, 29–30, 32, 34, 37, 112, 115–19, 128–30, 146–47, 154, 158, 160, 172, 193, 196, 198–200, 202, 204, 207, 219, 234–35, 285n22, 286n5, 288n20, 291n41; protection, 14, 41, 43, 60, 164; regimes, 3, 9, 11, 30–34, 37, 44–46, 64, 112–13, 116, 119, 125, 128, 130, 146, 153, 193–94, 200, 219, 231, 234, 287n7

Patent Act: 1911 (Indian), 115, 127, 207, 210; 1950 (Indian), 115, 127, 207; 1970 (Indian), 6, 10–11, 14, 112, 115, 126, 128, 138, 189, 194, 196–98, 200, 206–8, 210, 226, 236, 242, 280n45, 292n41; 1999 (Indian), 116, 128, 161–62, 280n45, 288n21; 2005 (India), 14, 34, 112–14, 116–19, 123, 128–30, 144, 146, 162, 164–65, 191, 200, 220, 229, 280nn45–46, 284n6, 286n5, 288n13

patient advocacy, 39, 119, 143, 148, 158, 185, 195, 246, 257n4

patient assistance program(s). *See* drug donation program(s)

Pegasys, 274n2, 276n10

people's health movement(s), 15, 251n30

people's science movement(s), 251n30

Pfizer, 56, 229, 267n58, 274n2, 280n47

pharmaceutical company(ies). *See* pharmaceutical industry

pharmaceutical industry, 38–39, 41–44, 50–54, 257n7, 257–58n11; Euro-American, 6, 9, 15, 23, 28–29, 35, 38–39, 44, 46–47, 50–52, 57, 59, 113, 154, 189, 194–95, 200, 204, 216, 219, 237, 250n26, 257n7, 281n51, 286n5, 290n38; generic, 10, 16, 31, 35, 38, 59, 112, 128, 148, 154, 161, 163, 168, 189, 193, 205, 208, 211, 215–16, 223–24, 232–34, 236, 254n44, 260n22, 285n14, 287n7, 290n41, 296n70; global, 11, 37, 194; Indian, 1 4, 15–16, 51, 64–65, 101, 128, 161, 165, 179, 183, 189, 195–96, 206–9, 211, 223, 227, 232, 236, 242, 277n16, 281n53, 286n4, 287n7, 289n33, 290n38, 291n41; literature, 257n8; marketing, 20; mergers and acquisitions (M&A)-based/driven, 43; multinational, 6–7, 11, 23, 29, 31–32, 35, 46–47, 64, 112, 114, 149–50, 153, 156, 158, 160, 165, 189, 191, 204, 210, 215–16, 232–33, 229, 232, 237, 248n11, 280n45, 280n47, 283n66, 290n39; national, 11, 38, 195, 199, 209; research and development (R&D)-based/driven, 6, 11, 15–16, 29, 32, 38, 40–41, 43–44, 47–51, 53, 57, 59, 154, 189, 195, 219, 257n7, 258n11, 258n13, 259n16, 286n5, 290nn38–39, 296n72

pharmaceuticalization, 149, 155, 180

pharmaceutical marketing. *See* pharmaceutical industry: marketing

Pharmaceutical Research and Manufacturers of America (PhRMA), 138

pharmacodynamics, 137

pharmacokinetics, 137

phase 1 (clinical) trials, 8, 142

phase 2 (clinical) trials, 8, 142, 268n63

phase 3 (clinical) trials, 8, 13, 69, 88, 95–98, 142

phase 4 (clinical) trials, 96–97, 186

Philadelphia chromosome, 140, 279n36

philanthropy/ic, 17, 19, 28, 86, 157, 161, 167–69, 178–79, 187–89, 191, 196, 227, 236, 238, 298n14 pipeline, 40–42, 54–55, 69

political society, 25

postlicensure observational study, 69, 72, 77, 79, 89, 95–97, 99

postmarketing surveillance, 183

power/knowledge, 27, 253n39

pregrant opposition, 119–20, 143, 220, 230

prescription maximization, 37

price control, 10, 44–45, 49, 147, 212, 246, 281n28

Program for Appropriate Technology in Health (PATH), 13, 15, 65, 68–69, 71–72, 74, 77–78, 81, 86, 87, 89–100, 103, 110–11, 237–38, 246, 263n8, 264n14

promise of justice, 151, 155, 240, 280n56, 298n15

Prozac, 41

public health, 4–6, 18, 23, 27–29, 33, 67–70, 72, 76, 86, 88–94, 99, 102–3, 106–7, 110–11, 113, 117–19, 123, 128–29, 136, 144–45, 147, 164, 169, 183, 190, 204–5, 208–9, 211, 214, 219–20, 229, 213–38, 247n8, 264n15, 265n28, 269n64, 273n95, 273nn4–5, 277n17, 286n30, 286n5, 288n13, 289n30, 291n42, 298n14; flexibility, 14, 22, 118–19, 128, 191

public interest, 129, 133–34, 146, 149, 155, 158, 160, 163–65, 169, 191, 194, 196, 198–200, 221, 225–26, 230, 236, 240–42, 277n17, 299n17; litigation (PIL), 155, 158, 240, 249n18, 270n79, 283n68

public-private partnership(s), 15, 33, 69, 86, 238, 255n49, 263n8

public scandal, 13–14, 29–30, 62, 67–70, 94, 98, 102–3, 107–11, 188, 236, 240–41, 248n12, 248n18, 270n79, 271n80

public sector, 158–59, 208, 210–11, 224, 233, 237, 291n42

Quintiles, 262n5

Ranbaxy, 47, 64, 208, 211, 216, 258n13, 263n7, 275n10

Reagan, Ronald, 123, 218, 293n54

reformulation, 210–11, 250n26

Report of the Committee on the Drugs and Pharmaceutical Industry. See Hathi Committee Report

research and development (R&D), 11, 23, 38–39, 41–43, 50–62, 139–40, 142–43, 147, 154, 189,

195, 198, 201, 219, 225, 257–58n11, 259n16, 261n29, 286n5, 290nn38–39, 296n72

responsibility without limit, 238–39

return on equity, 40, 257n7

reverse engineer(ing), 1, 4, 10, 23, 38, 47, 60, 161

right to health, 117, 153, 155, 162, 230

right to life, 117, 150, 162, 165, 168

Sama, 15, 72, 74–81, 256n51, 264n12, 265n24, 265n26, 266n31, 266n35, 269n66, 270n80, 272n86, 299n18

Sandoz, 141, 160, 177

Sanofi-Aventis, 47, 280n47

scandalous clinical trial. See unethical clinical trial

scandalous publicity. See public scandal

Schedule Y, 5, 14, 63, 67, 87, 100, 105, 263n5

Schumpeter, Joseph, 47–48, 133, 160, 200

Section 3(d), 14, 117–22, 124–26, 128–30, 133–38, 143, 145, 154, 158, 161, 191, 219, 234–35, 276n10, 280n42, 284n6, 288n13, 293n55

securitization, 53–55

securitized debt. See securitization

serviceable truths, 253n37

Shantha Biotechnics, 47, 172

shareholder value, 40

side effect(s), 44, 76

Singh, Manmohan, 199, 201, 206–7, 212, 215, 229, 280n45, 291n43, 292n44

situated analysis. See situated perspective

situated knowledge. See situated perspective

situated perspective, 30, 143, 170, 207, 216, 254n43, 269n66, 279n41, 287n7

social contract, 45, 124, 169

sofasbuvir. See Sovaldi

Sovaldi, 231–32, 297nn5–7

special investment vehicle, 53–54

speculative capital, 30, 32, 39–40, 42–43, 51–57, 60–61, 188, 194, 262n31

speculative markets/marketplace. See speculative capital

Sprycel, 235, 285n22

stock market, 40, 53, 56, 257n7

stock repurchases, 56, 260n26

subject constitution, 76, 106–7, 140, 150

surplus health, 20, 43–44, 46, 59, 91, 93, 107, 192, 238